ESSENTIALS OF ENVIRONMENTAL TOXICOLOGY

Edited by
Jurex Cuenca Gallo

ArclerPress

Essentials of Environmental Toxicology

Edited by Jurex Cuenca Gallo

Edition 2018

ArclerPress

Published by
Arcler Press LLC
708 3rd Avenue, 6th Floor
New York
NY 10017
United States of America
www.arclerpress.com

ISBN: 978-1-68094-622-2 (Hardback)

Printed in United States of America

Library of Congress Control Number: 2017933218

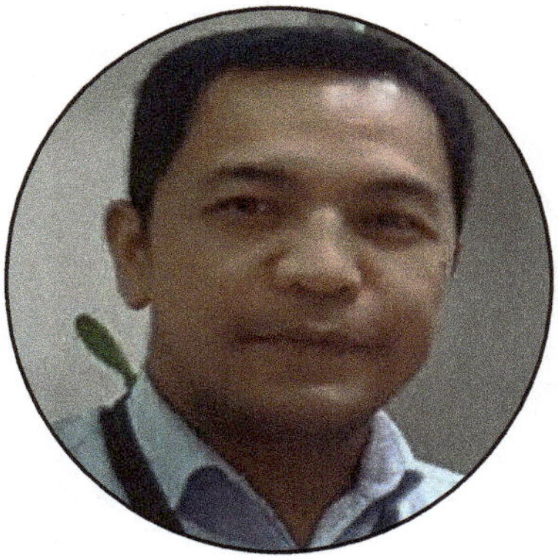

About the Editor

Jurex Cuenca Gallo

Dr. Jurex Gallo was conferred with his PhD degree in Chemical Engineering from De La Salle University – Manila in 2014. His expertise revolved in the fields of Material Science and Environmental Engineering focused on industrial and hazardous waste treatment and management. Presently, Dr. Gallo is affiliated as Senior Science Research Specialist of the Department of Science and Technology e-Asia Joint Research Program in the Philippines on developing functional carbon-based nanomaterials such as carbon nanotubes and graphene for energy and environmental applications.

Table of Contents

2 XENOBIOTIC METABOLISM

3 METAL TOXICITY

4 ENVIRONMENTAL IMPACT OF THE PETROLEUM INDUSTRY

5 PESTICIDE POISONING

6 AQUATIC TOXICOLOGY

7 RADIOACTIVE CONTAMINATION

8 AQUATIC TOXICOLOGY DATABASES

List of Abbreviations

AF	Application Factor
APHA	American Public Health Association
BCF	Bioconcentration Factor
CAIR	Clean Air Interstate Rule
CBR	Critical Body Residue
EC	Environment Canada
EPA	Environmental Protection Agency
EQS	Environmental Quality Standards
ERT	Environmental Research and Technology
LOEC	Lowest Observed Effect Concentration
LPO	Lipid Peroxides
MATC	Maximum Acceptable Toxicant Concentration
NAAQS	National Ambient Air Quality Standards
NAPAP	National Acidic Precipitation Assessment Program
NATA	National-Scale Air Toxics Assessment
NOAA	National Oceanic and Atmospheric Administration
NOEC	No Observed Effect Concentration
NPDES	National Pollutant Discharge Elimination System
NPSH	Nonprotein Sulfhydryl
OECD	Organization for Economic Co-operation and Development
PAH	Polycyclic Aromatic Hydrocarbons
PM	Particulate Matter
POP	Persistent Organic Pollutants

QSAR	Quantitative Structure-Activity Relationship
ROS	Reactive Oxygen Species
SCR	Selective Catalytic Reduction
SETAC	Society of Environmental Toxicology and Chemistry
SNCR	Selective Non-Catalytic Reduction
SQT	Sediment Quality Triad
THP	Total Petroleum Hydrocarbon
WHO	World Health Organization
WPCF	Water Pollution Control Federation

Preface

Environmental toxicology is a relatively new field, with its origins in the mid-20th century. The modern science of toxicology, on the other hand, was born in the early 19th century, and by the later decades of that century, some scientists had begun to consider the effects of toxic substances that had been released into the environment. Environmental toxicology is concerned with the assessment of toxic substances in the environment. Environmental toxicology draws heavily on principles and techniques from other fields, including biochemistry, cell biology, developmental biology, and genetics. Among its primary interests are the assessment of toxic substances in the environment, the monitoring of environments for the presence of toxic substances, the effects of toxins on biotic and abiotic components of ecosystems, and the metabolism and biological and environmental fate of toxins. Organisms can be introduced to toxicants at various stages of their life cycle. The degree of toxicity can vary depending on where the organism is found within its food web. Bioaccumulation occurs when molecular compounds are stored in an organism's fatty tissues. Over time, this leads to the establishment of a trophic cascade and the biomagnification of specific toxicants. Biodegradation releases CO_2 and water as by-products into the environment. This process is typically limited in areas affected by environmental toxicants. Harmful effects of chemical and biological agents can include toxicants from pollutants, insecticides, pesticides, and fertilizers, all of which can impact an organism and its community through shifts in species diversity and abundance. Resulting changes in population dynamics impact the ecosystem by altering its productivity and stability. Toxins affect the environment and organisms in a variety of ways, from having little negative impact on certain abiotic factors or resistant organisms to killing animals and destroying major components of ecosystems. The extent of damage depends on the type and structure of the toxic substance; the age, the size, and the species of the organism; and the temperature and the physical and chemical characteristics of the environment. Knowledge of how these factors interact is critical to understanding how best to prevent or reduce exposure or remove a toxin from the environment.

Content Coverage

Chapter One introduces the harmful effects of chemical, biological and physical agents in biological systems that establishes the extent of damage in living organisms. The relationship between dose and its effects on the exposed organism is of high significance in toxicology. Factors that influence chemical toxicity include the dosage; the route of exposure, the species, age, sex and environment.

Chapter Two is about metabolism of xenobiotics. It can be dangerous to the health. Some xenobiotics are resistant to degradation, such as, they may be synthetic organochlorides such as plastics and pesticides, or naturally occurring organic chemicals such as polyaromatic hydrocarbons (PAHs) and some fractions of crude oil and coal.

Chapter Three discusses about the metal toxicity or metal poisoning that affect in certain forms and doses on life. Some metals are toxic when they form poisonous soluble compounds.

Chapter Four focuses on the toxicity of petroleum. The environmental impact of petroleum is often negative because it is toxic to almost all forms of life and its extraction fuels climate change. Petroleum, commonly referred to as oil, is closely linked to virtually all aspects of present society, especially for transportation and heating for both homes and for commercial and industrial activities.

Chapter Five focuses on the toxicity of pesticides that occurs when chemicals intended to control a pest affect non-target organisms such as humans, wildlife, or bees.

Chapter Six covers the study of the effects of manufactured chemicals and other anthropogenic and natural materials and activities on aquatic organisms at various levels of organization, from subcellular through individual organisms to communities and ecosystems.

Chapter Seven highlights about the radioactive contamination that presents a hazard because of the radioactive decay of the contaminants, which emit harmful ionizing radiation such as alpha particles or beta particles, gamma rays or neutrons.

Chapter Eight focuses on the aquatic toxicological databases. These databases are invaluable resources in the field of aquatic toxicology because the likelihood of a chemical to cause toxicity is highly variable across the broad spectrum of contaminants in the environment.

CHAPTER 1

Understanding Toxicology

Chapter Contents

Toxicology is the scientific study of adverse effects that occur in living organisms due to chemicals. It involves observing and reporting symptoms, mechanisms, detection and treatments of toxic substances, in particular relation to the poisoning of humans.

INTRODUCTION

Toxicology (from the Ancient Greek words τοξικός *toxikos* "poisonous" and λόγος *logos*) is a branch of biology, chemistry, and medicine (more specifically pharmacology) concerned with the study of the adverse effects of chemicals on living organisms. It also studies the harmful effects of chemical, biological and physical agents in biological systems that establishes the extent of damage in living organisms. The relationship between dose and its effects on the exposed organism is of high significance in toxicology. Factors that influence chemical toxicity include the dosage (and whether it is acute or chronic); the route of exposure, the species, age, sex and environment.

HISTORY

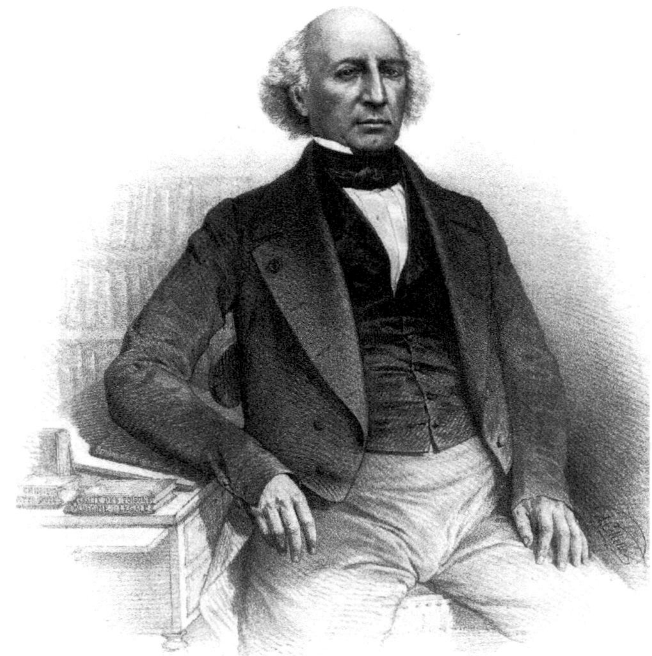

Lithograph of Mathieu Orfila.

Dioscorides, a Greek physician in the court of the Roman emperor Nero, made the first attempt to classify plants according to their toxic and therapeutic effect. Ibn Wahshiyya wrote the *Book on Poisons* in the 9th or 10th century. This was followed up in 1360 by Khagendra Mani Darpana.

Mathieu Orfila is considered the modern father of toxicology, having given the subject its first formal treatment in 1813 in his *Traité des poisons*, also called *Toxicologie générale*.

In 1850, Jean Stas became the first person to successfully isolate plant poisons from human tissue. This allowed him to identify the use of nicotine as a poison in the famous Bocarmé murder case, providing the evidence needed to convict the Belgian Count Hippolyte Visart de Bocarmé of killing his brother-in-law.

Theophrastus Phillipus Auroleus Bombastus von Hohenheim (1493–1541) (also referred to as Paracelsus, from his belief that his studies were above or beyond the work of Celsus – a Roman physician from the first century) is also considered "the father" of toxicology. He is credited with the classic toxicology maxim, "*Alle Dinge sind Gift und nichts ist ohne Gift; allein die Dosis macht, dass ein Ding kein Gift ist.*" which translates as, "All things are poisonous and nothing is without poison; only the dose makes a thing not poisonous." This is often condensed to: "The dose makes the poison" or in Latin "Sola dosis facit venenum".

Basic Toxicology

The goal of toxicity assessment is to identify adverse effects of a substance. Adverse effects depend on two main factors: i) routes of exposure (oral, inhalation, or dermal) and ii) dose (duration and concentration of exposure). To explore dose, substances are tested in both acute and chronic models. Generally, different sets of experiments are conducted to determine whether a substance causes cancer and to examine other forms of toxicity.

Factors that influence chemical toxicity:

- Dosage
- Both large single exposures (acute) and continuous small exposures (chronic) are studied.
- Route of exposure
- Ingestion, inhalation or skin absorption
- Other factors
- Species
- Age
- Sex
- Health
- Environment
- Individual characteristics

TESTING METHODS

Toxicity experiments may be conducted *in vivo* (using the whole animal) or *in vitro* (testing on isolated cells or tissues), or *in silico* (in a computer simulation).

Non-human Animals

The classic experimental tool of toxicology is testing on non-human animals. As of 2014, such animal testing provides information that is not available by other means about how substances function in a living organism.

Alternative Testing Methods

While testing in animal models remains as a method of estimating human effects, there are both ethical and technical concerns with animal testing.

Since the late 1950s, the field of toxicology has sought to reduce or eliminate animal testing under the rubric of "Three Rs" - reduce the number of experiments with animals to the minimum necessary; refine experiments to cause less suffering, and replace *in vivo* experiments with other types, or use more simple forms of life when possible.

Computer modeling is an example of alternative testing methods; using computer models of chemicals and proteins, structure-activity relationships can be determined, and chemical structures that are likely to bind to, and interfere with, proteins with essential functions, can be identified. This work requires expert knowledge in molecular modeling and statistics together with expert judgment in chemistry, biology and toxicology.

In 2007, the National Academy of Sciences published a report called Toxicity Testing in the 21st Century: A Vision and a Strategy which opened with a statement: Change often involves a pivotal event that builds on previous history and opens the door to a new era. Pivotal events in science include the discovery of penicillin, the elucidation of the DNA double helix, and the development of computers. ...Toxicity testing is approaching such a scientific pivot point. It is poised to take advantage of the revolutions in biology and biotechnology. Advances in toxicogenomics, bioinformatics, systems biology, epigenetics, and computational toxicology could transform toxicity testing from a system based on whole-animal testing to one founded primarily on in vitro methods that evaluate changes in biologic processes using cells, cell lines, or cellular components, preferably of human origin. As of 2014 that vision was still unrealized.

In some cases shifts away from animal studies has been mandated by law or regulation; the European Union (EU) prohibited use of animal testing for cosmetics in 2013.

DOSE RESPONSE COMPLEXITIES

Most chemicals display a classic dose response curve – at a low dose (below a threshold), no effect is observed. Some show a phenomenon known as sufficient challenge – a small exposure produces animals that "grow more rapidly, have better general appearance and coat quality, have fewer tumors, and live longer than the control animals". A few chemicals have no well-defined safe level of exposure. These are treated with special care. Some chemicals are subject to bioaccumulation as they are stored in rather than being excreted from the body; these also receive special consideration.

COMPUTATIONAL TOXICOLOGY

Computational toxicology is a discipline that develops mathematical and computer-based models to better understand and predict adverse health effects caused by chemicals, such as environmental pollutants and pharmaceuticals. Within the *Toxicology in the 21st Century* project, the best predictive models were identified to be Deep Neural Networks, Random Forest, and Support Vector Machines, which can reach the performance of in vitro experiments.

TOXICOLOGY AS A PROFESSION

A **toxicologist** is a scientist or medical personnel who specializes in the study of symptoms, mechanisms, treatments and detection of venoms and toxins; especially the poisoning of people. To work as a toxicologist one should obtain a degree in toxicology or a related degree like biology, chemistry or biochemistry. Toxicologists perform many different duties including research in the academic, nonprofit and industrial fields, product safety evaluation, consulting, public service and legal regulation.

Requirements

To work as a toxicologist one should obtain a degree in toxicology or a related degree like biology, chemistry or biochemistry. Bachelor's degree programs in toxicology cover the chemical makeup of toxins and their effects on biochemistry, physiology and ecology. After introductory life science courses are complete, students typically enroll in labs and apply toxicology principles to research and other studies. Advanced students delve into specific sectors, like the pharmaceutical industry or law enforcement, which apply methods of toxicology in their work. The Society of Toxicology (SOT) recommends that undergraduates in postsecondary schools that don't offer a bachelor's degree in toxicology consider attaining a degree in biology or chemistry. Additionally, the SOT advises aspiring toxicologists to take statistics and mathematics courses, as well as gain laboratory experience through lab courses, student research projects and internships.

Duties

Toxicologists perform many more duties including research in the academic, nonprofit and industrial fields, product safety evaluation, consulting, public service and legal regulation. In order to research and assess the effects of chemicals, toxicologists perform carefully designed studies and experiments. These experiments help identify the specific amount of a chemical that may cause harm and potential risks of being near or using products that contain certain chemicals. Research projects may range from assessing the effects of toxic pollutants on the environment to evaluating how the human immune system responds to chemical compounds within pharmaceutical drugs. While the basic duties of toxicologists are to determine the effects of chemicals on organisms and their surroundings, specific job duties may vary based on industry and employment. For example, forensic toxicologists may look for toxic substances in a crime scene, whereas aquatic toxicologists may analyze the toxicity level of wastewater.

Compensation

The salary for jobs in toxicology is dependent on several factors, including level of schooling, specialization, experience. The U.S. Bureau of Labor Statistics (BLS) notes that jobs for biological scientists, which generally include toxicologists, were expected to increase by 21% between 2008 and 2018. The BLS notes that this increase could be due to research and development growth in biotechnology, as well as budget increases for basic and medical research in biological science.

ECOTOXICOLOGY

Ecotoxicology is the study of the effects of toxic chemicals on biological organisms, especially at the population, community, ecosystem level. Ecotoxicology is a multidisciplinary field, which integrates toxicology and ecology.

The ultimate goal of this approach is to be able to *predict* the effects of pollution so that the most efficient and effective action to prevent or remediate any detrimental effect can be identified. In those ecosystems that are already impacted by pollution ecotoxicological studies can inform as to the best course of action to restore ecosystem services and functions efficiently and effectively.

Ecotoxicology differs from environmental toxicology in that it integrates the effects of stressors across all levels of biological organisation from the molecular to whole communities and ecosystems, whereas environmental toxicology focuses upon effects at the level of the individual and below.

The publication in 1962 of Rachel Carson's seminal volume, Silent Spring catalysed the separation of environmental toxicology - and, subsequently, ecotoxicology - from classical toxicology. The revolutionary element in Carson's work was her extrapolation from single-organism effects to effects at the whole ecosystem and the balance of nature

The term ecotoxicology was coined by René Truhaut in 1969 who defined it as "the branch of toxicology concerned with the study of toxic effects, caused by natural or synthetic pollutants, to the constituents of ecosystems, animal (including human), vegetable and microbial, in an integral context"

Although initially devoted to the study of anthropogenic toxicants, the term is now used to describe research into the ecological effects of diverse abiotic and biotic stresses, thereby integrating secondary effects of anthropogenic activities such as ocean acidification resulting from increased dissolution of carbon dioxide into the surface waters of the oceans It has been proposed that this broadening of focus from purely toxicological effects to the consideration of more general stressors moves beyond the definition of "ecotoxicology". Van Straalen (2003), in particular, argued that the field had diversified to become *Stress Ecology* and that, as the effects of anthropogenic toxicants compound existing, natural stressors, exclusive study of their effects in an ecological context was nonsensical. Whilst this proposal is well argued, it is odd of Van Straalen to have specified solely ecology as the field when the original field of ecotoxicology was intended to cover all levels of biological organisation from molecular-level causes to ecosystem-level effects. Therefore, the term *Stress Biology* would seem more appropriate.

Common environmental toxicants

- PCBs (polychlorinated biphenyls) - found in coolant and insulating fluids, pesticide extenders, adhesives, and hydraulic fluids.
- Pesticides - used widely for preventing, destroying, or repelling any organism that may be considered harmful. Commonly found in commercially grown fruits, vegetables, and meats. Methyl parathion is a commonly used pesticide used for agricultural reasons. Methyl parathion causes the formation of toxic mediums for humans, soil and water, fresh water fish, and other hydrophilous organisms in the ecosystem. Methyl parathion proposes numerous health risk factors that are life-threatening.

- Mold and other mycotoxins.
- Phthalates are found in plastic wrap, plastic bottles, and plastic food storage containers, all of which make up a considerable part of household plastic waste.
- VOCs (volatile organic compounds) - such as formaldehyde; can be found in drinking water and sewage systems.
- Dioxins are a class of chemical compounds that are formed as a result of combustion processes such as waste incineration and from burning fuels like wood, coal, and oil.
- Asbestos is found in the insulation of flows, ceilings, water pipes, and heating ducts.
- Heavy metals include arsenic, mercury, lead, aluminum, and cadmium, which are found in fish, and pesticides.
- Chloroform is used to make other chemicals.
- Chlorine is commonly found in household cleaners.

Exposure to toxic chemicals

- Chemicals propose the risk of killing off another animal's food supply that change the overall population of the prey
- Animals can go to the brink of extinction because of the food chain that exists through the different communities. For example, bald eagles, ospreys, and peregrine falcons were facing extinction because their food sources(fish and other birds) were contaminated with toxins.
- We are all connected between the communities of living things. Plants can absorb toxins through their roots and leaves. Animals and humans are always exposed to chemicals by the air we breathe, things we touch, and what we put in our mouth.
- Animals and humans can also eat other animals or plants that are already poisoned, which will continue the spread of chemicals, which is referred to as secondary poisoning
- Effects on individuals and entire population
- Direct effects- direct consumption of a toxin or something that has been contaminated with a toxin by breathing, eating, or drinking.
- Developmental and reproductive problems
- Indirect effects- organisms directly affected by the loss of food, which has declined due to toxins.
- Sub-lethal effects- toxins that do not kill but make the organism sick or make it change its behavior;
- With chronic use of pesticides, this runs the risk of causing abnormalities in chromosome structure in humans, as well as affecting the reproduction, nervous and cardiovascular system of any animals exposed.
- The genetics can be affected by toxicant exposure, direct changes can occur to the DNA, and if not repaired, the changes can lead to the appearance mutations

- Contaminants can modify the distribution of individuals in a population, effective population size, mutation rate and migration rate

Effects of Ecotoxicity on a Community

- Predator-prey relationships- either the predator is affected by the toxin resulting in a decline of predator population and thus increasing the prey population; or the prey population is affected by the toxin resulting in a decline in the prey population that, in essence, will cause a decline in the predator population due to lack of food resources
- Community ecotoxicology studies the effects of all contaminants on patterns and species abundance, diversity, community composition, and species interactions. Communities that rely heavily on competition and predation will have a difficult time responding and thriving in disturbances from contaminants. A community that is species-rich will have a better chance recovering from an exotoxin disturbance, rather than a community that is not species-rich. A species could be easily wiped out to the expense of a contamination from foreign chemicals. Protecting distinct community levels, such as species richness and diversity is essential for maintaining a healthy, well-balanced ecosystem

Overall Effects

Chemicals are shown to prohibit the growth of seed germination of an arrangement of different plant species. Plants are what make up the most vital trophic level of the biomass pyramids, known as the primary producers. Because they are at the bottom of the pyramid, every other organism in an ecosystem relies on the health and abundance of the primary producers in order to survive. If plants are battling problems with diseases relating to exposure to chemicals, other organisms will either die because of starvation or obtain the disease by eating the plants or animals already infected. So ecotoxicology is an ongoing battle that stems from many sources and can affect everything and everyone in an ecosystem

Ways of Prevention

Regulation:

- In the United States, the Environmental Protection Agency (EPA) reviews all pesticides before the products are registered for sale to ensure that the benefits will outweigh the risks.
- Food Quality Protection Act and the Safe Drinking Water Act were passed in 1996, which required EPA to screen pesticide chemical for potential to produce harmful effects.

- Keep close track of the labeling when using a fertilizer, or pesticide. Try to look for products that will have less of an impact on the environment
- There are many federal and state laws protecting birds, animals, and rare plants. But the first order of protection comes from us taking steps to avoid harm since we are the main source of all the toxins.
- Proper waste disposal

Ecotoxicity Testing

- Acute and chronic toxicity tests are performed for terrestrial organisms including avian, mammalian, nontarget arthropods, and earthworms.
- The Organization for Economic Cooperation and Development (OECD) test guideline has developed specific tests to test toxicity level in organisms. Ecotoxicological studies are generally performed in compliance with international guidelines, including EPA, OECD, EPPO, OPPTTS, SETAC, IOBC, and JMAFF.
- LC50 is the acute toxicity test that tests for the concentrate of tissue at which it is lethal to 50% within 96 hours. The test may start with eggs, embryos, or juveniles and last from 7 to 200 days.
- EC50 is the effective concentration at 50%, which is the concentration that causes adverse effects in 50% of the test organisms.
- Endocrine Disruptor Screening Program (EDSP)
- Tier 1 screening battery
- Endangered species assessments.
- Persistent, Bioaccumulative, and Inherently Toxic (PBiT) assessments using the Quantitative Structure-Activity Relationships (QSARs) to categorize regulated substances.
- Bioaccumulation in fish using the Bioconcentration Factor (BCF) methods.

Classification of Ecotoxicity

Total amount of acute toxicity is directly related to the classification of toxicity.

- < 1 part per million→ Class I
- 1-10 parts per million→ Class II
- 10-100 parts per million→ Class III

ECOTOXICITY

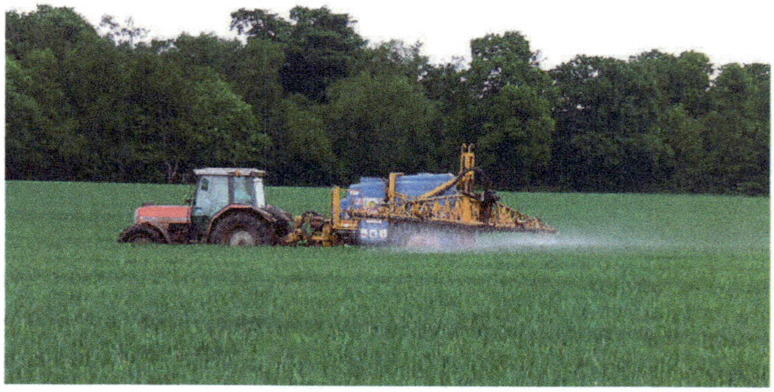

Pesticide distribution.

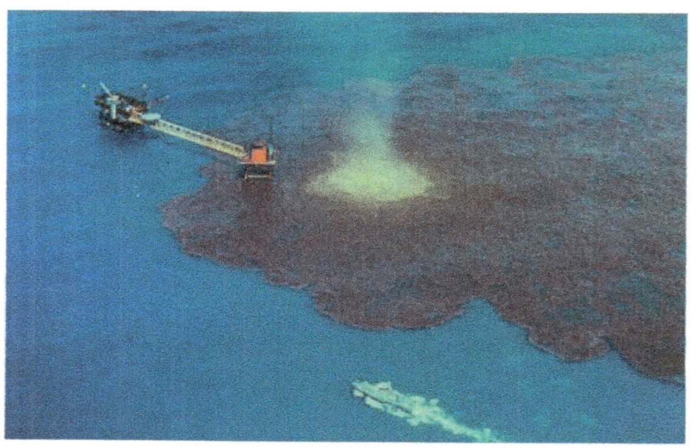

Oil spill

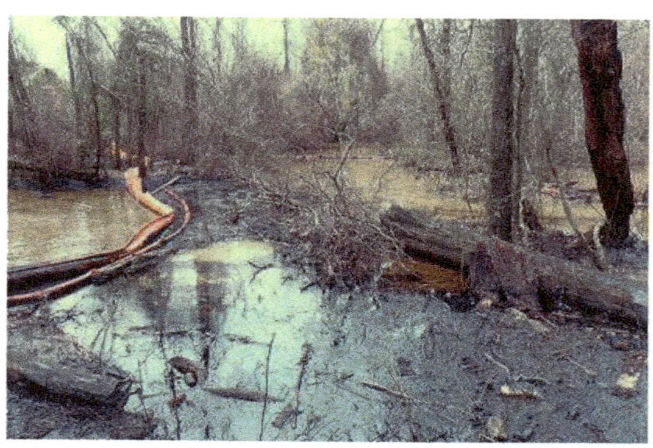

Oil spill creek.

Ecotoxicity, the subject of study of the field of ecotoxicology (a portmanteau of Ecology and Toxicology) refers to the potential for biological, chemical or physical stressors to affect ecosystems. Such stressors might occur in the natural environment at densities, concentrations or levels high enough to disrupt the natural biochemistry, physiology, behavior and interactions of the living organisms that comprise the ecosystem.

Ecotoxicology has been defined as, the branch of toxicology concerned with the study of toxic effects, caused by natural or synthetic pollutants, to the constituents of ecosystems, animal (including human), vegetable and microbial, in an integral context .

Common Environmental Toxicants

- Diethyl phthalate, that enter environments through industries manufacturing cosmetics, plastic and many other commercial products.
- Bisphenol A (BPA), found in many mass-produced products such as, medical devices, food packaging, cosmetics, children's toys, computers, CD's, etc.
- Pharmaceuticals such as Climbazole, a fungicide found in anti-dandruff shampoos.
- Pesticides
- Some but not all; cleaning products, laundry detergents, fabric softeners, oven cleaners, disinfectants
- Phosphates
- Oil. Petroleum Hydrocarbon

Everyday Hazards

In Canada, there is no law requiring manufacturers to state the health and environmental hazards associated with their cleaning products. Many people buy such products to support a clean and healthy home, often unaware of the products ability to harm both their own health and the surrounding environment. "Canadians spend more than $275 million on household cleaning products in a year" Chemicals from these cleaners enter our bodies through air passageways and absorption through the skin and when these cleaning products are washed down the drain they negatively affect aquatic ecosystems. There are also no regulations in place stating that the ingredients be listed on labels of cleaning products leading the users to be ultimately unaware of the chemicals they expose themselves and their surrounding environments to.

2-Butoxyethanol

The organic compound 2-Butoxyethanol, commonly found in glass cleaners, laundry stain removers, windshield wiper fluid, oven cleaners, and rust removers has been proven to cause reproductive problems in laboratory experiments.

Ammonia

The compound ammonia is found in many window cleaners, drain cleaners, bathroom cleaners, oven cleaners, car polish, and all-purpose cleaners. It's vapour is particularly harmful to people with asthma and it may also cause kidney and liver damage. When ammonia is mixed with products containing chlorine bleach, highly poisonous chloramine gas is formed. This poisonous gas often forms when cleaners are mixed in the home forming strong irritants.

Fragrance Chemicals

Fragrance chemicals are found in most cleaning products, perfumes, and personal care products. More than 3000 chemicals are used in these fragrance mixtures. The synthetic musks used in detergents accumulate in the environment and are harmful to aquatic organisms. Certain musks are possible endocrine disruptors that interfere with hormone functioning. Phthalates are a common ingredient in these fragrance mixtures found in laundry detergents and fabric softeners. These phthalates are suspected endocrine disrupters that affect reproduction rates including reduced sperm count in males. Certain glass cleaners and floor polishes contain dibutyl phthalate (DBP). The European Union classifies DBP as very toxic to aquatic organisms, posing a huge danger as these cleaners, especially the floor polishes are often rinsed down the drain and into aquatic environments.

Phosphates

Phosphates are found in many dishwasher detergents, laundry detergents, and bathroom cleaners. They act as a fertilizer in water and in high concentrations can promote algae blooms and increase weed growth. When water containing phosphates are washed into water areas they carry with them fertilizers, nutrients, and wastes from the land. Phytoplankton and algae flourish at the surface due to increased phosphates. Dead phytoplankton and other organisms sink to the bottom giving rise to large numbers of decomposers due to increased food supply (dead organisms, phytoplankton). Due to the increased number of decomposers that use more oxygen, fish and shrimp at the lower layers of the ocean become oxygen-starved and hypoxic zones become apparent.

Quaternary Ammonium Compounds (Quats)

Quats are anti-microbial agents that are found in bathroom cleaners, fabric softeners, and degreasers. They are a class of irritants and sensitizers that negatively affect people who suffer from asthma. Chemicals in this class are persistent in aquatic environments, and toxic to the organisms that live in these environments. Many researchers are concerned that their widespread use in everyday household disinfectants and cosmetics are contributing to antibiotic resistant bacteria, thus limiting microbial infection treatment options.

Trisodium Nitrilotriacetate

Trisodium nitrilotriacetate is found in bathroom cleaners and possibly some laundry detergents although more actively used in industrial formulations. Small amounts add up in the environment and add to an overall toxic issue. In aquatic ecosystems these chemicals cause heavy metals in sediment to redisolve and many of these metals are toxic to fish and other wildlife.

Plasticizers

Phthalates and BPA date back to the 1920s and 1930s. Phthalates have been applied as polyvinyl chloride (PVC) additives since 1926, but were also used for health care purposes as insect repellents and cercaricides. BPA is present in most aquatic environments, entering water systems through landfills and sewage treatment plant runoff allowing for bioaccumulation in aquatic organisms. These endocrine disrupters are a large group of chemicals that enter into the aquatic environment through the manufacturing of various industrial and consumer products, agriculture and food/drug processing, waste water treatment plants and human wastes. Phthalate esters are common additives that soften and make PVC more flexible. It is used in many everyday items such as medical devices, packaging for fragrances and cosmetics, ropes and varnishes, in plastic used to wrap food, and shower curtains. These Phthalate esters have been found in areas of water, air, sediment,and in gulfs and rivers around the world, Giam et al. as cited by. Phalates and BPA affect reproduction in animal groups such as Molluscs, crustaceans, amphibians and fish. Most of these plasticizers affect hormone systems, and some phthalates have even larger pathways of disruption. Phthalates and BPA have been proven to affect development and reproduction in a variety of species. Disturbances include changes in the number of offspring produced and reduced hatching success. In amphibians for example, phthalates and BPA disrupt thyroid functioning which in turn impacts larval development. Molluscs, crustaceans and amphibians appear to be more responsive than fish, with most effects being induced in low concentration ranges with the exception of disrupted spermatogenesis in fish in the low range. A Phthalate referred to as diethyl phthalate (DEP) enters the aquatic environment through industries that manufacture cosmetics, plastics and many commercial products that pose hazards to aquatic organisms and human health. Through exposing an adult male common Carp (Cyprinus carpio) to LC50 doses it was evident that a bioaccumulation of DEP in testis, liver, brain, gills and muscle tissue was present. Fish exposed to 20 ppm of DEP became drowsy and discolored during the onset of the fourth week. Sources of DEP contamination and accumulation in humans include cosmetic products and dietary meat of fish, Persky et al. This DEP acts as a cosmetic ingredient and vehicle for fragrances, both which come in contact with the skin. Many countries around the world including India practice sewage fed fisheries where waste waters are used for the purpose of culturing fish. Endocrine disruption and a presence of phthalate residue is highly likely to be observable in these sewage fed fish. This is the case as waste water from various industries and garbage containing DEP are released into these waters. Through a DEP treatment with Cyprinus carpio, liver size was observed to increase and testis size decreased. In fish, muscle ALT and AST activities decreased as it was effected by DEP treatment. Like many toxic chemicals DEP has been known to affect metabolic enzyme profiles and activities of phosphatases and transaminases, Ghorpade et al. as cited by. A decrease in immunity of M. rosenbergii after exposure to DEP was also noted. Given that biological effect concentrations for plasticizers used in the laboratory coincide with concentrations present in the environment, it seems that some wildlife species must be negatively impacted.

Personal Hygiene Products

Personal care products can reach the environment through drainage from waste water treatment plants and digested sludge. Recently, the anti-dandruff and antimycotic, Climbazole, was detected in waste water treatment drainages. Climbazole is readily used in cosmetics, and is an ingredient in anti-dandruff shampoos. Shampoos contain formulations of up to 2.0% which is the equivalent of approximately 15g/L. Climbazole is classified as very toxic to aquatic organisms. It affects the growth of green algae Pseudokirchneriella subcapitata at very low concentrations. Zebrafish experienced lethal effects after exposure to climbazole in laboratory testing. Effects included thickening of fertilized eggs, lack of somite formation, lack of detachment of the tail bud from the yolk sac, and lack of a heartbeat were evaluated after 48 hours. Along with Danio rerio, Lemna minor, Navicula pelliculosa, Pseudokirchneriella subcapitata, and Daphnia magna were tested and all were found to be negatively affected by climbazole in a concentration-dependant manner with highest toxicity observed in L. minor. Effects included stunted colony growth and darkening in color. Effects of climbazole on oats and turnip included retarded, stunted growth of the leaves and shoot as well as turning darker in color. The aquatic ecotoxicity of climbazole can be classified as very toxic to Lemna and algae, toxic to fish and harmful to Daphnia.

Pesticides

Pesticides often pose serious problems as they kill not only targeted organisms but also non-targeted organisms in the process. They are released into the natural environment intentionally by people who are often unaware that the chemicals will travel further than anticipated, Hatakeyama et al. as cited in.Thus the pesticides largely affect the natural communities in which they are used. They negatively effect multiple levels ranging from molecules to tisues to organs to individuals to populations and onto communities. In the natural environment, a combination of pesticide exposure and natural stressors such as fluctuating temperature, food shortage or decreased oxygen availability are worse than when presented alone. Pesticides can affect the feeding rates of zoo-plankton. In the presence of pesticides zoo-plankton display lower feeding rates which result in reduced growth and reproduction. Swimming may also be affected by pesticides which poses a life-threatening issue for zoo-plankton as they swim to obtain food and nutrients and avoid predators. Such changes may alter predator-prey relationships. A spinning behavior became apparent in Daphnia induced by carbaryl which increased the probability of the Daphnia being eaten by other fish, Dodson et al. as cited by. The toxicant pentachlorophenol increases swimming speed in the rotifer Brachionus calyciflorus, in turn increasing the encounter rate of the prey with their predators, Preston et al. as cited by.

Oil Spills

One of the major environmental impacts of oil exploration on the environment is the contamination of aquatic ecosystems from oil spills and oil seepages from pits. Oftentimes, as is the case in the Ecuadorian Amazon, oil is used to control dust on roadways, causing the precipitation runoff from these roads to also be contaminated. Direct human health hazards occur since many people, including children walk barefoot on these oiled roads putting them in direct contact with the crude oil. Other hazards to humans include seepages into ponds that provide drinking water for the population. During the exploration for oil, mud that has been drilled is deposited into pits. These production pits are often not lined risking the possibility for contaminants to leak into the surrounding environment. Environmental concerns are primarily focused on a group of polycyclic aromatic hydrocarbons (PAHs). “PAHs accumulate on particles and sediments, which tend to protect them from biodegrading processes , Green and Trett as cited in. During the exploration for oil, mud that has been drilled is deposited into pits. These production pits are often not lined risking the possibility for contaminants to leak into the surrounding environment. Samples were collected from four sites (13 stations) in the Ecuadorian Amazon where crude oil was the main pollutant. The water collected from Site B, a drinking water pond located 100m from an in use pit, had the highest total petroleum hydrocarbon (THP) concentration. Sediments were found to be acutely phototoxic. This area which has poorly developed infrastructure is one where residents collect water for drinking, cooking and bathing from the rivers and ponds nearby. “A recent study observed excess cancer rates in a village in this region” Sebastian et. Al, as cited in. Not only were excess cancer rates apparent but many people in this area that were consuming the water for drinking purposes became ill. In Wernersson’s study, toxicity of water and sediment samples were studied on Daphnia magna (a crustacean zoo-plankton species) and Hyalella azteca (an amphipod). These samples were collected from four sites where crude oil was the main source of pollution. 1-4 day old organisms of both species were used in the tests. Immobility of D. magna was recorded after 24 hours of exposure indoors. They were then moved outdoors where they were exposed to sunlight. After 1–2 hours the samples were removed from the sunlight and it was found that D. Magna often recovered within an hour after UV exposure. Hyalella azteca was cultured in the same medium as was used for the D. Magna species. To minimize stress shade was provided. 16 hours of light and 8 hours of darkness were provided. Lethality was recorded after 96 hours of exposure.

REFERENCES

1. Altenburger, Rolf (2011). “Chapter 1. Understanding combined effects for metal co-exposure in ecotoxicology”. Metal ions in toxicology: effects, interactions, interdependencies. pp. 1–26. doi:10.1039/9781849732116-00001.
2. Agency, United States Environmental Protection. “Office of Chemical Safety and Pollution Prevention.” 5 October 2011. U.S Environmental Protection Agency. 9 December 2011.
3. An J, Zhou Q, Sun Y, Xu Z. “Ecotoxicological effects of typical personal care

products on seed germination and seedling development of wheat (Triticum aestivum L.)." Chemosphere (2009): p1428-1434.

4. Bazerman, Charles and René Agustin De los Santos. "Measuring Incommensurability: Are toxicology and ecotoxicology blind to what the other sees?" 9 January 2006.
5. *Chapman P. M. (2002). "Integrating toxicology and ecology: putting the "eco" into ecotoxicology". Marine Pollution Bulletin.* ***44*** *(1): 7–15. doi:10.1016/s0025-326x(01)00253-3.*
6. Clements, William and Jason Rohr. "Community Responses to Contaminants: Using Basic Ecological Principles to Predict Ecotoxicological Events." Environmental Toxicology and Chemistry (2009): p1789-1800.
7. Erkan Kalipci*, Celalettin Özdemir, Fulya Öztas and Serkan Sahinkaya. Ecotoxicological effects of Methyl parathion on living. *African Journal of Agricultural Research* (2010): p712-718.
8. *Fritsch C, Cœurdassier M, Giraudoux P, Raoul F, Douay F, Rieffel D, de Vaufleury A, Scheifler R (2011). Spatially explicit analysis of metal transfer to biota: influence of soil contamination and landscape; . PLOS ONE.* ***6*** *(5): e20682. doi:10.1371/journal.pone.0020682. PMC 3105103. PMID 21655187.*
9. Harley et al. (2006). The impacts of climate change in coastal marine systems. Ecology Letters Vol. 9 Issue 2, Pages 228 - 241
10. The Humane Society of the United States. (2011). Ecotoxicity. Retrieved December 12, 2011, from Procter & Gamble website: http://alttox.org/ttrc/toxicity-tests/ecotoxicity/
11. Maltby L., Naylor C. (1990). Preliminary Observations on the Ecological Relevance of the Gammarus `Scope for Growth' Assay: Effect of Zinc on Reproduction - Functional Ecology, Vol. 4, No. 3, New Horizons in Ecotoxicology (1990), pp. 393–397
12. Mercola, J. (2007). 10 most common environmental toxins. Retrieved December 6, 2011, from Encognitive.com website: http://www.encognitive.com/node/1670
13. Newman, M. C., & Clements, W. H. (2008). Ecotoxicology: a Comprehensive Treatment. Retrieved from https://books.google.com/books?id=y11sdkzQLKkC&pg=PA355&lpg= PA355&dq=ecotoxicology+affecting+population&source=bl&ots=WADQOnWEKb&sig=wkhTGGdYOL4O1mYRg8gAT9iRU&hl=en&ei=snDeTvnbI-L20gGisPC0Bw&sa=X&oi=book_result&ct=result&resnum= 1&ved=0CCIQ6AEwAA#v=onepage&q=ecotoxicology%20affecting%20population&f=false19.2.5
14. Newman, M. C., & Jagoe, C. H. (1996). Ecotoxicology: a Hierarchical Treatment. Retrieved from https://books.google.com/books?hl=en&lr=&id=I1i9SvR4wcMC&oi=fnd&pg=PA197&dq=ecotoxicology+affecting+population&ots=H6rxvWZ9BI&sig=hNJszO7dKkXyL1uf28xF9_VUPJw#v=onepage&q&f=false
15. Oregon State University. (2011, March). Ecotoxicology topic fact sheet. Retrieved December 6, 2011, from National Pesticide Information Center website: http://npic.orst.edu/factsheets/ecotox.pdf

16. Relyea R.; Hoverman J. (2006). "Assessing the ecology in ecotoxicology: a review and synthesis in freshwater systems". Ecology Letters. 9: 1157–1171. doi:10.1111/j.1461-0248.2006.00966.x.

17. Truhaut R (1977). "Eco-Toxicology - Objectives, Principles and Perspectives". Ecotoxicology and Environmental Safety. 1 (2): 151–173. doi:10.1016/0147-6513(77)90033-1.

18. Van Straalen N (2003). Ecotoxicology becomes Stress Ecology . Environmental Science & Technology. 37: 324A–329A. doi:10.1021/es0325720.

CHAPTER 2

Xenobiotic Metabolism

Chapter Contents

- Introduction
- Xenobiotic Metabolism
- Xenobiotics in the Environment
- Inter-Species Organ Transplantation
- Environmental Xenobiotic
- Drug Metabolism
- Cytochrome P450
- Flavin-Containing Monooxygenase
- Alcohol Dehydrogenase
- Peroxidase

A **xenobiotic** is a foreign chemical substance found within an organism that is not normally naturally produced by or expected to be present within. It can also cover substances that are present in much higher concentrations than are usual. Specifically, drugs such as antibiotics are xenobiotics in humans because the human body does not produce them itself, nor are they part of a normal food.

Natural compounds can also become xenobiotics if they are taken up by another organism, such as the uptake of natural human hormones by fish found downstream of sewage treatment plant outfalls, or the chemical defenses produced by some organisms as protection against predators.

INTRODUCTION

The term **xenobiotics**, however, is very often used in the context of pollutants such as dioxins and polychlorinated biphenyls and their effect on the biota, because xenobiotics are understood as substances foreign to an entire biological system, i.e. artificial substances, which did not exist in nature before their synthesis by humans. The term xenobiotic is derived from the Greek words ξένος (xenos) = foreigner, stranger and βίος (bios, vios) = life, plus the Greek suffix for adjectives -τικός, -ή, -ό (tic).

Xenobiotics may be grouped as carcinogens, drugs, environmental pollutants, food additives, hydrocarbons, and pesticides.

XENOBIOTIC METABOLISM

The body removes xenobiotics by xenobiotic metabolism. This consists of the deactivation and the excretion of xenobiotics, and happens mostly in the liver. Excretion routes are urine, feces, breath, and sweat. Hepatic enzymes are responsible for the metabolism of xenobiotics by first activating them (oxidation, reduction, hydrolysis and/or hydration of the xenobiotic), and then conjugating the active secondary metabolite with glucuronic acid, sulphuric acid, or glutathione, followed by excretion in bile or urine. An example of a group of enzymes involved in xenobiotic metabolism is hepatic microsomal cytochrome P450. These enzymes that metabolize xenobiotics are very important for the pharmaceutical industry, because they are responsible for the breakdown of medications.

Organisms can also evolve to tolerate xenobiotics. An example is the co-evolution of the production of tetrodotoxin in the rough-skinned newt and the evolution of tetrodotoxin resistance in its predator, the Common Garter Snake. In this predator–prey pair, an evolutionary arms race has produced high levels of toxin in the newt and correspondingly high levels of resistance in the snake. This evolutionary response is based on the snake evolving modified forms of the ion channels that the toxin acts upon, so becoming resistant to its effects.

XENOBIOTICS IN THE ENVIRONMENT

Xenobiotic substances are an issue for sewage treatment systems, since they are many in number, and each will present its own problems as to how to remove them (and whether it is worth trying to). It can be dangerous to the health.

Some xenobiotics are resistant to degradation. For example, they may be synthetic organochlorides such as plastics and pesticides, or naturally occurring organic chemicals such as polyaromatic hydrocarbons (PAHs) and some fractions of crude oil and coal. However, it is believed that microorganisms are capable of degrading almost all the different complex and resistant xenobiotics found on the earth. Many xenobiotics produce a variety of biological effects, which is used when they are characterized using bioassay. Before they can be registered for sale in most countries, xenobiotic pesticides must undergo extensive evaluation for risk factors, such as toxicity to humans, ecotoxicity, or persistence in the environment. For example, during the registration process, the herbicide, cloransulam-methyl was found to degrade relatively quickly in soil.

INTER-SPECIES ORGAN TRANSPLANTATION

The term **xenobiotic** is also used to refer to organs transplanted from one species to another. For example, some researchers hope that hearts and other organs could be transplanted from pigs to humans. Many people die every year whose lives could have been saved if a critical organ had been available for transplant. Kidneys are currently the most commonly transplanted organ. Xenobiotic organs would need to be developed in such a way that they would not be rejected by the immune system.

ENVIRONMENTAL XENOBIOTIC

Environmental xenobiotic are xenobiotic compounds with a biological activity that are found as pollutants in the natural environment.

Pharmaceuticals

Pharmaceutical drug is a chemical used for the alteration, diagnosis, prevention and treatment of disease, health conditions or structure/function of the human body. **Pharmaceutically active compounds (PhACs)** are those pharmaceuticals that have by one route or another entered the environment as the parent compound or as pharmacologically active metabolites. Drugs are developed with the intention of having a beneficial biological effect on the organism to which they are administered, but many such compounds all too often pass into the environment where they may exert an unwanted biological effect.

For many years PhACs have been all but ignored as environmental researchers concentrated on the well known environmentally dangerous chemicals that were/are largely used in agriculture and industry. But with increasing technology to help in the separation and identification of multiple compounds in a mixture, PhACs and their effects have received increasing attention. PhACs have not (until relatively recently) been seen as potentially toxic because regulations associated with pharmaceuticals are typically overseen by human health organizations which have limited experience with environmental issues.

Nearly all categories of pharmaceuticals including pain killers (analgesics and anti-inflammatory), antibiotics (antibacterial), anticonvulsant drugs, Beta-blockers, blood lipid regulators, X-ray contrast media, cytostatic drugs (Chemotherapy), oral contraceptives, and veterinary pharmaceuticals among many others have been found in the environment.

Sources and Origins

PhACs can be entered into the environment in two main ways; direct and indirect. Indirect sources are PhACs that have performed their biologically intended effect and are passed onto the environment in either their complete or a modified state.

PhAC's can be discharged directly by manufacturers of the pharmaceuticals or effluents from hospitals. However with increasing regulation by local, state and federal regulating agencies, direct discharge is becoming much less of an issue.

There are also several indirect sources of PhACs into the environment. One common indirect source of PhACs into the environment is the passing of antibiotics, anesthetics and growth promoting hormones by domesticated animals in urine and manure. This is often stored in large pits before being pumped and applied to fields as fertilizers where many of the PhACs can be washed away by rainfall to aquatic environments.

Family pets can also be an indirect source of PhACs into the environment.

Most of the PhACs in the environment however come from human sources. A direct human source is leachate from a landfill. Often the pharmaceuticals that are located in landfills are found in their original, most chemically active state.

Most pharmaceuticals are administered and passed through the human body in one of three ways:

- Metabolized partially or completely within the body and made inactive (Ideal)
- Partially metabolized and passed through the system
- Passed through the body unmodified (Worst Case Scenario). In any manner PhACs are then passed to sewage treatment plants (STPs), where facilities are designed to break down natural human waste by microbial degradation. However, many PhACs are of very complex structure and are incompletely broken down in STPs before they are passed into the environment.

Fate in Environment

Once PhACs are entered into the environment they suffer one of three fates:

- Biodegradation into carbon dioxide and water.
- Undergo some form of degradation and form metabolites.
- Persist in the environment unmodified. The amount of the compound that is broken down depends on several factors such as bioavailability and compound structure among many others.

Effects

Because PhACs have come into the limelight relatively recently their effects on the environment are not completely understood. PhACs are also not generally intended to come in contact with the environment, and therefore are not typically tested environmentally prior to release. Therefore several tests are required to determine the different mechanisms and side effects of PhACs in the environment making testing largely impractical.

Many PhACs have very broad modes of action in humans. Similar, subtle reactions may occur in organisms in the environment that are not easily seen by humans. Highly specific mechanisms in humans may solicit profound effects at extremely low concentrations. Many effects may not necessarily be readily detectable and lead to ecological change that would be erroneously attributed to natural change. This said there are several effects that have been identified in the literature.

One long term, possibly irreversible effect is microbiological resistance to antibiotics (antibiotic resistance). Some bacteria may be able to survive when administered antibiotics (especially at low concentrations). Those colonies will multiply and produce new colonies that are resistant to that particular antibiotic and will not succumb the next time antibiotics are administered. Because rivers and streams are ever flowing objects they are an ideal pathway for antibiotics to reach bacteria and therefore provide a source and reservoir for resistant strains to develop and establish themselves.

Another recent discovery is endocrine disruptors. Endocrine disruptors can replace or disturb the balance of hormones within an organism and have been found to be occurring in waters with a concentration in the ng/L level for certain compounds. Some possible effects of endocrine disruptors are male and female sterility, feminization of males, masculinization of females and abnormal testes growth among many others. The exact pathway of occurrence of endocrine disruptors is not completely certain, however several pathways have been proposed.

Typically PhACs are found in low concentrations, (<1 ug/L) making acute toxicity effects fairly unlikely. However, because of their continual input to the environment it is possible for chronic toxicity effects to occur. One major area of concern with several compounds being present at low levels at the same time is what happens when the compounds mix? It is possible and truly likely that these mixtures will have additive, neutralistic or synergistic effects. But again testing would be both time consuming and very expensive to test all of the combined effects.

Common PhACs Found in the Environment

Analgesics (anti-inflammatory and antipyretic)

- Acetaminophen
- Acetylsalicylic Acid
- Diclofenac
- Codeine
- Ibuprofen

Antibiotics

- Macrolide Antibiotics
- Sulfonamides
- Fluoroquinolones
- Chloraphenicol
- Tylosin
- Trimethoprim
- Erythromycin
- Lincomycin
- Sulfamethoxazole
- Trimethoprim

Anticonvulsant

- Carbamazepine
- Primidone

Beta-blockers

- Metoprolol
- Propanolol
- Betaxolol
- Bisoprolol
- Nadolol

X-ray Media

- Iopromide
- Iopamidol
- Iohexol
- Diatrizoate

Cytostatics (Chemotherapy Drugs)

Steroids and hormones

- 17α-ethinylestradiol
- Mestranol
- 19-norethisterone

DRUG METABOLISM

Drug metabolism is the metabolic breakdown of drugs by living organisms, usually through specialized enzymatic systems. More generally, **xenobiotic metabolism** (from the Greek xenos "stranger" and biotic "related to living beings") is the set of metabolic pathways that modify the chemical structure of xenobiotics, which are compounds foreign to an organism's normal biochemistry, such any drug or poison. These pathways are a form of biotransformation present in all major groups of organisms, and are considered to be of ancient origin. These reactions often act to detoxify poisonous compounds (although in some cases the intermediates in xenobiotic metabolism can themselves cause toxic effects). The study of drug metabolism is called pharmacokinetics.

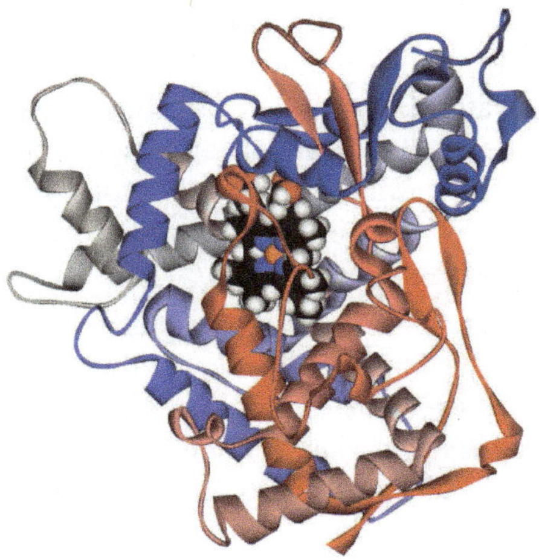

Cytochrome P450 oxidases are important enzymes in xenobiotic metabolism.

The metabolism of pharmaceutical drugs is an important aspect of pharmacology and medicine. For example, the rate of metabolism determines the duration and intensity of a drug's pharmacologic action. Drug metabolism also affects multidrug resistance in infectious diseases and in chemotherapy for cancer, and the actions of some drugs as substrates or inhibitors of enzymes involved in xenobiotic metabolism are a common reason for hazardous drug interactions. These pathways are also important in environmental science, with the xenobiotic metabolism of microorganisms determining whether a pollutant will be broken down during bioremediation, or persist in the environment. The enzymes of xenobiotic metabolism, particularly the glutathione S-transferases are also important in agriculture, since they may produce resistance to pesticides and herbicides.

Drug metabolism is divided into three phases. In phase I, enzymes such as cytochrome P450 oxidases introduce reactive or polar groups into xenobiotics. These modified compounds are then conjugated to polar compounds in phase II reactions. These reactions are catalysed by transferase enzymes such as glutathione S-transferases. Finally, in phase III, the conjugated xenobiotics may be further processed, before being recognised by efflux transporters and pumped out of cells. Drug metabolism often converts lipophilic compounds into hydrophilic products that are more readily excreted.

Permeability Barriers and Detoxification

The exact compounds an organism is exposed to will be largely unpredictable, and may differ widely over time; these are major characteristics of xenobiotic toxic stress. The major challenge faced by xenobiotic detoxification systems is that they must be able to remove the almost-limitless number of xenobiotic compounds from the complex mixture of chemicals involved in normal metabolism. The solution that has evolved to address this problem is an elegant combination of physical barriers and low-specificity enzymatic systems.

All organisms use cell membranes as hydrophobic permeability barriers to control access to their internal environment. Polar compounds cannot diffuse across these cell membranes, and the uptake of useful molecules is mediated through transport proteins that specifically select substrates from the extracellular mixture. This selective uptake means that most hydrophilic molecules cannot enter cells, since they are not recognised by any specific transporters. In contrast, the diffusion of hydrophobic compounds across these barriers cannot be controlled, and organisms, therefore, cannot exclude lipid-soluble xenobiotics using membrane barriers.

However, the existence of a permeability barrier means that organisms were able to evolve detoxification systems that exploit the hydrophobicity common to membrane-permeable xenobiotics. These systems therefore solve the specificity problem by possessing such broad substrate specificities that they metabolise almost any non-polar compound. Useful metabolites are excluded since they are polar, and in general contain one or more charged groups.

The detoxification of the reactive by-products of normal metabolism cannot be achieved by the systems outlined above, because these species are derived from normal cellular constituents and usually share their polar characteristics. However, since these compounds are few in number, specific enzymes can recognize and remove them. Examples of these specific detoxification systems are the glyoxalase system, which removes the reactive aldehyde methylglyoxal, and the various antioxidant systems that eliminate reactive oxygen species.

Phases of Detoxification

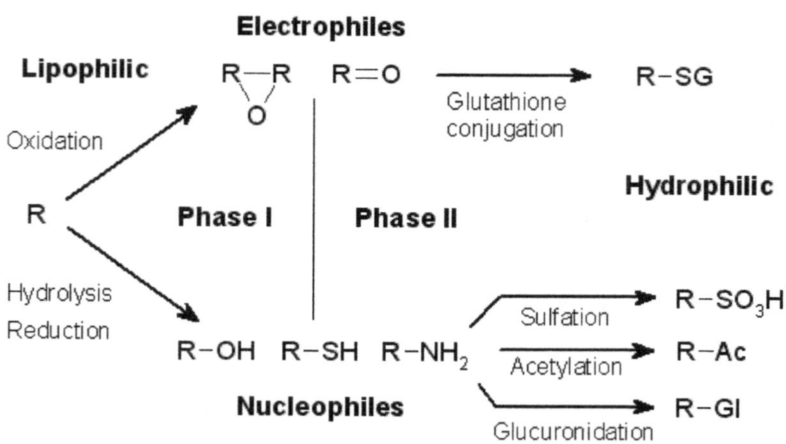

Phases I and II of the metabolism of a lipophilic xenobiotic.

The metabolism of xenobiotics is often divided into three phases:- modification, conjugation, and excretion. These reactions act in concert to detoxify xenobiotics and remove them from cells.

Phase I – Modification

In phase I, a variety of enzymes act to introduce reactive and polar groups into their substrates. One of the most common modifications is hydroxylation catalysed by the cytochrome P-450-dependent mixed-function oxidase system. These enzyme complexes act to incorporate an atom of oxygen into nonactivated hydrocarbons, which can result in either the introduction of hydroxyl groups or N-, O- and S-dealkylation of substrates. The reaction mechanism of the P-450 oxidases proceeds through the reduction of cytochrome-bound oxygen and the generation of a highly-reactive oxyferryl species, according to the following scheme:

$$O_2 + NADPH + H^+ + RH \rightarrow NADP^+ + H_2O + ROH$$

Phase I reactions (also termed nonsynthetic reactions) may occur by oxidation, reduction, hydrolysis, cyclization, decyclization, and addition of oxygen or removal of hydrogen, carried out by mixed function oxidases, often in the liver. These oxidative reactions typically involve a cytochrome P450 monooxygenase (often abbreviated CYP), NADPH and oxygen. The classes of pharmaceutical drugs that utilize this method for their metabolism include phenothiazines, paracetamol, and steroids. If the metabolites of phase I reactions are sufficiently polar, they may be readily excreted at this point. However, many phase I products are not eliminated rapidly and undergo a subsequent reaction in which an endogenous substrate combines with the newly incorporated functional group to form a highly polar conjugate.

A common Phase I oxidation involves conversion of a C-H bond to a C-OH. This reaction sometimes converts a pharmacologically inactive compound (a prodrug) to a pharmacologically active one. By the same token, Phase I can turn a nontoxic molecule into a poisonous one (toxification). Simple hydrolysis in the stomach is normally an innocuous reaction, however there are exceptions. For example, phase I metabolism converts acetonitrile to $HOCH_2CN$, which rapidly dissociates into formaldehyde and hydrogen cyanide, both of which are toxic.

Phase I metabolism of drug candidates can be simulated in the laboratory using non-enzyme catalysts.This example of a biomimetic reaction tends to give products that often contains the Phase I metabolites. As an example, the major metabolite of the pharmaceutical trimebutine, desmethyltrimebutine (nor-trimebutine), can be efficiently produced by in vitro oxidation of the commercially available drug. Hydroxylation of an N-methyl group leads to expulsion of a molecule of formaldehyde, while oxidation of the O-methyl groups takes place to a lesser extent.

Oxidation

- Cytochrome P450 monooxygenase system
- Flavin-containing monooxygenase system

- Alcohol dehydrogenase and aldehyde dehydrogenase
- Monoamine oxidase
- Co-oxidation by peroxidases

Reduction

- NADPH-cytochrome P450 reductase

Cytochrome P450 reductase, also known as NADPH:ferrihemoprotein oxidoreductase, NADPH:hemoprotein oxidoreductase, NADPH:P450 oxidoreductase, P450 reductase, POR, CPR, CYPOR, is a membrane-bound enzyme required for electron transfer to cytochrome P450 in the microsome of the eukaryotic cell from a FAD- and FMN-containing enzyme NADPH:cytochrome P450 reductase The general scheme of electron flow in the POR/ P450 system is: NADPH → FAD → FMN → P450 → O_2

- Reduced (ferrous) cytochrome P450

During reduction reactions, a chemical can enter *futile cycling*, in which it gains a free-radical electron, then promptly loses it to oxygen (to form a superoxide anion).

Hydrolysis

- Esterases and amidase
- Epoxide hydrolase

Phase II – conjugation

In subsequent phase II reactions, these activated xenobiotic metabolites are conjugated with charged species such as glutathione (GSH), sulfate, glycine, or glucuronic acid. Sites on drugs where conjugation reactions occur include carboxyl (-COOH), hydroxyl (-OH), amino (NH_2), and sulfhydryl (-SH) groups. Products of conjugation reactions have increased molecular weight and tend to be less active than their substrates, unlike Phase I reactions which often produce active metabolites. The addition of large anionic groups (such as GSH) detoxifies reactive electrophiles and produces more polar metabolites that cannot diffuse across membranes, and may, therefore, be actively transported.

These reactions are catalysed by a large group of broad-specificity transferases, which in combination can metabolise almost any hydrophobic compound that contains nucleophilic or electrophilic groups.One of the most important classes of this group is that of the glutathione S-transferases (GSTs).

Mechanism	Involved enzyme	Co-factor	Location
methylation	methyltransferase	S-adenosyl-L-methionine	liver, kidney, lung, CNS
sulphation	sulfotransferases	3'-phosphoadenosine-5'-phosphosulfate	liver, kidney, intestine

acetylation	• N-acetyltransferases • bile acid-CoA:amino acid N-acyltransferases	acetyl coenzyme A	liver, lung, spleen, gastric mucosa, RBCs, lymphocytes
glucuronidation	UDP-glucuronosyltransferases	UDP-glucuronic acid	liver, kidney, intestine, lung, skin, prostate, brain
glutathione conjugation	glutathione S-transferases	glutathione	liver, kidney
glycine conjugation	acetyl Co-enzyme As	glycine	liver, kidney

Phase III – Further Modification and Excretion

After phase II reactions, the xenobiotic conjugates may be further metabolised. A common example is the processing of glutathione conjugates to acetylcysteine (mercapturic acid) conjugates. Here, the γ-glutamate and glycine residues in the glutathione molecule are removed by Gamma-glutamyl transpeptidase and dipeptidases. In the final step, the cystine residue in the conjugate is acetylated.

Conjugates and their metabolites can be excreted from cells in phase III of their metabolism, with the anionic groups acting as affinity tags for a variety of membrane transporters of the multidrug resistance protein (MRP) family. These proteins are members of the family of ATP-binding cassette transporters and can catalyse the ATP-dependent transport of a huge variety of hydrophobic anions, and thus act to remove phase II products to the extracellular medium, where they may be further metabolised or excreted.

Endogenous Toxins

The detoxification of endogenous reactive metabolites such as peroxides and reactive aldehydes often cannot be achieved by the system described above. This is the result of these species' being derived from normal cellular constituents and usually sharing their polar characteristics. However, since these compounds are few in number, it is possible for enzymatic systems to utilize specific molecular recognition to recognize and remove them. The similarity of these molecules to useful metabolites therefore means that different detoxification enzymes are usually required for the metabolism of each group of endogenous toxins. Examples of these specific detoxification systems are the glyoxalase system, which acts to dispose of the reactive aldehyde methylglyoxal, and the various antioxidant systems that remove reactive oxygen species.

Sites

Quantitatively, the smooth endoplasmic reticulum of the liver cell is the principal organ of drug metabolism, although every biological tissue has some ability to metabolize drugs. Factors responsible for the liver's contribution to drug metabolism include that it is a large organ, that it is the first organ perfused by chemicals absorbed in the gut, and that there are very high concentrations of most drug-metabolizing enzyme systems relative to other organs. If a drug is taken into the GI tract, where it enters hepatic circulation through the portal vein, it becomes well-metabolized and is said to show the *first pass effect.*

Other sites of drug metabolism include epithelial cells of the gastrointestinal tract, lungs, kidneys, and the skin. These sites are usually responsible for localized toxicity reactions.

Factors Affecting Drug Metabolism

The duration and intensity of pharmacological action of most lipophilic drugs are determined by the rate they are metabolized to inactive products. The Cytochrome P450 monooxygenase system is the most important pathway in this regard. In general, anything that *increases* the rate of metabolism (*e.g.*, enzyme induction) of a pharmacologically active metabolite will *decrease* the duration and intensity of the drug action. The opposite is also true (*e.g.*, enzyme inhibition). However, in cases where an enzyme is responsible for metabolizing a pro-drug into a drug, enzyme induction can speed up this conversion and increase drug levels, potentially causing toxicity.

Various *physiological* and *pathological* factors can also affect drug metabolism. Physiological factors that can influence drug metabolism include age, individual variation (*e.g.*, pharmacogenetics), enterohepatic circulation, nutrition, intestinal flora, or sex differences.

In general, drugs are metabolized more slowly in fetal, neonatal and elderly humans and animals than in adults.

Genetic variation (polymorphism) accounts for some of the variability in the effect of drugs. With N-acetyltransferases (involved in *Phase II* reactions), individual variation creates a group of people who acetylate slowly (*slow acetylators*) and those who acetylate quickly, split roughly 50:50 in the population of Canada. This variation may have dramatic consequences, as the slow acetylators are more prone to dose-dependent toxicity.

Cytochrome P450 monooxygenase system enzymes can also vary across individuals, with deficiencies occurring in 1 – 30% of people, depending on their ethnic background.

Pathological factors can also influence drug metabolism, including liver, kidney, or heart diseases.

In silico modelling and simulation methods allow drug metabolism to be predicted in virtual patient populations prior to performing clinical studies in human subjects. This can be used to identify individuals most at risk from adverse reaction.

Studies on how people transform the substances that they ingest began in the mid-nineteenth century, with chemists discovering that organic chemicals such as benzaldehyde could be oxidized and conjugated to amino acids in the human body. During the remainder of the nineteenth century, several other basic detoxification reactions were discovered, such as methylation, acetylation, and sulfonation.

In the early twentieth century, work moved on to the investigation of the enzymes and pathways that were responsible for the production of these metabolites. This field became defined as a separate area of study with the publication by Richard Williams of the book *Detoxication mechanisms* in 1947. This modern biochemical research resulted in the identification of glutathione *S*-transferases in 1961,followed by the discovery of cytochrome P450s in 1962, and the realization of their central role in xenobiotic metabolism in 1963.

CYTOCHROME P450

Cytochromes P450 (CYPs) are proteins of the superfamily containing heme as a cofactor and, therefore, are hemoproteins. CYPs use a variety of small and large molecules as substrates in enzymatic reactions. They are, in general, the terminal oxidase enzymes in electron transfer chains, broadly categorized as P450-containing systems. The term *P450* is derived from the spectrophotometric peak at the wavelength of the absorption maximum of the enzyme (450 nm) when it is in the reduced state and complexed with carbon monoxide.

CYP enzymes have been identified in all kingdoms of life: animals, plants, fungi, protists, bacteria, archaea, and even in viruses. However, they are not omnipresent; for example, they have not been found in *Escherichia coli*. More than 200,000 distinct CYP proteins are known.

Most CYPs require a protein partner to deliver one or more electrons to reduce the iron (and eventually molecular oxygen). Based on the nature of the electron transfer proteins, CYPs can be classified into several groups:

- **Microsomal P450 systems**, in which electrons are transferred from NADPH via cytochrome P450 reductase (variously CPR, POR, or CYPOR). Cytochrome b5 (cyb5) can also contribute reducing power to this system after being reduced by cytochrome b5 reductase (CYB5R).
- **Mitochondrial P450 systems**, which employ adrenodoxin reductase and adrenodoxin to transfer electrons from NADPH to P450.
- **Bacterial P450 systems**, which employ a ferredoxin reductase and a ferredoxin to transfer electrons to P450.
- **CYB5R/cyb5/P450 systems**, in which both electrons required by the CYP come from cytochrome b5.
- **FMN/Fd/P450 systems**, originally found in *Rhodococcus* species, in which a FMN-domain-containing reductase is fused to the CYP.
- **P450 only** systems, which do not require external reducing power. Notable ones include thromboxane synthase (CYP5), prostacyclin synthase (CYP8), and CYP74A (allene oxide synthase).

The most common reaction catalyzed by cytochromes P450 is a monooxygenase reaction, e.g., insertion of one atom of oxygen into the aliphatic position of an organic substrate (RH) while the other oxygen atom is reduced to water:

$$RH + O_2 + NADPH + H^+ \rightarrow ROH + H_2O + NADP^+$$

Many hydroxylation reactions (insertion of hydroxyl groups) use CYP enzymes.

Nomenclature

Genes encoding CYP enzymes, and the enzymes themselves, are designated with the root symbol **CYP** for the superfamily, followed by a number indicating the gene family, a capital letter indicating the subfamily, and another numeral for the individual gene. The convention is to *italicise* the name when referring to the gene. For example, *CYP2E1* is the gene that encodes the enzyme CYP2E1—one of the enzymes involved in paracetamol (acetaminophen) metabolism. The **CYP** nomenclature is the official naming convention, although occasionally **CYP450** or **CYP$_{450}$** is used synonymously. However, some gene or enzyme names for CYPs may differ from this nomenclature, denoting the catalytic activity and the name of the compound used as substrate. Examples include CYP5A1, thromboxane A_2 synthase, abbreviated to TBXAS1 (**T**hrom**B**o**X**ane **A**$_2$ **S**ynthase **1**), and CYP51A1, lanosterol 14-α-demethylase, sometimes unofficially abbreviated to LDM according to its substrate (**L**anosterol) and activity (**D**e**M**ethylation).

The current nomenclature guidelines suggest that members of new CYP families share at least 40% amino acid identity, while members of subfamilies must share at least 55% amino acid identity. There are nomenclature committees that assign and track both base gene names (Cytochrome P450 Homepage) and allele names (CYP Allele Nomenclature Committee).

Mechanism

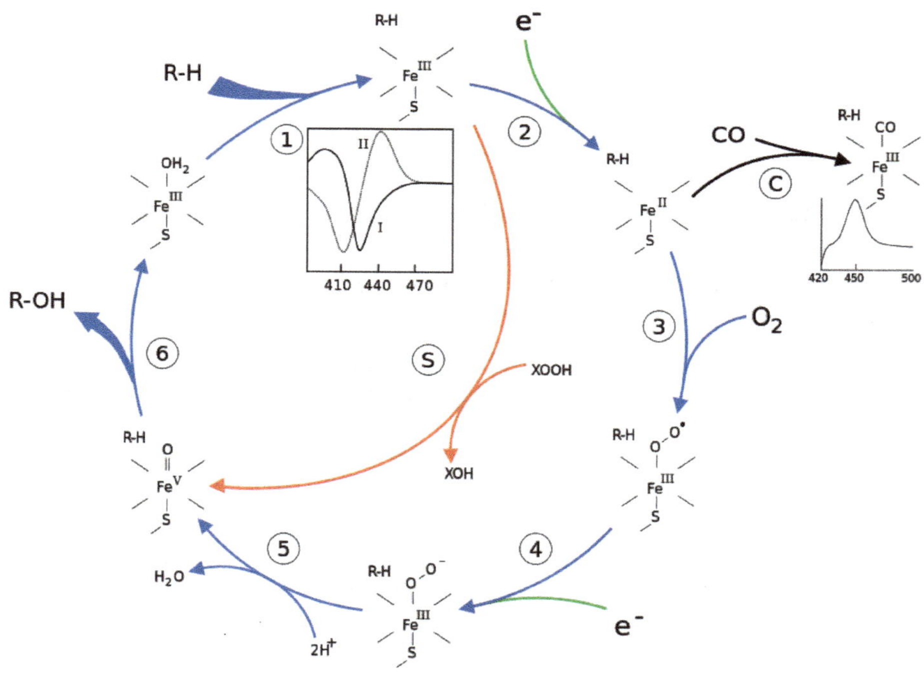

The "Fe(V) intermediate" at the bottom left is a simplification: it is an Fe(IV) with a radical heme ligand.

Structure

The active site of cytochrome P450 contains a heme-iron center. The iron is tethered to the protein via a cysteine thiolate ligand. This cysteine and several flanking residues are highly conserved in known CYPs and have the formal PROSITE signature consensus pattern [FW] - [SGNH] - x - [GD] - {F} - [RKHPT] - {P} - C - [LIVMFAP] - [GAD]. Because of the vast variety of reactions catalyzed by CYPs, the activities and properties of the many CYPs differ in many aspects. In general, the P450 catalytic cycle proceeds as follows:

Catalytic Cycle

- Substrate binds in proximity to the heme group, on the side opposite to the axial thiolate. Substrate binding induces a change in the conformation of the active site, often displacing a water molecule from the distal axial coordination position of the heme iron, and changing the state of the heme iron from low-spin to high-spin.
- Substrate binding induces electron transfer from NAD(P)H via cytochrome P450 reductase or another associated reductase.
- Molecular oxygen binds to the resulting ferrous heme center at the distal axial coordination position, initially giving a dioxygen adduct not unlike oxy-myoglobin.
- A second electron is transferred, from either cytochrome P450 reductase, ferredoxins, or cytochrome b5, reducing the Fe-O_2 adduct to give a short-lived peroxo state.
- The peroxo group formed in step 4 is rapidly protonated twice, releasing one molecule of water and forming the highly reactive species referred to as **P450 Compound 1** (or just Compound I). This highly reactive intermediate was isolated in 2010, P450 Compound 1 is an iron(IV) oxo (or ferryl) species with an additional oxidizing equivalent delocalized over the porphyrin and thiolate ligands. Evidence for the alternative perferryl iron(V)-oxo is lacking.
- Depending on the substrate and enzyme involved, P450 enzymes can catalyze any of a wide variety of reactions. A hypothetical hydroxylation is shown in this illustration. After the product has been released from the active site, the enzyme returns to its original state, with a water molecule returning to occupy the distal coordination position of the iron nucleus.

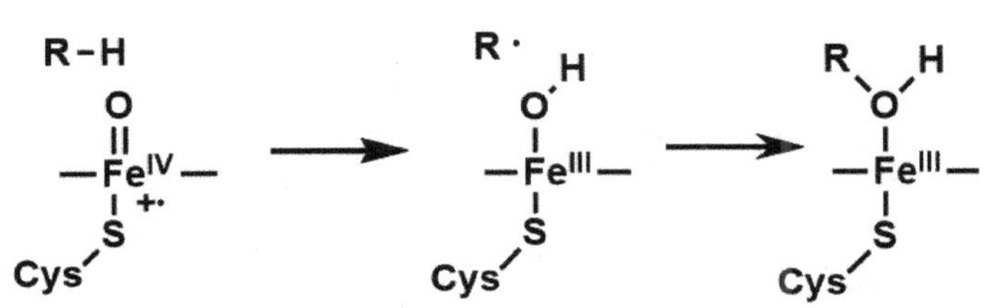

Oxygen rebound mechanism utilized by cytochrome P450 for conversion of hydrocarbons to alcohols via the action of "compound I", an iron(IV) oxide bound to a radical heme.

- An alternative route for mono-oxygenation is via the "peroxide shunt" (path "S" in figure). This pathway entails oxidation of the ferric-substrate complex with oxygen-atom donors such as peroxides and hypochlorites. A hypothetical peroxide "XOOH" is shown in the diagram.

Spectroscopy

Binding of substrate is reflected in the spectral properties of the enzyme, with an increase in absorbance at 390 nm and a decrease at 420 nm. This can be measured by difference spectrometry and is referred to as the "type I" difference spectrum (see inset graph in figure). Some substrates cause an opposite change in spectral properties, a "reverse type I" spectrum, by processes that are as yet unclear. Inhibitors and certain substrates that bind directly to the heme iron give rise to the type II difference spectrum, with a maximum at 430 nm and a minimum at 390 nm (see inset graph in figure). If no reducing equivalents are available, this complex may remain stable, allowing the degree of binding to be determined from absorbance measurements *in vitro* C: If carbon monoxide (CO) binds to reduced P450, the catalytic cycle is interrupted. This reaction yields the classic CO difference spectrum with a maximum at 450 nm.

P450s in Humans

Human CYPs are primarily membrane-associated proteins located either in the inner membrane of mitochondria or in the endoplasmic reticulum of cells. CYPs metabolize thousands of endogenous and exogenous chemicals. Some CYPs metabolize only one (or a very few) substrates, such as *CYP19* (aromatase), while others may metabolize multiple substrates. Both of these characteristics account for their central importance in medicine. Cytochrome P450 enzymes are present in most tissues of the body, and play important roles in hormone synthesis and breakdown (including estrogen and testosterone synthesis and metabolism), cholesterol synthesis, and vitamin D metabolism. Cytochrome P450 enzymes also function to metabolize potentially toxic compounds, including drugs and products of endogenous metabolism such as bilirubin, principally in the liver.

The Human Genome Project has identified 57 human genes coding for the various cytochrome P450 enzymes.

Drug Metabolism

CYPs are the major enzymes involved in drug metabolism, accounting for about 75% of the total metabolism. Most drugs undergo deactivation by CYPs, either directly or by facilitated excretion from the body. Also, many substances are bioactivated by CYPs to form their active compounds.

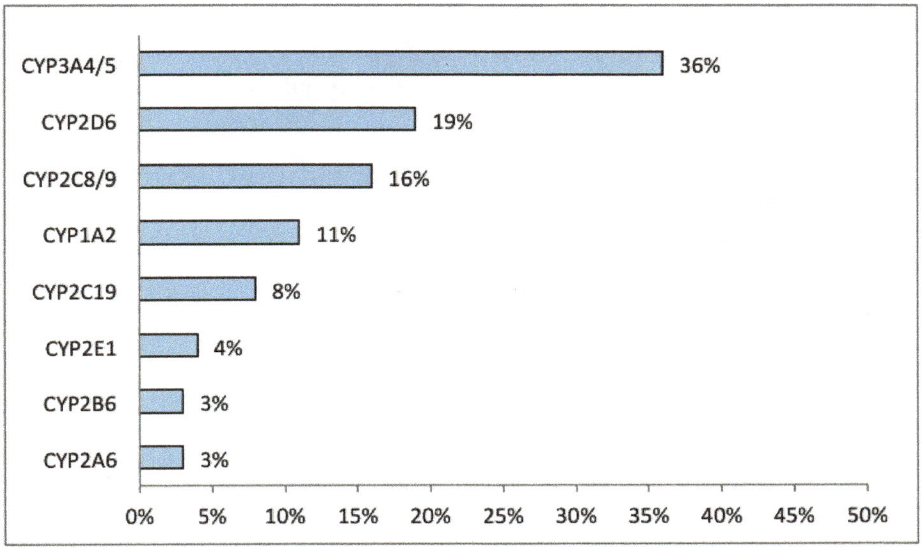

Proportion of antifungal drugs metabolized by different families of CYPs.

Drug Interaction

Many drugs may increase or decrease the activity of various CYP isozymes either by inducing the biosynthesis of an isozyme (enzyme induction) or by directly inhibiting the activity of the CYP (enzyme inhibition). This is a major source of adverse drug interactions, since changes in CYP enzyme activity may affect the metabolism and clearance of various drugs. For example, if one drug inhibits the CYP-mediated metabolism of another drug, the second drug may accumulate within the body to toxic levels. Hence, these drug interactions may necessitate dosage adjustments or choosing drugs that do not interact with the CYP system. Such drug interactions are especially important to take into account when using drugs of vital importance to the patient, drugs with important side-effects and drugs with small therapeutic windows, but any drug may be subject to an altered plasma concentration due to altered drug metabolism.

A classical example includes anti-epileptic drugs. Phenytoin, for example, induces CYP1A2, CYP2C9, CYP2C19, and CYP3A4. Substrates for the latter may be drugs with critical dosage, like amiodarone or carbamazepine, whose blood plasma concentration may either increase because of enzyme inhibition in the former, or decrease because of enzyme induction in the latter.

Interaction of other Substances

Naturally occurring compounds may also induce or inhibit CYP activity. For example, bioactive compounds found in grapefruit juice and some other fruit juices, including bergamottin, dihydroxybergamottin, and paradicin-A, have been found to inhibit CYP3A4-

mediated metabolism of certain medications, leading to increased bioavailability and, thus, the strong possibility of overdosing.Because of this risk, avoiding grapefruit juice and fresh grapefruits entirely while on drugs is usually advised.

Other examples:

- Saint-John's wort, a common herbal remedy induces CYP3A4, but also inhibits CYP1A1, CYP1B1, and CYP2D6.
- Tobacco smoking induces CYP1A2 (example CYP1A2 substrates are clozapine, olanzapine, and fluvoxamine)
- At relatively high concentrations, starfruit juice has also been shown to inhibit CYP2A6 and other CYPs. Watercress is also a known inhibitor of the cytochrome P450 CYP2E1, which may result in altered drug metabolism for individuals on certain medications (e.g., chlorzoxazone).
- Tributyltin has been found to inhibit the function of Cytochrome P450, leading to masculinization of mollusks.
- Goldenseal, with its two notable alkaloids berberine and hydrastine, has been shown to alter P450-marker enzymatic activities (involving CYP2C9, CYP2D6, and CYP3A4).

Other specific CYP Functions

Steroid Hormones

A subset of cytochrome P450 enzymes play important roles in the synthesis of steroid hormones (steroidogenesis) by the adrenals, gonads, and peripheral tissue:

- CYP11A1 (also known as P450scc or P450c11a1) in adrenal mitochondria affects "the activity formerly known as 20,22-desmolase (steroid 20α-hydroxylase, steroid 22-hydroxylase, cholesterol side-chain scission).
- CYP11B1 (encoding the protein P450c11β) found in the inner mitochondrial membrane of adrenal cortex has steroid 11β-hydroxylase, steroid 18-hydroxylase, and steroid 18-methyloxidase activities.
- CYP11B2 (encoding the protein P450c11AS), found only in the mitochondria of the adrenal zona glomerulosa, has steroid 11β-hydroxylase, steroid 18-hydroxylase, and steroid 18-methyloxidase activities.
- CYP17A1, in endoplasmic reticulum of adrenal cortex has steroid 17α-hydroxylase and 17,20-lyase activities.
- CYP21A1 (P450c21) in adrenal cortex conducts 21-hydroxylase activity.
- CYP19A (P450arom, aromatase) in endoplasmic reticulum of gonads, brain, adipose tissue, and elsewhere catalyzes aromatization of androgens to estrogens.

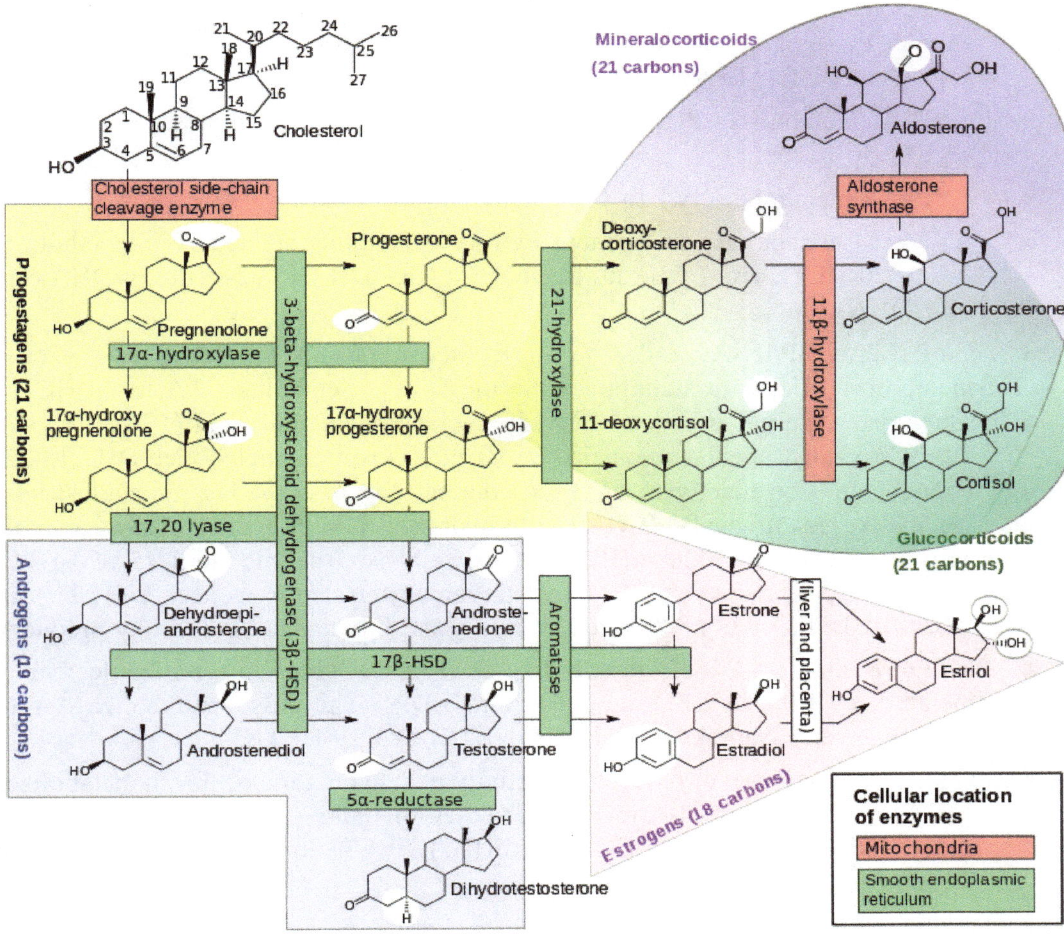

Steroidogenesis, showing many of the enzyme activities that are performed by cytochrome P450 enzymes. HSD: Hydroxysteroid dehydrogenase.

Polyunsaturated Fatty Acids And Eicosanoids

Certain cytochrome P450 enzymes are critical in metabolizing polyunstaturated fatty acids (PUFAs) to biologically active, intercellular cell signaling molecules (eicosanoids) and/or metabolize biologically active metabolites of the PUFA to less active or inactive products. These CYPs possess Cytochrome P450 omega hydroxylase and/or epoxygenase enzyme activity.

- CYP1A1, CYP1A2, and CYP2E1 metabolize endogenous PUFAs to signaling molecules: they metabolize arachidonic acid (i.e. AA) to 19-hydroxyeicosatetraenoic acid (i.e. 19-HETE; see 20-Hydroxyeicosatetraenoic acid); eicosapentaenoic acid (i.e. EPA) to epoxyeicosatetraenoic acids (i.e. EEQs); and docosahexaenoic acid (i.e. DHA) to epoxydocosapentaenoic acids (i.e. EDPs).

- CYP2C8, CYP2C9, CYP2C18, CYP2C19, and CYP2J2 metabolize endogenous PUFAs to signaling molecules: they metabolize AA to epoxyeicosatetraenoic acids (i.e. EETs); EPA to EEQs; and DHA to EDPs.
- CYP2S1 metabolizes PUFA to signaling molecules: it metabolizes AA to EETs ad EPA to EEQs.
- CYP3A4 metabolizes AA to EET signaling molecules.
- CYP4A11 metabolizes endogenous PUFAs to signaling molecules: it metabolizes AA to 20-HETE and EETs; it also hydroxylates DHA to 22-hydroxy-DHA (i.e. 12-HDHA).
- CYP4F2, CYP4F3A, and CYP4F3B (see CYP4F3 for latter two CYPs) metabolize PUFAs to signaling molecules: they metabolizes AA to 20-HETE. They also metabolize EPA to 19-hydroxyeicosapentaenoic acid (19-HEPE) and 20-hydroxyeicosapentaenoic acid (20-HEPE) as well as metabolize DHA to 22-HDA. They also inactivate or reduce the activity of signaling molecules: they metabolize leukotriene B4 (LTB4) to 20-hydroxy-LTB4, 5-hydroxyeicosatetraenoic acid (5-HETE) to 5,20-diHETE, 5-oxo-eicosatetraenoic acid (5-oxo-ETE) to 5-oxo,20-hydroxy-ETE, 12-hydroxyeicosatetraenoic acid (12-HETE) to 12,20-diHETE, EETs to 20-hydroxy-EETs, and lipoxins to 20-hydroxy products.
- CYP4F8 and CYP4F12 metabolize PUFAs to signaling molecules: they metabolizes EPA to EEQs and DHA to EDPs. They also metabolize AA to 18-hydroxyeicosatetraenoic acid (18-HETE) and 19-HETE.
- CYP4F11 inactivates or reduces the activity of signaling molecules: it metabolizes LTB4 to 20-hydroxy-LTB4, (5-HETE) to 5,20-diHETE, (5-oxo-ETE) to 5-oxo,20-hydroxy-ETE, (12-HETE) to 12,20-diHETE, EETs to 20-hydroxy-EETs, and lipoxins to 20-hydroxy products.
- CYP4F22 ω-hydroxylates extremely long "very long chain fatty acids, i.e. fatty acids that are 28 or more carbons long. The ω-hydroxylation of these special fatty acids is critical to creating and maintaining the skins water barrier function; autosomal recessive inactivating mutations of CYP4F22 are associated with the Lamellar ichthyosis subtype of Congenital ichthyosiform erythrodema in humans.

CYP Families in Humans

Humans have 57 genes and more than 59 pseudogenes divided among 18 families of cytochrome P450 genes and 43 subfamilies. This is a summary of the genes and of the proteins they encode. See the homepage of the Cytochrome P450 Nomenclature Committee for detailed information.

Family	Function	Members	Names
CYP1	drug and steroid (especially estrogen) metabolism, benzo[*a*] pyrene toxification (forming (+)-benzo[*a*] pyrene-7,8-dihydrodiol-9,10-epoxide)	3 subfamilies, 3 genes, 1 pseudogene	CYP1A1, CYP1A2, CYP1B1
CYP2	drug and steroid metabolism	13 subfamilies, 16 genes, 16 pseudogenes	CYP2A6, CYP2A7, CYP2A13, CYP2B6, CYP2C8, CYP2C9, CYP2C18, CYP2C19, CYP2D6, CYP2E1, CYP2F1, CYP2J2, CYP2R1, CYP2S1, CYP2U1, CYP2W1
CYP3	drug and steroid (including testosterone) metabolism	1 subfamily, 4 genes, 2 pseudogenes	CYP3A4, CYP3A5, CYP3A7, CYP3A43
CYP4	arachidonic acid or fatty acid metabolism	6 subfamilies, 12 genes, 10 pseudogenes	CYP4A11, CYP4A22, CYP4B1, CYP4F2, CYP4F3, CYP4F8, CYP4F11, CYP4F12, CYP4F22, CYP4V2, CYP4X1, CYP4Z1
CYP5	thromboxane A_2 synthase	1 subfamily, 1 gene	CYP5A1
CYP7	bile acid biosynthesis 7-alpha hydroxylase of steroid nucleus	2 subfamilies, 2 genes	CYP7A1, CYP7B1
CYP8	*varied*	2 subfamilies, 2 genes	CYP8A1 (prostacyclin synthase), CYP8B1 (bile acid biosynthesis)
CYP11	steroid biosynthesis	2 subfamilies, 3 genes	CYP11A1, CYP11B1, CYP11B2
CYP17	steroid biosynthesis, 17-alpha hydroxylase	1 subfamily, 1 gene	CYP17A1
CYP19	steroid biosynthesis: aromatase synthesizes estrogen	1 subfamily, 1 gene	CYP19A1
CYP20	unknown function	1 subfamily, 1 gene	CYP20A1
CYP21	steroid biosynthesis	2 subfamilies, 1 gene, 1 pseudogene	CYP21A2
CYP24	vitamin D degradation	1 subfamily, 1 gene	CYP24A1
CYP26	retinoic acid hydroxylase	3 subfamilies, 3 genes	CYP26A1, CYP26B1, CYP26C1
CYP27	*varied*	3 subfamilies, 3 genes	CYP27A1 (bile acid biosynthesis), CYP27B1 (vitamin D_3 1-alpha hydroxylase, activates vitamin D_3), CYP27C1 (unknown function)
CYP39	7-alpha hydroxylation of 24-hydroxycholesterol	1 subfamily, 1 gene	CYP39A1
CYP46	cholesterol 24-hydroxylase	1 subfamily, 1 gene	CYP46A1
CYP51	cholesterol biosynthesis	1 subfamily, 1 gene, 3 pseudogenes	CYP51A1 (lanosterol 14-alpha demethylase)

P450s in Other Species

Animals

Many animals have as many or more CYP genes than humans do. Reported numbers range from 35 genes in the sponge *Amphimedon queenslandica* to 235 genes in the cephalochordate *Branchiostoma floridae*. Mice have genes for 101 CYPs, and sea urchins have even more (perhaps as many as 120 genes). Most CYP enzymes are presumed to have monooxygenase activity, as is the case for most mammalian CYPs that have been investigated (except for, e.g., CYP19 and CYP5). Gene and genome sequencing is far outpacing biochemical characterization of enzymatic function, though many genes with close homology to CYPs with known function have been found, giving clues to their functionality.

The classes of CYPs most often investigated in non-human animals are those either involved in development (e.g., retinoic acid or hormone metabolism) or involved in the metabolism of toxic compounds (such as heterocyclic amines or polyaromatic hydrocarbons). Often there are differences in gene regulation or enzyme function of CYPs in related animals that explain observed differences in susceptibility to toxic compounds (ex. canines inability to metabolize xanthines such as caffeine). Some drugs undergo metabolism in both species via different enzymes, resulting in different metabolites, while other drugs are metabolized in one species but excreted unchanged in another species. For this reason, one species's reaction to a substance is not a reliable indication of the substance's effects in humans.

CYPs have been extensively examined in mice, rats, dogs, and less so in zebrafish, in order to facilitate use of these model organisms in drug discovery and toxicology. Recently CYPs have also been discovered in avian species, in particular turkeys, that may turn out to be a great model for cancer research in humans. CYP1A5 and CYP3A37 in turkeys were found to be very similar to the human CYP1A2 and CYP3A4 respectively, in terms of their kinetic properties as well as in the metabolism of aflatoxin B1.

CYPs have also been heavily studied in insects, often to understand pesticide resistance. For example, CYP6G1 is linked to insecticide resistance in DDT-resistant Drosophila melanogaster and CYP6Z1 in the mosquito malaria vector Anopheles gambiae is capable of directly metabolizing DDT.

Microbial

Microbial cytochromes P450 are often soluble enzymes and are involved in diverse metabolic processes. In bacteria the distribution of P450s is very variable with many bacteria having no identified P450s (e.g. E.coli). Some bacteria, predominantly actinomycetes, have numerous P450s (e.g.,). Those so far identified are generally involved in either biotransformation of xenobiotic compounds (e.g. CYP105A1 from Streptomyces griseolus metabolizes sulfonylurea herbicides to less toxic derivatives,) or are part of specialised metabolite biosynthetic pathways (e.g. CYP170B1 catalyses production of the sesquiterpenoid albaflavenone in Streptomyces albus,). Although no P450 has yet been shown to be essential in a microbe, the CYP105 family is highly conserved with a representative in every streptomycete genome sequenced so far (). Due to the solubility of bacterial P450 enzymes, they are generally regarded as easier to work with than the predominantly membrane bound eukaryotic P450s. This, combined with the remarkable chemistry they catalyse, has led to many studies using the heterologously expressed proteins in vitro. Few studies have investigated what P450s do in vivo, what the natural substrate(s) are and how P450s contribute to survival of the bacteria in the natural environment.Three examples that have contributed significantly to structural and mechanistic studies are listed here, but many different families exist.

- Cytochrome P450cam (CYP101) originally from *Pseudomonas putida* has been used as a model for many cytochromes P450 and was the first cytochrome P450 three-dimensional protein structure solved by X-ray crystallography. This enzyme is part of a camphor-hydroxylating catalytic cycle consisting of two electron transfer steps from putidaredoxin, a 2Fe-2S cluster-containing protein cofactor.
- Cytochrome P450 eryF (CYP107A1) originally from the actinomycete bacterium *Saccharopolyspora erythraea* is responsible for the biosynthesis of the antibiotic erythromycin by C6-hydroxylation of the macrolide 6-deoxyerythronolide B.
- Cytochrome P450 BM3 (CYP102A1) from the soil bacterium *Bacillus megaterium* catalyzes the NADPH-dependent hydroxylation of several long-chain fatty acids at the ω–1 through ω–3 positions. Unlike almost every other known CYP (except CYP505A1, cytochrome P450 foxy), it constitutes a natural fusion protein between the CYP domain and an electron donating cofactor. Thus, BM3 is potentially very useful in biotechnological applications.
- Cytochrome P450 119 (CYP119) isolated from the thermophillic archea *Sulfolobus acidocaldarius* has been used in a variety of mechanistic studies. Because thermophillic enzymes evolved to function at high temperatures, they tend to function more slowly at room temperature (if at all) and are therefore excellent mechanistic models.

Fungi

The commonly used azole class antifungal drugs work by inhibition of the fungal cytochrome P450 14α-demethylase. This interrupts the conversion of lanosterol to ergosterol, a component of the fungal cell membrane. (This is useful only because humans' P450 have a different sensitivity; this is how this class of antifungals work.)

Significant research is ongoing into fungal P450s, as a number of fungi are pathogenic to humans (such as Candida yeast and Aspergillus) and to plants.

Cunninghamella elegans is a candidate for use as a model for mammalian drug metabolism.

Plants

Plant cytochrome P450s are involved in a wide range of biosynthetic reactions and target a diverse range of biomolecules. These reactions lead to various fatty acid conjugates, plant hormones, secondary metabolites, lignins, and a variety of defensive compounds. Plant genome annotations suggest that Cytochrome P450 genes make up as much as 1% of the plant genes. The number and diversity of P450 genes is responsible, in part, for the multitude of bioactive compounds.

P450s in Biotechnology

The remarkable reactivity and substrate promiscuity of P450s have long attracted the attention of chemists. Recent progress towards realizing the potential of using P450s towards difficult oxidations have included: (i) eliminating the need for natural co-factors by replacing them with inexpensive peroxide containing molecules, (ii) exploring the compatibility of p450s with organic solvents, and (iii) the use of small, non-chiral auxiliaries to predictably direct P450 oxidation.

InterPro Subfamilies

InterPro subfamilies:

- Cytochrome P450, B-class InterPro: *IPR002397*
- Cytochrome P450, mitochondrial InterPro: *IPR002399*
- Cytochrome P450, E-class, group I InterPro: *IPR002401*
- Cytochrome P450, E-class, group II InterPro: *IPR002402*
- Cytochrome P450, E-class, group IV InterPro: *IPR002403*
- Aromatase

Clozapine, imipramine, paracetamol, phenacetin Heterocyclic aryl amines Inducible and CYP1A2 5-10% deficient oxidize uroporphyrinogen to uroporphyrin (CYP1A2) in heme metabolism, but they may have additional undiscovered endogenous substrates. are inducible by some polycyclic hydrocarbons, some of which are found in cigarette smoke and charred food.

These enzymes are of interest, because in assays, they can activate compounds to carcinogens. High levels of CYP1A2 have been linked to an increased risk of colon cancer. Since the 1A2 enzyme can be induced by cigarette smoking, this links smoking with colon cancer.

FLAVIN-CONTAINING MONOOXYGENASE

The **flavin-containing monooxygenase (FMO)** protein family specializes in the oxidation of xeno-substrates in order to facilitate the excretion of these compounds from living organisms. These enzymes can oxidize a wide array of heteroatoms, particularly soft nucleophiles, such as amines, sulfides, and phosphites. This reaction requires an oxygen, an NADPH cofactor, and an FAD prosthetic group. FMOs share several structural features, such as a NADPH binding domain, FAD binding domain, and a conserved arginine residue present in the active site. Recently, FMO enzymes have received a great deal of attention from the pharmaceutical industry both as a drug target for various diseases and as a means to metabolize pro-drug compounds into active pharmaceuticals. These monooxygenases are often misclassified because they share activity profiles similar to those of cytochrome P450 (CYP450), which is the major contributor to oxidative xenobiotic metabolism. However, a key difference between the two enzymes lies in how they proceed to oxidize their respective substrates; CYP enzymes make use of an oxygenated heme prosthetic group, while the FMO family utilizes FAD to oxidize its substrates.

Prior to the 1960s, the oxidation of xenotoxic materials was thought to be completely accomplished by CYP450. However, in the early 1970s, Dr. Daniel Ziegler from the University of Texas at Austin discovered a hepatic flavoprotein isolated from pig liver that was found to oxidize a vast array of various amines to their corresponding nitro state. This flavoprotein named Ziegler's enzyme exhibited unusual chemical and spectrometric properties. Upon further spectroscopic characterization and investigation of the substrate pool of this enzyme, Dr. Ziegler discovered that this enzyme solely bound FAD molecule that could form a C4a-hydroxyperoxyflavin intermediate, and that this enzyme could oxidize a wide variety of substrates with no common structural features, including phosphines, sulfides, selenium compounds, amongst others. Once this was noticed, Dr. Ziegler's enzyme was reclassified as a broadband flavin monooxygenase.

In 1984, the first evidence for multiple forms of FMOs was elucidated by two different laboratories when two distinct FMOs were isolated from rabbit lungs. Since then, over 150 different FMO enzymes have been successfully isolated from a wide variety of organisms. Up until 2002, only 5 FMO enzymes were successfully isolated from mammals. However, a group of researchers found a sixth FMO gene located on human chromosome 1. In addition to the sixth FMO discovered as of 2002, the laboratories of Dr. Ian Philips and Elizabeth Sheppard discovered a second gene cluster in humans that consists of 5 additional pseudogenes for FMO on human chromosome 1.

Evolution of FMO Gene Family

The FMO family of genes is conserved across all phyla that have been studied so far, therefore some form of the FMO gene family can be found in all studied eukaryotes. FMO genes are characterized by specific structural and functional constraints, which led to the evolution of different types of FMO's in order to perform a variety of functions. Divergence between the functional types of FMO's (FMO 1–5) occurred before the amphibians and mammals diverged into separate classes. FMO5 found in vertebrates appears to be evolutionarily older than other types of FMO's, making FMO5 the first functionally distinct member of the FMO family. Phylogenetic studies suggest that FMO1 and FMO3 are the most recent FMO's to evolve into enzymes with distinct functions. Although FMO5 was the first distinct FMO, it is not clear what function it serves since it does not oxygenate the typical FMO substrates involved in first-pass metabolism.

Analyses of FMO genes across several species have shown extensive silent DNA mutations, which indicate that the current FMO gene family exists because of selective pressure at the protein level rather than the nucleotide level. FMO's found in invertebrates are found to have originated polyphyletically; meaning that a phenotypically similar gene evolved in invertebrates which was not inherited from a common ancestor.

Classification and characterization

FMOs are one subfamily of class B external flavoprotein monooxygenases (EC 1.14.13), which belong to the family of monooxygenase oxidoreductases, along with the other subfamilies Baeyer-Villiger monooxygenases and microbial N-hydroxylating monooxygenases. FMO's are found in fungi, yeast, plants, mammals, and bacteria.

Mammals

Developmental and tissue specific expression has been studied in several mammalian species, including humans, mice, rats, and rabbits. However, because FMO expression is unique to each animal species, it is difficult to make conclusions about human FMO regulation and activity based on other mammalian studies. It is likely that species-specific expression of FMO's contributes to differences in susceptibility to toxins and xenobiotics as well as the efficiency with excreting among different mammals.

Six functional forms of human FMO genes have been reported. However, FMO6 is considered to be a pseudogene. FMOs 1–5 share between 50–58% amino acid identity across the different species. Recently, five more human FMO genes were discovered, although they fall in the category of pseudogenes.

- FMO1, FMO2, FMO3, FMO4, FMO5, FMO6

Yeast

Unlike mammals, yeast (*Saccharomyces cerevisiae*) do not have several isoforms of FMO, but instead only have one called yFMO. This enzyme does not accept xenobiotic compounds. Instead, yFMO helps to fold proteins that contain disulfide bonds by catalyzing O_2 and NADPH-dependent oxidations of biological thiols, just like mammalian FMO's. An example is the oxidation of glutathione to glutathione disulfide, both of which form a redox buffering system in the cell between the endoplasmic reticulum and the cytoplasm. yFMO is localized in the cytoplasm in order to maintain the optimum redox buffer ratio necessary for proteins containing disulfide bonds to fold properly. This non-xenobiotic role of yFMO may represent the original role of the FMO's before the rise of the modern FMO family of enzymes found in mammals.

Plants

Plant FMO's play a role in defending against pathogens and catalyze specific steps in the biosynthesis of auxin, a plant hormone. Plant FMO's also play a role in the metabolism of glucosinolates. These non-xenobiotic roles of plant FMO's suggest that other FMO functions could be identified in non-plant organisms.

Structure

Crystal structures have been determined for yeast (*Schizosaccharomyces pombe*) FMO (PDB: 1VQW) and bacterial (*Methylophaga aminisulfidivorans*) FMO (PDB: 2XVH). The crystal structures are similar to each other and they share 27% sequence identity. These enzymes share 22% and 31% sequence identity with human FMOs, respectively.

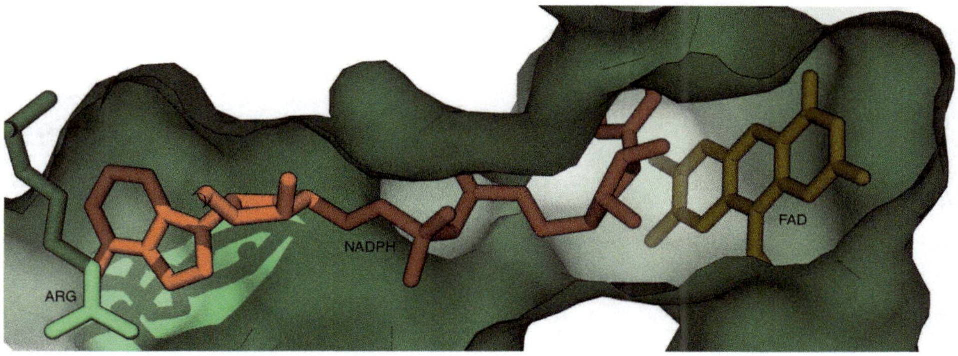

Channel and active site of bacterial FMO with bound NADPH and FAD (PDB: 2XVH).

FMOs have a tightly bound FAD prosthetic group and a binding NADPH cofactor. Both dinucleotide binding motifs form Rossmann folds. The yeast FMO and bacterial FMO are dimers, with each monomer consisting of two structural domains: the smaller NADPH binding domain and the larger FAD-binding domain. The two domains are connected by a double linker. A channel between the two domains leads to the active site where NADPH binds both domains and occupies a cleft that blocks access to the flavin group of FAD, which is bound to the large domain along the channel together with a water molecule. The nicotinamide group of NADPH interacts with the flavin group of FAD, and the NADPH binding site overlaps with the substrate binding site on the flavin group.

FMOs contain several sequence motifs that are conserved across all domains:

- FAD-binding motif (GXGXXG)
- FMO identifying motif (FXGXXXHXXXF/Y)
- NADPH-binding motif (GXSXXA)
- F/LATGY motif
- arginine residue in the active site

The FMO identifying motif interacts with the flavin of FAD. The F/LATGY motif is a sequence motif common in *N*-hydroxylating enzymes. The arginine residue interacts with the phosphate group of NADPH.

Function

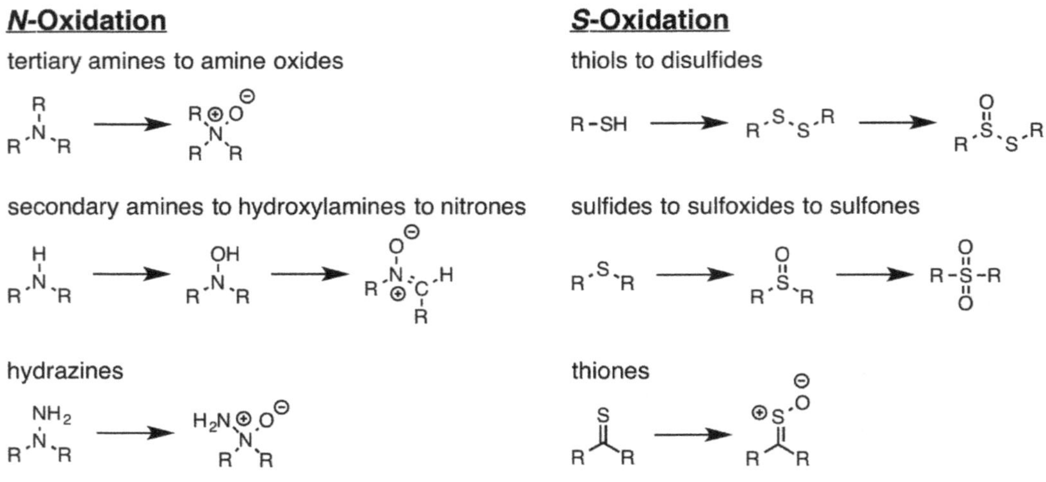

Reactions catalyzed by FMOs.

The general function of these enzymes is to metabolisexenobiotics. Hence, they are considered to be xenobiotic detoxication catalysts. These proteins catalyze the oxygenation of multiple heteroatom-containing compounds that are present in our diet, such as amine-, sulfide-, phosphorus-, and other nucleophilic heteroatom-containing compounds. FMOs have been implicated in the metabolism of a number of pharmaceuticals, pesticides and toxicants, by converting the lipophilic xenobiotics into polar, oxygenated, and readily excreted metabolites.

Substrate Diversity

FMO substrates are structurally diverse compounds. However, they all share similar characteristics:

- Soft nucleophiles (basic amines, sulfides, Se- or P-containing compounds)
- Neutral or single-positively charged

Zwitterions, anions and dications are considered to be unfavorable substrates. There are several drugs reported to be typical substrates for FMOs.

Typical Drug Substrates		
Albendazole	Clindamycin	Pargyline
Benzydamine	Fenbendazole	Ranitidine
Chlorpheniramine	Itopride	Thioridazine
Cimetidine	Olopatadine	Sulindac sulfide
Xanomeline	Zimeldine	

The majority of drugs function as alternate substrate competitive inhibitors to FMOs (i.e. good nucleophiles that compete with the drug for FMO oxygenation), since they are not likely to serve as FMO substrates. Only a few true FMO competitive inhibitors have been reported. Those include indole-3-carbinol and *N,N*-dimethylamino stilbene carboxylates. A well-known FMO inhibitor is methimazole (MMI).

Mechanism

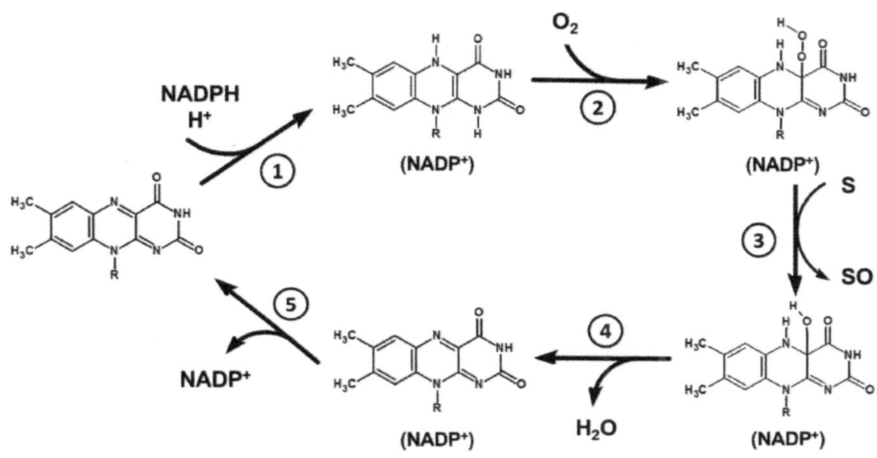

Catalytic cycle of FMOs together with the redox state of the FAD prosthetic group.

The FMO catalytic cycle proceeds as follows:

- The cofactor NADPH binds to the oxidized state of the FADprosthetic group, reducing it to $FADH_2$.
- Molecular oxygen binds to the formed $NADP^+$-$FADH_2$-enzyme complex and is reduced, resulting in 4a-hydroperoxyflavin (4a-HPF or FADH-OOH). This specie is stabilized by $NADP^+$ in the catalytic site of the enzyme. These first two steps in the cycle are fast.
- In the presence of a substrate (S), a nucleophilic attack occurs on the distal O-atom of the prosthetic group. The substrate is oxygenated to SO, forming the 4a-hydroxyflavin (FADH-OH). Only when the flavin is in the hydroperoxy form is when the xenobiotic substrate will react.
- The flavin product then breaks down with release of water to reform FAD.
- Due to the low dissociation constant of the $NADP^+$-enzyme complex, $NADP^+$ is released by the end of the cycle and the enzyme returns to its original state. The rate-limiting step involves either the breakdown of FADH-OH to water or the release of $NADP^+$.
- Quantum mechanics simulations showed the N-hydroxylation catalyzed by flavin-containing monooxygenases initiated by homolysis of the O-O bond in

the C4a-hydroperoxyflavin intermediate resulting in the formation of an internal hydrogen bonded hydroxyl radical.

Cellular Expression in Humans

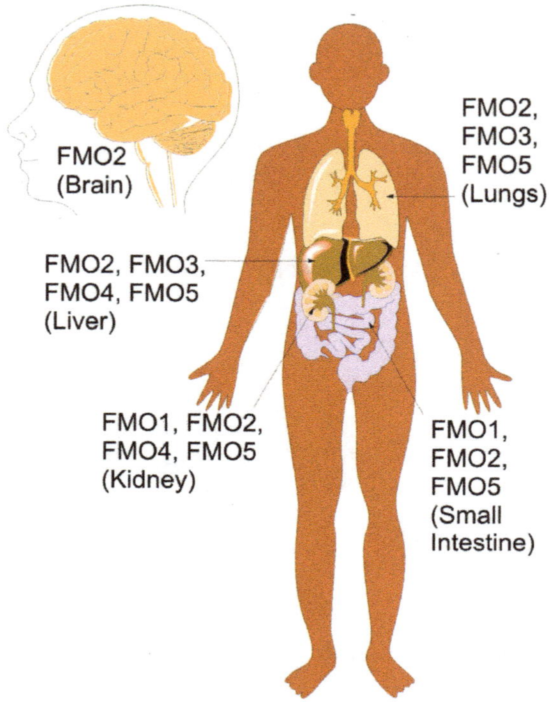

Main distributions of different types of Flavin-containing Monooxygenases (FMO) in adult human tissues.

Expression of each type of FMO relies on several factors including, cofactor supply, physiological & environmental factors, as well as diet. Because of these factors, each type of FMO is expressed differently depending on the species and tissue. In humans, expression of FMO's is mainly concentrated to the human liver, lungs, and kidneys, where most of the metabolism of xenobiotics occur. However, FMO's can also be found in the human brain and small intestine. While FMO1-5 can be found in the brain, liver, kidneys, lungs, and small intestine, the distribution of each type of FMO differs depending on the tissue and the developmental stage of the person.

Expression in Adult Tissues

In an adult, FMO1 is predominately expressed in the kidneys and to a lesser extent in the lungs and small intestine. FMO2 is the most abundant of the FMO's and is mostly expressed in the lungs and kidneys, with lower expression in the liver and small intestine. FMO3 is highly concentrated in the liver, but is also expressed in the lungs. FMO4 is expressed mostly in the liver and kidneys. FMO5 is highly expressed in the liver, but also has substantial expression in the lungs and small intestine. Though FMO2 is the most expressed FMO in the brain, it only constitutes about 1% of that found in the lungs, making FMO expression in the brain fairly low.

Expression in Fetal Tissues

The distribution of FMO's in various types of tissues changes as a person continues to develop, making the fetal distribution of FMO's quite different than adult distribution of FMO's. While the adult liver is dominated by the expression of FMO3 and FMO5, the fetal liver is dominated by the expression of FMO1 and FMO5. Another difference is in the brain, where adults mostly express FMO2 and fetuses mostly express FMO1.

Clinical Significance

Drug Development

Drug metabolism is one of the most important factors to consider when developing new drugs for therapeutic applications. The degradation rate of these new drugs in an organism's system determines the duration and intensity of their pharmacological action. During the past few years, FMOs have gained a lot of attention in drug development since these enzymes are not readily induced or inhibited by the chemicals or drugs surrounding their environment. CYPs are the primary enzymes involved in drug metabolism. However, recent efforts have been directed towards the development of drug candidates that incorporate functional groups that can be metabolized by FMOs. By doing this, the number of potential adverse drug-drug interactions is minimized and the reliance on CYP450 metabolism is decreased. Several approaches have been made to screen potential drug interactions. One of them includes human FMO3 (hFMO3), which is described as the most vital FMO regarding drug interactions. In order to successfully screen hFMO3 in a high throughput fashion hFMO3 was successfully fixed to graphene oxide chips in order to measure the change in electrical potential generated as a result of the drug being oxidized when it interacts with the enzyme.

Hypertension

There is evidence that FMOs are associated to the regulation of blood pressure. FMO3 is involved in the formation of TMA N-oxides (TMAO). Some studies indicate that hypertension can develop when there are no organic osmolytes (i.e. TMAO) that can counteract an increase in osmotic pressure and peripheral resistance. Individuals with deficient FMO3 activity have a higher prevalence of hypertension and other cardiovascular diseases, since there is a decrease in formation of TMA N-oxides to counterbalance the effects of a higher osmotic pressure and peripheral resistance.

Fish odor Syndrome

The trimethylaminuria disorder, also known as fish odor syndrome, causes abnormal FMO3-mediated metabolism or a deficiency of this enzyme in an individual. A person with this disorder has a low capacity to oxidize the trimethylamine (TMA) that comes from their diet to its odourless metabolite TMAO.When this happens, large amounts of TMA are excreted through the individual's urine, sweat, and breath, with a strong fish-like odor. As of today, there is no known cure or treatment for this disorder. However, doctors recommend patients to avoid foods containing choline, carnitine, nitrogen, sulfur and lecithin.

Other Diseases

FMOs have also been associated with other diseases, such as cancer and diabetes. Yet, additional studies are imperative to elucidate what is the relationship between FMO function and these diseases, as well as to define these enzymes' clinical relevance.

ALCOHOL DEHYDROGENASE

Alcohol dehydrogenases (ADH) (EC 1.1.1.1) are a group of dehydrogenase enzymes that occur in many organisms and facilitate the interconversion between alcohols and aldehydes or ketones with the reduction of nicotinamide adenine dinucleotide (NAD^+ to NADH). In humans and many other animals, they serve to break down alcohols that otherwise are toxic, and they also participate in generation of useful aldehyde, ketone, or alcohol groups during biosynthesis of various metabolites. In yeast, plants, and many bacteria, some alcohol dehydrogenases catalyze the opposite reaction as part of fermentation to ensure a constant supply of NAD^+.

Evolution

Genetic evidence from comparisons of multiple organisms showed that a glutathione-dependent formaldehyde dehydrogenase, identical to a class III alcohol dehydrogenase (ADH-3/ADH5), is presumed to be the ancestral enzyme for the entire ADH family. Early on in evolution, an effective method for eliminating both endogenous and exogenous formaldehyde was important and this capacity has conserved the ancestral ADH-3 through time. Gene duplication of ADH-3, followed by series of mutations, the other ADHs evolved.

The ability to produce ethanol from sugar (which is the basis of how alcoholic beverages are made) is believed to have initially evolved in yeast. Though this feature is not adaptive from an energy point of view, by making alcohol in such high concentrations so that they would be toxic to other organisms, yeast cells could effectively eliminate their competition. Since rotting fruit can contain more than 4% of ethanol, animals eating the fruit needed a system to metabolize exogenous ethanol. This was thought to explain the conservation of ethanol active ADH in other species than yeast, though ADH-3 is now known to also have a major role in nitric oxide signaling.

In humans, sequencing of the ADH1B gene (responsible for production of an alcohol dehydrogenase polypeptide) shows two variants, in which there is an SNP (single nucleotide polymorphism) that leads to either a Histidine or an Arginine residue in the enzyme catalyzing the conversion of ethanol into acetaldehyde. In the Histidine variant, the enzyme is much more effective at the aforementioned conversion. The enzyme responsible for the conversion of acetaldehyde to acetate, however, remains unaffected, which leads to differential rates of substrate catalysis and causes a buildup of toxic acetaldehyde, causing cell damage. In humans, various haplotypes arising from this mutation are more concentrated in regions near Eastern China, a region also known for its low alcohol tolerance and dependence. A study was conducted in order to find a correlation between allelic distribution and alcoholism, and the results suggest that the allelic distribution arose along with rice cultivation in the region between 12,000 and 6,000 years ago. In regions where rice was cultivated, rice was also fermented into ethanol. The results of increased alcohol availability led to alcoholism and abuse by those able to acquire it, resulting in lower reproductive fitness. Those with the variant allele have little tolerance for alcohol, thus lowering chance of dependence and abuse. The hypothesis posits that those individuals with the His variant enzyme were sensitive enough to the effects of alcohol that differential reproductive success arose and the corresponding alleles were passed through the generations.

Classical Darwinian evolution would act to select against the detrimental form of the enzyme (Arg variant) because of the lowered reproductive success of individuals carrying the allele. The result would be a higher frequency of the allele responsible for the His-variant enzyme in regions that had been under selective pressure the longest. The distribution and frequency of the His variant follows the spread of rice cultivation to inland regions of Asia, with higher frequencies of the His variant in regions that have cultivated rice the longest. The geographic distribution of the alleles seems to therefore be a result of natural selection against individuals with lower reproductive success, namely, those who carried the Arg variant allele and were more susceptible to alcoholism.

Discovery

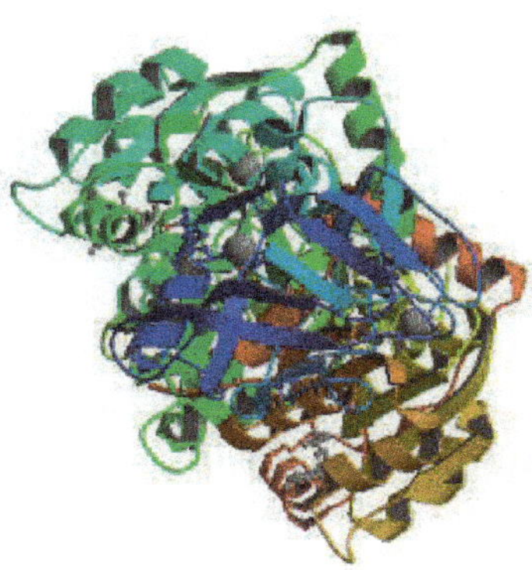

Horse LADH (Liver Alcohol Dehydrogenase).

The first-ever isolated alcohol dehydrogenase (ADH) was purified in 1937 from *Saccharomyces cerevisiae* (brewer's yeast). Many aspects of the catalytic mechanism for the horse liver ADH enzyme were investigated by Hugo Theorell and coworkers. ADH was also one of the first oligomeric enzymes that had its amino acid sequence and three-dimensional structure determined.

In early 1960, it was discovered in fruit flies of the genus *Drosophila*.

Properties

The alcohol dehydrogenases comprise a group of several isozymes that catalyse the oxidation of primary and secondary alcohols to aldehydes and ketones, respectively, and also can catalyse the reverse reaction. In mammals this is a redox (reduction/oxidation) reaction involving the coenzyme nicotinamide adenine dinucleotide (NAD^+).

Alcohol dehydrogenase is a dimer with a mass of 80 kDa.

Oxidation of Alcohol

Mechanism of Action in Humans

Steps

- Binding of the coenzyme NAD^+
- Binding of the alcohol substrate by coordination to zinc
- Deprotonation of His-51
- Deprotonation of nicotinamide ribose
- Deprotonation of Thr-48
- Deprotonation of the alcohol
- Hydride transfer from the alkoxide ion to NAD^+, leading to NADH and a zinc bound aldehyde or ketone
- Release of the product aldehyde.

The mechanism in yeast and bacteria is the reverse of this reaction. These steps are supported through kinetic studies.

Involved Subunits

The substrate is coordinated to the zinc and this enzyme has two zinc atoms per subunit. One is the active site, which is involved in catalysis. In the active site, the ligands are Cys-46, Cys-174, His-67, and one water molecule. The other subunit is involved with structure. In this mechanism, the hydride from the alcohol goes to NAD^+. Crystal structures indicate that the His-51 deprotonates the nicotinamide ribose, which deprotonates Ser-48. Finally, Ser-48 deprotonates the alcohol, making it an aldehyde. From a mechanistic perspective, if the enzyme adds hydride to the re face of NAD^+, the resulting hydrogen is incorporated into the pro-R position. Enzymes that add hydride to the re face are deemed Class A dehydrogenases.

Active Site

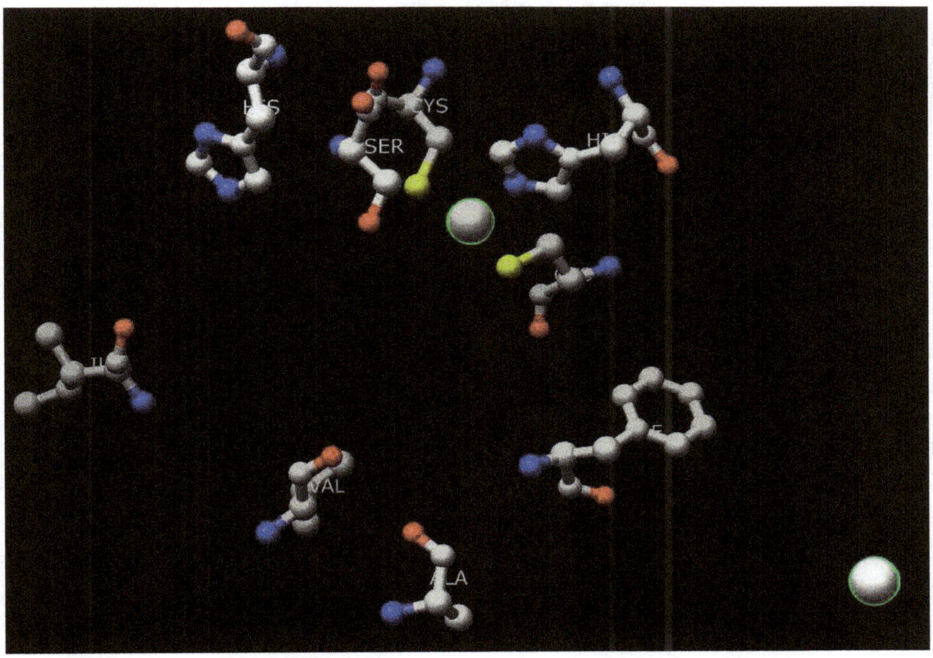

The active site of alcohol dehydrogenase.

The active site of human ADH1 (PDB:1HSO) consists of a zinc atom, His-67, Cys-174, Cys-46, Thr-48, His-51, Ile-269, Val-292, Ala-317, and Leu-319. In the commonly studied horse liver isoform, Thr-48 is a Ser, and Leu-319 is a Phe. The zinc coordinates the substrate (alcohol). The zinc is coordinated by Cys-46, Cys-174, and His-67. Leu-319, Ala-317, His-51, Ile-269 and Val-292 stabilize NAD^+ by forming hydrogen bonds. His-51 and Ile-269 form hydrogen bonds with the alcohols on nicotinamide ribose. Phe-319, Ala-317 and Val-292 form hydrogen bonds with the amide on NAD^+.

Structural Zinc Site

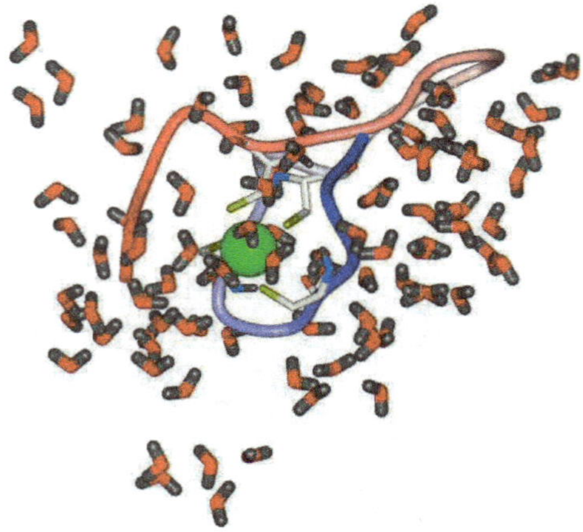

The structural zinc binding motif in alcohol dehydrogenase from a MD simulation.

Mammalian alcohol dehydrogenases also have a structural zinc site. This Zn ion plays a structural role and is crucial for protein stability. The structures of the catalytic and structural zinc sites in horse liver alcohol dehydrogenase (HLADH) as revealed in crystallographic structures, which has been studied computationally with quantum chemical as well as with classical molecular dynamics methods. The structural zinc site is composed of four closely spaced cysteine ligands (Cys97, Cys100, Cys103, and Cys111 in the amino acid sequence) positioned in an almost symmetric tetrahedron around the Zn ion. A recent study showed that the interaction between zinc and cysteine is governed by primarily an electrostatic contribution with an additional covalent contribution to the binding.

Types

Human

In humans, ADH exists in multiple forms as a dimer and is encoded by at least seven different genes. There are five classes (I-V) of alcohol dehydrogenase, but the hepatic form that is used primarily in humans is class 1. Class 1 consists of α, β, and γ subunits that are encoded by the genes ADH1A, ADH1B, and ADH1C. The enzyme is present at high levels in the liver and the lining of the stomach. It catalyzes the oxidation of ethanol to acetaldehyde (ethanal):

$$CH_3CH_2OH + NAD^+ \rightarrow CH_3CHO + NADH + H^+$$

This allows the consumption of alcoholic beverages, but its evolutionary purpose is probably the breakdown of alcohols naturally contained in foods or produced by bacteria in the digestive tract.

Another evolutionary purpose may be metabolism of the endogenous alcohol vitamin A (retinol), which generates the hormone retinoic acid, although the function here may be primarily the elimination of toxic levels of retinol.

alcohol dehydrogenase 1A, α polypeptide	
Identifiers	
Symbol	ADH1A
Alt. symbols	ADH1
Entrez	124
HUGO	249
OMIM	103700
RefSeq	NM_000667
UniProt	P07327
Other data	
EC number	1.1.1.1
Locus	Chr. 4 *q23*

alcohol dehydrogenase 1B, β polypeptide	
Identifiers	
Symbol	ADH1B
Alt. symbols	ADH2
Entrez	125
HUGO	250
OMIM	103720
RefSeq	NM_000668
UniProt	P00325
Other data	
EC number	1.1.1.1
Locus	Chr. 4 *q23*

alcohol dehydrogenase 1C, γ polypeptide	
Identifiers	
Symbol	ADH1C
Alt. symbols	ADH3
Entrez	126
HUGO	251
OMIM	103730
RefSeq	NM_000669
UniProt	P00326
Other data	

EC number	1.1.1.1
Locus	Chr. 4 *q23*

Alcohol dehydrogenase is also involved in the toxicity of other types of alcohol: For instance, it oxidizes methanol to produce formaldehyde and ethylene glycol to ultimately yield glycolic and oxalic acids. Humans have at least six slightly different alcohol dehydrogenases. Each is a dimer (i.e., consists of two polypeptides), with each dimer containing two zinc ions Zn^{2+}. One of those ions is crucial for the operation of the enzyme: It is located at the catalytic site and holds the hydroxyl group of the alcohol in place.

Alcohol dehydrogenase activity varies between men and women, between young and old, and among populations from different areas of the world. For example, young women are unable to process alcohol at the same rate as young men because they do not express the alcohol dehydrogenase as highly, although the inverse is true among the middle-aged. The level of activity may not be dependent only on level of expression but also on allelic diversity among the population.

The human genes that encode class II, III, IV, and V alcohol dehydrogenases are ADH4, ADH5, ADH7, and ADH6, respectively.

alcohol dehydrogenase 4 (class II), π polypeptide	
Identifiers	
Symbol	ADH4
Entrez	127
HUGO	252
OMIM	103740
RefSeq	NM_000670
UniProt	P08319
Other data	
EC number	1.1.1.1
Locus	Chr. 4 *q22*

alcohol dehydrogenase 5 (class III), χ polypeptide	
Identifiers	
Symbol	ADH5
Entrez	128
HUGO	253
OMIM	103710
RefSeq	NM_000671
UniProt	P11766
Other data	
EC number	1.1.1.1

Locus	Chr. 4 *q23*

alcohol dehydrogenase 6 (class V)	
Identifiers	
Symbol	ADH6
Entrez	130
HUGO	255
OMIM	103735
RefSeq	NM_000672
UniProt	P28332
Other data	
EC number	1.1.1.1
Locus	Chr. 4 *q23*

alcohol dehydrogenase 7 (class IV), μ or σ polypeptide	
Identifiers	
Symbol	ADH7
Entrez	131
HUGO	256
OMIM	600086
RefSeq	NM_000673
UniProt	P40394
Other data	
EC number	1.1.1.1
Locus	Chr. 4 *q23-q24*

Yeast and Bacteria

Unlike humans, yeast and bacteria (except lactic acid bacteria, and *E. coli* in certain conditions) do not ferment glucose to lactate. Instead, they ferment it to ethanol and CO_2. The overall reaction can be seen below:

Glucose + 2 ADP + 2 Pi → 2 ethanol + 2 CO_2 + 2 ATP + 2 H_2O

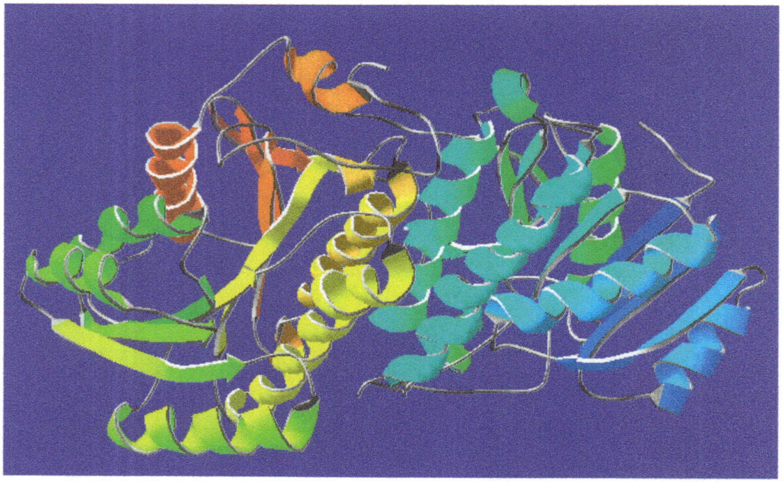

Alcohol Dehydrogenase.

In yeast and many bacteria, alcohol dehydrogenase plays an important part in fermentation: Pyruvate resulting from glycolysis is converted to acetaldehyde and carbon dioxide, and the acetaldehyde is then reduced to ethanol by an alcohol dehydrogenase called ADH1. The purpose of this latter step is the regeneration of NAD^+, so that the energy-generating glycolysis can continue. Humans exploit this process to produce alcoholic beverages, by letting yeast ferment various fruits or grains. It is interesting to note that yeast can produce and consume their own alcohol.

The main alcohol dehydrogenase in yeast is larger than the human one, consisting of four rather than just two subunits. It also contains zinc at its catalytic site. Together with the zinc-containing alcohol dehydrogenases of animals and humans, these enzymes from yeasts and many bacteria form the family of "long-chain"-alcohol dehydrogenases.

Brewer's yeast also has another alcohol dehydrogenase, ADH2, which evolved out of a duplicate version of the chromosome containing the ADH1 gene. ADH2 is used by the yeast to convert ethanol back into acetaldehyde, and it is expressed only when sugar concentration is low. Having these two enzymes allows yeast to produce alcohol when sugar is plentiful (and this alcohol then kills off competing microbes), and then continue with the oxidation of the alcohol once the sugar, and competition, is gone.

Plants

In plants, ADH catalyses the same reaction as in yeast and bacteria to ensure that there is a constant supply of NAD^+. Maize has two versions of ADH - ADH1 and ADH2, *Arabidopsis thaliana* contains only one ADH gene. The structure of *Arabidopsis* ADH is 47%-conserved, relative to ADH from horse liver. Structurally and functionally important residues, such as the seven residues that provide ligands for the catalytic and noncatalytic zinc atoms, however, are conserved, suggesting that the enzymes have a similar structure. ADH is constitutively expressed at low levels in the roots of young plants grown on agar. If the roots lack oxygen, the expression of *ADH* increases significantly. Its expression is also increased in response to dehydration, to low temperatures, and to abscisic acid, and it plays an important role in fruit ripening, seedlings development, and pollen development. Differences in the sequences of *ADH* in different species have been used to create phylogenies showing how closely related different species of plants are. It is an ideal gene to use due to its convenient size (2–3 kb in length with a ~1000 nucleotide coding sequence) and low copy number.

Iron-containing

Iron-containing alcohol dehydrogenase	
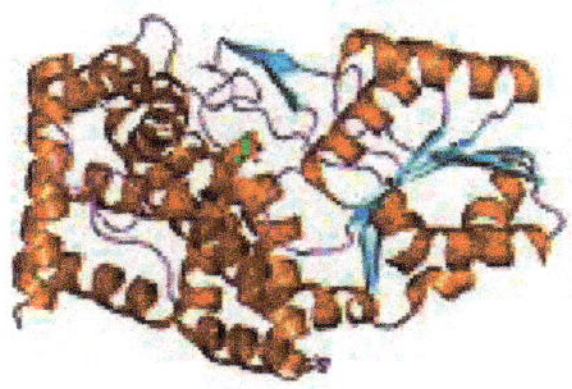 bacillus stearothermophilus glycerol dehydrogenase complex with glycerol	
Identifiers	
Symbol	Fe-ADH
Pfam	PF00465
Pfam clan	CL0224
InterPro	IPR001670
PROSITE	PDOC00059
SCOP	1jqa
SUPERFAMILY	1jqa

A third family of alcohol dehydrogenases, unrelated to the above two, are iron-containing ones. They occur in bacteria and fungi. In comparison to enzymes the above families, these enzymes are oxygen-sensitive. Members of the iron-containing alcohol dehydrogenase family include:

- *Saccharomyces cerevisiae* alcohol dehydrogenase 4 (gene ADH4)
- *Zymomonas mobilis* alcohol dehydrogenase 2 (gene adhB)
- *Escherichia coli* propanediol oxidoreductase EC1.1.1.77 (gene fucO), an enzyme involved in the metabolism of fucose and which also seems to contain ferrous ion(s).

- *Clostridium acetobutylicum* NADPH- and NADH-dependent butanol dehydrogenases EC 1.1.1.-(genes adh1, bdhA and bdhB), enzymes that have activity using butanol and ethanol as substrates.
- *E. coli* adhE, an iron-dependent enzyme that harbours three different activities: alcohol dehydrogenase, acetaldehyde dehydrogenase (acetylating) EC 1.2.1.10 and pyruvate-formate-lyase deactivase.
- Bacterial glycerol dehydrogenase EC 1.1.1.6 (gene gldA or dhaD).
- *Clostridium kluyveri* NAD-dependent 4-hydroxybutyrate dehydrogenase (4hbd) EC 1.1.1.61
- *Citrobacter freundii* and *Klebsiella pneumoniae* 1,3-propanediol dehydrogenase EC 1.1.1.202(gene dhaT)
- *Bacillus methanolicus* NAD-dependent methanol dehydrogenase EC 1.1.1.244
- *E. coli* and *Salmonella typhimurium* ethanolamine utilization protein eutG.
- *E. coli* hypothetical protein yiaY.

Other Types

A further class of alcohol dehydrogenases belongs to quinoenzymes and requires quinoid cofactors (e.g., pyrroloquinoline quinone, PQQ) as enzyme-bound electron acceptors. A typical example for this type of enzyme is methanol dehydrogenase of methylotrophic bacteria.

Applications

In biotransformation, alcohol dehydrogenases are often used for the synthesis of enantiomerically pure stereoisomers of chiral alcohols. Often, high chemo- and enantioselectivity can be achieved. One example is the alcohol dehydrogenase from *Lactobacillus brevis* (*Lb*ADH), which is described to be a versatile biocatalyst. The high chemospecificity has been confirmed also in the case of substrates presenting two potential redox sites. For instance cinnamaldehyde presents both aliphatic double bond and aldehyde function. Unlike conventional catalysts, alcohol dehydrogenases are able to selectively act only on the latter, yielding exclusively cinnamyl alcohol.

In fuel cells, alcohol dehydrogenases can be used to catalyze the breakdown of fuel for an ethanol fuel cell. Scientists at Saint Louis University have used carbon-supported alcohol dehydrogenase with poly(methylene green) as an anode, with a nafion membrane, to achieve about 50 $\mu A/cm^2$.

In 1949, E. Racker defined one unit of alcohol dehydrogenase activity as the amount that causes a change in optical density of 0.001 per minute under the standard conditions of assay. Recently, the international definition of enzymatic unit (E.U.) has been more common: one unit of Alcohol Dehydrogenase will convert 1.0 μmole of ethanol to acetaldehyde per minute at pH 8.8 at 25 °C.

Clinical Significance

Alcoholism

There have been studies showing that ADH may have an influence on the dependence on ethanol metabolism in alcoholics. Researchers have tentatively detected a few genes to be associated with alcoholism. If the variants of these genes encode slower metabolizing forms of ADH2 and ADH3, there is increased risk of alcoholism. The studies have found that mutations of ADH2 and ADH3 are related to alcoholism in Northeast Asian populations. However, research continues in order to identify the genes and their influence on alcoholism.

Drug Dependence

Drug dependence is another problem associated with ADH, which researchers think might be linked to alcoholism. One particular study suggests that drug dependence has seven ADH genes associated with it. These results may lead to treatments that target these specific genes. However, more research is necessary.

Poisoning

Fomepizole, a drug that inhibits alcohol dehydrogenase, can be used in the setting of acute methanolor ethylene glycol toxicity. This prevents the conversion of methanol to its toxic metabolites, formic acid and formaldehyde.

PEROXIDASE

Peroxidases (EC number 1.11.1.x) are a large family of enzymes that typically catalyze a reaction of the form:

$$\mathrm{ROOR'} + \overbrace{2\,\mathrm{e}^-}^{\text{electron donor}} + 2\,\mathrm{H}^+ \xrightarrow{\text{Peroxidase}} \mathrm{ROH} + \mathrm{R'OH}$$

For many of these enzymes the optimal substrate is hydrogen peroxide, but others are more active with organic hydroperoxides such as lipid peroxides. Peroxidases can contain a heme cofactor in their active sites, or alternately redox-active cysteine or selenocysteine residues.

The nature of the electron donor is very dependent on the structure of the enzyme.

- For example, horseradish peroxidase can use a variety of organic compounds as electron donors and acceptors. Horseradish peroxidase has an accessible active site, and many compounds can reach the site of the reaction.
- Because there is a very closed active site, for an enzyme such as cytochrome c peroxidase, the compounds that donate electrons are very specific.

While the exact mechanisms have yet to be determined, peroxidases are known to play a part in increasing a plant's defenses against pathogens. Peroxidases are sometimes used as histological marker. Cytochrome c peroxidase is used as a soluble, easily purified model for cytochrome c oxidase.

The glutathione peroxidase family consists of 8 known human isoforms. Glutathione peroxidases use glutathione as an electron donor and are active with both hydrogen peroxide and organic hydroperoxide substrates. Gpx1, Gpx2, Gpx3, and Gpx4 have been shown to be selenium-containing enzymes, whereas Gpx6 is a selenoprotein in humans with cysteine-containing homologues in rodents.

Amyloid beta, when bound to heme, has been shown to have peroxidase activity.

A typical group of peroxidases are the haloperoxidases. This group is able to form reactive halogen species and, as a result, natural organohalogen substances.

A majority of peroxidase protein sequences can be found in the PeroxiBase database.

Applications

Peroxidase can be used for treatment of industrial waste waters. For example, phenols, which are important pollutants, can be removed by enzyme-catalyzed polymerization using horseradish peroxidase. Thus phenols are oxidized to phenoxy radicals, which participate in reactions where polymers and oligomers are produced that are less toxic than phenols. It also can be used to convert toxic materials into less harmful substances.

There are many investigations about the use of peroxidase in many manufacturing processes like adhesives, computer chips, car parts, and linings of drums and cans. Other studies have shown that peroxidases may be used successfully to polymerize anilines and phenols in organic solvent matrices.

REFERENCES

1. PDB: 1m6h; Sanghani PC, Robinson H, Bosron WF, Hurley TD (September 2002). Human glutathione-dependent formaldehyde dehydrogenase. Structures of apo, binary, and inhibitory ternary complexes. Biochemistry. **41** *(35): 10778–86.* doi:10.1021/bi0257639. PMID 12196016.
2. Gutheil WG, Holmquist B, Vallee BL (Jan 1992). Purification, characterization, and partial sequence of the glutathione-dependent formaldehyde dehydrogenase from Escherichia coli: a class III alcohol dehydrogenase. Biochemistry. **31** *(2): 475–81.* doi:10.1021/bi00117a025. PMID 1731906.
3. Danielsson O, Jörnvall H (Oct 1992). Enzymogenesis: classical liver alcohol dehydrogenase origin from the glutathione-dependent formaldehyde dehydrogenase line. Proceedings of the National Academy of Sciences of the United States of America. **89** *(19): 9247–51. doi:10.1073/pnas.89.19.9247. PMC 50103. PMID 1409630.*
4. Persson B, Hedlund J, Jörnvall H (Dec 2008). Medium- and short-chain dehydrogenase/reductase gene and protein families : the MDR superfamily. Cellular and Molecular Life Sciences. **65** *(24): 3879–94.* doi:10.1007/s00018-008-8587-z. PMC 2792335. PMID 19011751.

5. Staab CA, Hellgren M, Höög JO (Dec 2008). Medium- and short-chain dehydrogenase/reductase gene and protein families : Dual functions of alcohol dehydrogenase 3: implications with focus on formaldehyde dehydrogenase and S-nitrosoglutathione reductase activities. Cellular and Molecular Life Sciences. **65** *(24): 3950–60.* doi:10.1007/s00018-008-8592-2. PMID 19011746.

6. Godoy L, Gonzàlez-Duarte R, Albalat R (2006). S-Nitrosogluthathione reductase activity of amphioxus ADH3: insights into the nitric oxide metabolism. International Journal of Biological Sciences. **2** *(3): 117–24. doi:10.7150/ijbs.2.117. PMC 1458435. PMID 16763671.*

7. Whitfield, John B. ADH and ALDH genotypes in relation to alcohol metabolic rate and sensitivity(PDF). Alcohol & Alcoholism.

8. Peng Y, Shi H, Qi XB, Xiao CJ, Zhong H, Ma RL, Su B (2010). The ADH1B Arg47His polymorphism in east Asian populations and expansion of rice domestication in history. BMC Evolutionary Biology. **10**: 15. doi:10.1186/1471-2148-10-15. PMC 2823730. PMID 20089146.

9. Eng, Mimi Y. (2007-01-01). Alcohol Research and Health. U.S. Government Printing Office. ISSN 1535-7414.

10. Negelein E, Wulff HJ (1937). Biochem. Z. **293**: 351.

11. Theorell H, McKEE JS (Oct 1961). Mechanism of action of liver alcohol dehydrogenase. Nature. **192** *(4797): 47–50.* doi:10.1038/192047a0. PMID 13920552.

12. Jörnvall H, Harris JI (Apr 1970). Horse liver alcohol dehydrogenase. On the primary structure of the ethanol-active isoenzyme. European Journal of Biochemistry / FEBS. **13** *(3): 565–76. doi:10.1111/j.1432-1033.1970.tb00962.x. PMID 5462776.*

13. Brändén CI, Eklund H, Nordström B, Boiwe T, Söderlund G, Zeppezauer E, Ohlsson I, Akeson A (Aug 1973). Structure of liver alcohol dehydrogenase at 2.9-angstrom resolution. Proceedings of the National Academy of Sciences of the United States of America. **70** *(8): 2439–42. doi:10.1073/pnas.70.8.2439. PMC 433752. PMID 4365379.*

14. Hellgren M (2009). Enzymatic studies of alcohol dehydrogenase by a combination of in vitro and in silico methods, Ph.D. thesis (PDF). Stockholm, Sweden: Karolinska Institutet. p. 70. ISBN 978-91-7409-567-8.

15. Sofer W, Martin PF (1987). Analysis of alcohol dehydrogenase gene expression in Drosophila. Annual Review of Genetics. **21**: 203–25. doi:10.1146/annurev.ge.21.120187.001223. PMID 3327463.

16. Hammes-Schiffer S, Benkovic SJ (2006). Relating protein motion to catalysis. Annual Review of Biochemistry. **75**: 519–41. doi:10.1146/annurev.biochem.75.103004.142800. PMID 16756501.

17. Brandt EG, Hellgren M, Brinck T, Bergman T, Edholm O (Feb 2009). Molecular dynamics study of zinc binding to cysteines in a peptide mimic of the alcohol dehydrogenase structural zinc site. Physical Chemistry Chemical Physics. **11** *(6): 975–83.* doi:10.1039/b815482a. PMID 19177216.

18. Sultatos LG, Pastino GM, Rosenfeld CA, Flynn EJ (Mar 2004). Incorporation of the genetic control of alcohol dehydrogenase into a physiologically based pharmacokinetic model for ethanol in humans. Toxicological Sciences. **78** *(1): 20–31. doi:10.1093/*toxsci/kfh057. PMID 14718645.
19. Farrés J, Moreno A, Crosas B, Peralba JM, Allali-Hassani A, Hjelmqvist L, Jörnvall H, Parés X (Sep 1994). Alcohol dehydrogenase of class IV (sigma sigma-ADH) from human stomach. cDNA sequence and structure/function relationships. European Journal of Biochemistry / FEBS. **224** *(2): 549–57. doi:10.1111/j.1432-1033.1994.00549.x. PMID 7925371.*
20. Kovacs B, Stöppler MC. Alcohol and Nutrition. MedicineNet, Inc. Archived from the original on 23 June 2011. Retrieved 2011-06-07.
21. Duester G (Sep 2008). Retinoic acid synthesis and signaling during early organogenesis. Cell. **134** *(6): 921–31. doi:10.1016/j.cell.2008.09.002. PMC 2632951. PMID 18805086.*
22. Hellgren M, Strömberg P, Gallego O, Martras S, Farrés J, Persson B, Parés X, Höög JO (Feb 2007). Alcohol dehydrogenase 2 is a major hepatic enzyme for human retinol metabolism. Cellular and Molecular Life Sciences. **64** *(4): 498–505.* doi:10.1007/s00018-007-6449-8. PMID 17279314.
23. Parlesak A, Billinger MH, Bode C, Bode JC (2002). Gastric alcohol dehydrogenase activity in man: influence of gender, age, alcohol consumption and smoking in a caucasian population. Alcohol and Alcoholism. **37** *(4): 388–93. doi:10.1093/* alcalc/37.4.388. PMID 12107043.
24. Cox, Michael; Nelson, David R.; Lehninger, Albert L (2005). Lehninger Principles of Biochemistry. San Francisco: W. H. Freeman. p. 180. ISBN 0-7167-4339-6.
25. Leskovac V, Trivić S, Pericin D (Dec 2002). The three zinc-containing alcohol dehydrogenases from baker's yeast, Saccharomyces cerevisiae. FEMS Yeast Research. **2** *(4): 481–94. doi:10.1111/j.1567-1364.2002.tb00116.x. PMID 12702265.*
26. Coghlan A (23 December 2006). Festive special: The brewer's tale - life. New Scientist. Archivedfrom the original on 15 September 2008. Retrieved 2009-04-27.
27. Chang C, Meyerowitz EM (Mar 1986). Molecular cloning and DNA sequence of the Arabidopsis thaliana alcohol dehydrogenase gene. Proceedings of the National Academy of Sciences of the United States of America. **83** *(5): 1408–12. doi:10.1073/pnas.83.5.1408. PMC 323085. PMID 2937058.*
28. Chung HJ, Ferl RJ (Oct 1999). Arabidopsis alcohol dehydrogenase expression in both shoots and roots is conditioned by root growth environment. Plant Physiology. **121** *(2): 429–36. doi:10.1104/pp.121.2.429. PMC 59405. PMID 10517834.*
29. Thompson CE, Fernandes CL, de Souza ON, de Freitas LB, Salzano FM (May 2010). Evaluation of the impact of functional diversification on Poaceae, Brassicaceae, Fabaceae, and Pinaceae alcohol dehydrogenase enzymes. Journal of Molecular Modeling. **16** *(5): 919–28.* doi:10.1007/s00894-009-0576-0. PMID 19834749.

30. Järvinen P, Palmé A, Orlando Morales L, Lännenpää M, Keinänen M, Sopanen T, Lascoux M (Nov 2004). Phylogenetic relationships of Betula species (Betulaceae) based on nuclear ADH and chloroplast matK sequences. American Journal of Botany. Amjbot.org. **91** *(11): 1834–45. doi:10.3732/ajb.91.11.1834. PMID 21652331. Archived from the original on 26 May 2010.*

31. Williamson VM, Paquin CE (Sep 1987). Homology of Saccharomyces cerevisiae ADH4 to an iron-activated alcohol dehydrogenase from Zymomonas mobilis. Molecular & General Genetics. **209** *(2): 374–81.* doi:10.1007/bf00329668. PMID 2823079.

32. Conway T, Sewell GW, Osman YA, Ingram LO (Jun 1987). Cloning and sequencing of the alcohol dehydrogenase II gene from Zymomonas mobilis. Journal of Bacteriology. **169** *(6): 2591–7. PMC 212129. PMID 3584063.*

33. Conway T, Ingram LO (Jul 1989). Similarity of Escherichia coli propanediol oxidoreductase (fucO product) and an unusual alcohol dehydrogenase from Zymomonas mobilis and Saccharomyces cerevisiae. Journal of Bacteriology. **171** *(7): 3754–9. PMC 210121. PMID 2661535.*

34. Walter KA, Bennett GN, Papoutsakis ET (Nov 1992). Molecular characterization of two Clostridium acetobutylicum ATCC 824 butanol dehydrogenase isozyme genes. Journal of Bacteriology. **174** *(22): 7149–58. PMC 207405. PMID 1385386.*

35. Kessler D, Leibrecht I, Knappe J (Apr 1991). Pyruvate-formate-lyase-deactivase and acetyl-CoA reductase activities of Escherichia coli reside on a polymeric protein particle encoded by adhE. FEBS Letters. **281** *(1-2): 59–63.* doi:10.1016/0014-5793(91)80358-A. PMID 2015910.

36. Truniger V, Boos W (Mar 1994). Mapping and cloning of gldA, the structural gene of the Escherichia coli glycerol dehydrogenase. Journal of Bacteriology. **176** *(6): 1796–800. PMC 205274. PMID 8132480.*

37. de Vries GE, Arfman N, Terpstra P, Dijkhuizen L (Aug 1992). Cloning, expression, and sequence analysis of the Bacillus methanolicus C1 methanol dehydrogenase gene. Journal of Bacteriology. **174** *(16): 5346–53. PMC 206372. PMID 1644761.*

38. Leuchs S, Greiner L (2011). Alcohol dehydrogenase from Lactobacillus brevis: A versatile catalyst for enenatioselective reduction (PDF). CABEQ: 267–281.

39. Zucca P, Littarru M, Rescigno A, Sanjust E (May 2009). Cofactor recycling for selective enzymatic biotransformation of cinnamaldehyde to cinnamyl alcohol. Bioscience, Biotechnology, and Biochemistry. **73** *(5): 1224–6. doi:10.1271/bbb.90025. PMID 19420690.*

40. Moore CM, Minteer SD, Martin RS (Feb 2005). Microchip-based ethanol/oxygen biofuel cell. Lab on a Chip. **5** *(2): 218–25.* doi:10.1039/b412719f. PMID 15672138.

41. Racker E (1950). Crystalline alcohol dehydrogenase from baker's yeast. J. Biol. Chem. **184** *(1): 313–9. PMID 15443900.*

42. Enzymatic Assay of Alcohol Dehydrogenase (EC 1.1.1.1). Sigma Aldrich. Retrieved 13 July 2015.

43. Sher KJ, Grekin ER, Williams NA (2005). The development of alcohol use disorders. Annual Review of Clinical Psychology. **1**: 493–523. doi:10.1146/annurev.clinpsy.1.102803.144107. PMID 17716097.

44. Luo X, Kranzler HR, Zuo L, Wang S, Schork NJ, Gelernter J (Feb 2007). Multiple ADH genes modulate risk for drug dependence in both African- and European-Americans. Human Molecular Genetics. **16** *(4): 380–90. doi:10.1093/* hmg/ddl460. PMC 1853246. PMID 17185388.

45. International Programme on Chemical Safety (IPCS): Methanol (PIM 335), , retrieved on March 1, 2008

46. Velez LI, Shepherd G, Lee YC, Keyes DC (September 2007). Ethylene glycol ingestion treated only with fomepizole (PDF). J Med Toxicol. **3** *(3): 125–8.* doi:10.1007/BF03160922. PMID 18072148.

Metal Toxicity

Chapter Contents

The toxicity of heavy metals depends on a number of factors. Specific symptomatology varies according to the metal in question, the total dose absorbed, and whether the exposure was acute or chronic. The age of the person can also influence toxicity. For example, young children are more susceptible to the effects of lead exposure because they absorb several times the percent ingested compared with adults and because their brains are more plastic and even brief exposures may influence developmental processes. The route of exposure is also important. Elemental mercury is relatively inert in the gastrointestinal tract and also poorly absorbed through intact skin, yet inhaled or injected elemental mercury may have disastrous effects.

INTRODUCTION

Metal toxicity or metal poisoning is the toxic effect of certain metals in certain forms and doses on life. Some metals are toxic when they form poisonous soluble compounds. Certain metals have no biological role, i.e. are not essential minerals, or are toxic when in a certain form. In the case of lead, any measurable amount may have negative health effects. Often heavy metals are thought as synonymous, but lighter metals may also be toxic in certain circumstances, such as beryllium and lithium. Not all heavy metals are particularly toxic, and some are essential, such as iron. The definition may also include trace elements when considered in abnormally high, toxic doses. An option for treatment of metal poisoning may be chelation therapy, which is a technique which involves the administration of chelation agents to remove metals from the body.

Toxic metals sometimes imitate the action of an essential element in the body, interfering with the metabolic process to cause illness. Many metals, particularly heavy metals are toxic, but some heavy metals are essential, and some, such as bismuth, have a low toxicity. Most often the definition of toxic metals includes at least cadmium, manganese, lead, mercury and the radioactive metals.Metalloids (arsenic, polonium) may be included in the definition. Radioactive metals have both radiological toxicity and chemical toxicity. Metals in an oxidation state abnormal to the body may also become toxic: chromium(III) is an essential trace element, but chromium(VI) is a carcinogen.

Toxicity is a function of solubility. Insoluble compounds as well as the metallic forms often exhibit negligible toxicity. The toxicity of any metal depends on its ligands. In some cases, organometallic forms, such as methylmercury and tetraethyl lead, can be extremely toxic. In other cases, organometallic derivatives are less toxic such as the cobaltocenium cation.

Decontamination for toxic metals is different from organic toxins: because toxic metals are elements, they cannot be destroyed. Toxic metals may be made insoluble or collected, possibly by the aid of chelating agents. Alternatively, they can be diluted into a sufficiently large reservoir, such as the sea, because immediate toxicity is a function of concentration rather than amount. However, bioaccumulation has the potential to reverse this.

Toxic metals can bioaccumulate in the body and in the food chain. Therefore, a common characteristic of toxic metals is the chronic nature of their toxicity. This is particularly notable with radioactive heavy metals such as radium, which imitates calcium to the point of being incorporated into human bone, although similar health implications are found in lead or mercury poisoning. The exceptions to this are barium and aluminium, which can be removed efficiently by the kidneys.

TESTING FOR POISONING

People are continually exposed to metals in the environment. Medical tests can detect metals often, but this is to be expected and alone is not evidence that a person is poisoned. Metal screening tests should not be used unless there is reason to believe that a person has had excessive exposure to metals. People should seek medical testing for poisoning only if they are concerned for a particular reason, and physicians should consider a patient's history and physical examination before conducting tests to detect metals.

TREATMENT FOR POISONING

Chelation therapy is a medical procedure that involves the administration of chelating agents to remove heavy metals from the body. Chelating agents are molecules that have multiple electron-donating groups, which can form stable coordination complexes with metal ions. Complexation prevents the metal ions from reacting with molecules in the body, and enable them to be dissolved in blood and eliminated in urine. It should only be used in people who have a diagnosis of metal intoxication. That diagnosis should be validated with tests done in appropriate biological samples.

Chelation therapy is administered under very careful medic+al supervision due to various inherent risks.When the therapy is administered properly, the chelation drugs have significant side effects. Chelation administered inappropriately can cause neurodevelopmental toxicity, increase risk of developing cancer, and cause death; chelation also removes essential metal elements and requires measures to prevent their loss.

SPECIFIC TYPES OF POISONING

Aluminium Phosphide Poisoning

Aluminium has no known biological role and its classification into toxic metals is controversial. Significant toxic effects and accumulation to tissues have been observed in renally impaired patients.

Acute aluminium phosphide poisoning (AAlPP) is a large, though under-reported, problem in the Indian subcontinent. Aluminium phosphide (AlP), which is readily available as a fumigant for stored cereal grains, sold under various brand names such as *QuickPhos* and *Celphos*, is highly toxic, especially when consumed from a freshly opened container. Death results from profound shock, myocarditis and multi-organ failure. Aluminium phosphide has a fatal dose of between 0.15 and 0.5 grams (0.0053 and 0.0176 oz). It has been reported to be the most common cause of suicidal death in North India. The very high toxicity of aluminium phosphide is attributed to the phosphine content and is not related to aluminium. Calcium phosphide and zinc phosphide are similar poisons.

Beryllium Poisoning

Beryllium poisoning is illness resulting from the toxic effect of beryllium in its elemental form or in various chemical compounds. The toxicity of beryllium depends upon the duration, intensity and frequency of exposure (features of dose), as well as the form of beryllium and the route of exposure (i.e. inhalation, dermal, ingestion). According to the International Agency for Research on Cancer (IARC), beryllium and beryllium compounds are Category 1 carcinogens; they are carcinogenic to both animals and humans.

Cadmium Poisoning

Cadmium is an extremely toxic metal commonly found in industrial workplaces. Due to its low permissible exposure limit, overexposures may occur even in situations where trace quantities of cadmium are found. Cadmium is used extensively in electroplating, although the nature of the operation does not generally lead to overexposures. Cadmium is also found in some industrial paints and may represent a hazard when sprayed. Operations involving removal of cadmium paints by scraping or blasting may pose a significant hazard. Cadmium is also present in the manufacturing of some types of batteries. Exposures to cadmium are addressed in specific standards for the general industry, shipyard employment, construction industry, and the agricultural industry.

Iron Poisoning

Iron poisoning is an iron overload caused by a large excess of iron intake and usually refers to an acute overload rather than a gradual one. The term has been primarily associated with young children who consumed large quantities of iron supplement pills, which resemble sweets and are widely used, including by pregnant women—see overnutrition (approximately 3 grams is lethal for a 2 year old). Targeted packaging restrictions in the US for supplement containers with over 250 mg elemental iron have existed since 1978, and recommendations for unit packaging have reduced the several iron poisoning fatalities per year to almost nil since 1998. No known cases of iron poisoning have been identified that are associated with iron mining.

Lithium Poisoning

Lithium is used in some medications, specifically to treat bipolar disorder. The level of "sufficient" medication is thought by many physicians to be close to toxic tolerance for kidney function. Therefore, the patient is often monitored for this purpose.

Manganese Poisoning, or Manganism

Manganism or manganese poisoning is a toxic condition resulting from chronic exposure to manganese and first identified in 1837 by James Couper.

Silver Poisoning, or Argyria

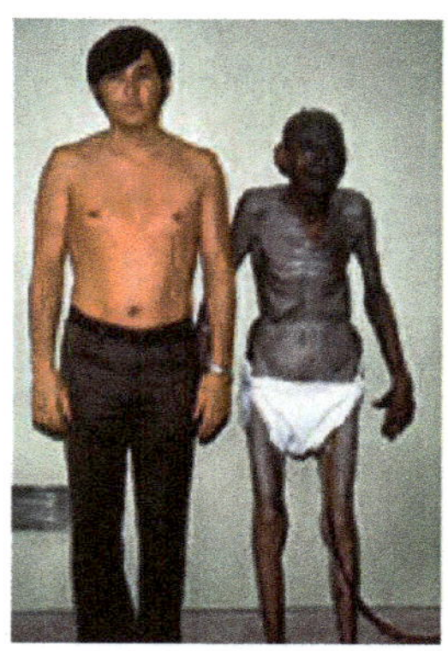

A 92-year-old Caucasian man (right) with pigmentary changes had used nose drops containing silver for many years. His skin biopsy showed silver deposits in the dermis, confirming the diagnosis of generalized argyria.

Argyria or argyrosis is a condition caused by inappropriate exposure to chemical compounds of the element silver, or to silver dust. The most dramatic symptom of argyria is that the skin turns blue or bluish-grey. It may take the form of *generalized argyria* or *local argyria*. Generalized argyria affects large areas over much of the visible surface of the body. Local argyria shows in limited regions of the body, such as patches of skin, parts of the mucous membrane or the conjunctiva.

Thallium Poisoning

Thallium and its compounds are often highly toxic. Contact with skin is dangerous, and adequate ventilation should be provided when melting this metal. Many thallium(I) compounds are highly soluble in water and are readily absorbed through the skin. Exposure to them should not exceed 0.1 mg per m^2 of skin in an 8-hour time-weighted average (40-hour work week). Thallium is a suspected human carcinogen.

Tin Poisoning

Tin poisoning refers to the toxic effects of tin and its compounds. Cases of poisoning from tin metal, its oxides, and its salts are "almost unknown"; on the other hand certain organotin compounds are almost as toxic as cyanide.

Zinc Toxicity

Even though zinc is an essential requirement for a healthy body, excess zinc can be harmful, and cause **zinc toxicity**. Such toxicity levels have been seen to occur at ingestion of greater than 225 mg of Zinc. Excessive absorption of zinc can suppress copper and iron absorption. The free zinc ion in solution is highly toxic to bacteria, plants, invertebrates, and even vertebrate fish.

SOCIETY AND CULTURE

It is difficult to differentiate the effects of low level metal poisoning from the environment with other kinds of environmental harms, including nonmetal pollution. Generally, increased exposure to heavy metals in the environment increases risk of developing cancer.

Without a diagnosis of metal toxicity and outside of evidence-based medicine, but perhaps because of worry about metal toxicity, some people seek chelation therapy to treat autism, cardiovascular disease, Alzheimer's disease, or any sort of neurodegeneration. Chelation therapy does not improve outcomes for those diseases.

MERCURY POISONING

Mercury poisoning is a type of metal poisoning, due to exposure to mercury. Symptoms may include muscle weakness, poor coordination, numbness in the hands and feet, skin rashes, memory problems, trouble speaking, trouble hearing, or trouble seeing.Symptoms depend upon the type, dose, method, and duration of exposure. The effects of long term low dose exposure to methylmercury is unclear. High level exposure to methylmercury is known as Minamata disease. Exposure in children may result in acrodynia (pink's disease) in which the skin becomes pink and peels. Long term complications may include kidney problems and decreased intelligence.

Mercury (chemical symbol Hg) exposure may occur in number of forms including: metal, vapor, salt, and organic compound. Most exposure is from eating fish, amalgam based dental fillings, or exposure at work. In fish, those higher up in the food chain generally have higher levels of mercury. Less commonly poisoning may occur as an attempt to end one's life. Human activities that release mercury into the environment include the burning of coal and mining of gold. Tests of the blood, urine, and hair for mercury are available but do not relate well to the amount in the body.

Prevention includes eating a diet low in mercury, removing mercury from medical and other devices, proper disposal of mercury, and not mining further mercury. In those with acute poisoning from inorganic mercury salts, chelation with either dimercaptosuccinic acid (DMSA) or dimercaptopropane sulfonate (DMPS) appears to improve outcomes if given within a few hours of exposure. Chelation for those with long term exposure is of unclear benefit. In certain communities which survive on fishing, rates of mercury poisoning among children are as high as 1.7 per 100.

Signs and Symptoms

Common symptoms of mercury poisoning include peripheral neuropathy, presenting as paresthesia or itching, burning, pain, or even a sensation that resembles small insects crawling on or under the skin (formication); skin discoloration (pink cheeks, fingertips and toes); swelling; and desquamation (shedding or peeling of skin).

Mercury irreversibly inhibits selenium-dependent enzymes (see below) and may also inactivate *S*-adenosyl-methionine, which is necessary for catecholamine catabolism by catechol-*O*-methyl transferase. Due to the body's inability to degrade catecholamines (e.g. epinephrine), a person suffering from mercury poisoning may experience profuse sweating, tachycardia (persistently faster-than-normal heart beat), increased salivation, and hypertension (high blood pressure).

Affected children may show red cheeks, nose and lips, loss of hair, teeth, and nails, transient rashes, hypotonia (muscle weakness), and increased sensitivity to light. Other symptoms may include kidney dysfunction (e.g. Fanconi syndrome) or neuropsychiatric symptoms such as emotional lability, memory impairment, or insomnia.

Thus, the clinical presentation may resemble pheochromocytoma or Kawasaki disease. Desquamation (skin peeling) can occur with severe mercury poisoning acquired by handling elemental mercury.

Causes

The consumption of fish is by far the most significant source of ingestion-related mercury exposure in humans, although plants and livestock also contain mercury due to bioconcentration of mercury from seawater, freshwater, marine and lacustrine sediments, soils, and atmosphere, and due to biomagnification by ingesting other mercury-containing organisms. Exposure to mercury can occur from breathing contaminated air, from eating foods that have acquired mercury residues during processing, from exposure to mercury vapor in mercury amalgam dental restorations, and from improper use or disposal of mercury and mercury-containing objects, for example, after spills of elemental mercury or improper disposal of fluorescent lamps.

All of these, except elemental liquid mercury produce toxicity or death with less than a gram. Mercury's zero oxidation state (Hg^0) exists as vapor or as liquid metal, its mercurous state (Hg^+) exists as inorganic salts, and its mercuric state (Hg^{2+}) may form either inorganic salts or organomercury compounds.

Consumption of whale and dolphin meat, as is the practice in Japan, is a source of high levels of mercury poisoning. Tetsuya Endo, a professor at the Health Sciences University of Hokkaido, has tested whale meat purchased in the whaling town of Taiji and found mercury levels more than 20 times the acceptable Japanese standard.

Human-generated sources, such as coal-burning power plants emit about half of atmospheric mercury, with natural sources such as volcanoes responsible for the remainder. An estimated two-thirds of human-generated mercury comes from stationary combustion, mostly of coal. Other important human-generated sources include gold production, nonferrous metal production, cement production, waste disposal, human crematoria, caustic soda production, pig iron and steel production, mercury production (mostly for batteries), and biomass burning.

Small independent gold-mining operation workers are at higher risk of mercury poisoning because of crude processing methods. Such is the danger for the galamsey in Ghana and similar workers known as *orpailleurs* in neighboring francophone countries. While no official government estimates of the labor force have been made, observers believe 20,000-50,000 work as galamseys in Ghana, a figure including many women, who work as porters. Similar problems have been reported amongst the gold miners of Indonesia.

Mercury and many of its chemical compounds, especially organomercury compounds, can also be readily absorbed through direct contact with bare, or in some cases (such as methylmercury) insufficiently protected, skin. Mercury and its compounds are commonly used in chemical laboratories, hospitals, dental clinics, and facilities involved in the production of items such as fluorescent light bulbs, batteries, and explosives.

No scientific data support the claim that mercury compounds in vaccine preservatives cause autismor its symptoms.

Sources

Compounds of mercury tend to be much more toxic than either the elemental or the salts. These compounds have been implicated in causing brain and liver damage. The most dangerous mercury compound, dimethylmercury, is so toxic that even a few microliters spilled on the skin, or even on a latex glove, can cause death, as in the case of Karen Wetterhahn.

Methylmercury and Related Organomercury Compounds

Methylmercury is the major source of organic mercury for all individuals. Due to bioaccumulation it works its way up through the food web and thus biomagnifies, resulting in high concentrations among populations of some species. Top predatory fish, such as tuna or swordfish, are usually of greater concern than smaller species. The US FDA and the EPA advise women of child-bearing age, nursing mothers, and young children to completely avoid swordfish, shark, king mackerel and tilefish from the Gulf of Mexico, and to limit consumption of albacore (white) tuna to no more than 6 oz (170 g) per week, and of all other fish and shellfish to no more than 12 oz (340 g) per week. A 2006 review of the risks and benefits of fish consumption found, for adults, the benefits of one to two servings of fish per week outweigh the risks, even (except for a few fish species) for women of childbearing age, and that avoidance of fish consumption could result in significant excess coronary heart disease deaths and suboptimal neural development in children.

The period between exposure to methylmercury and the appearance of symptoms in adult poisoning cases is long. The longest recorded latent period is five months after a single exposure, in the Dartmouth case (see History); other latent periods in the range of weeks to months have also been reported. No explanation for this long latent period is known. When the first symptom appears, typically paresthesia (a tingling or numbness in the skin), it is followed rapidly by more severe effects, sometimes ending in coma and death. The toxic damage appears to be determined by the peak value of mercury, not the length of the exposure.

Methylmercury exposure during rodent gestation, a developmental period that approximately models human neural development during the first two trimesters of gestation, has long-lasting behavioral consequences that appear in adulthood and, in some cases, may not appear until aging. Prefrontal cortex or dopamine neurotransmission could be especially sensitive to even subtle gestational methylmercury exposure and suggests that public health assessments of methylmercury based on intellectual performance may underestimate the impact of methylmercury in public health.

Ethylmercury is a breakdown product of the antibacteriological agent ethylmercurithiosalicylate, which has been used as a topical antiseptic and a vaccine preservative (further discussed under Thiomersal below). Its characteristics have not been studied as extensively as those of methylmercury. It is cleared from the blood much more rapidly, with a half-life of seven to 10 days, and it is metabolized much more quickly than methylmercury. It is presumed not to have methylmercury's ability to cross the blood–brain barrier via a transporter, but instead relies on simple diffusion to enter the brain. Other exposure sources of organic mercury include phenylmercuric acetate and phenylmercuric nitrate. These compounds were used in indoor latex paints for their antimildew properties, but were removed in 1990 because of cases of toxicity.

Inorganic Mercury Compounds

Mercury occurs as salts such as mercuric chloride ($HgCl_2$) and mercurous chloride (Hg_2Cl_2), the latter also known as calomel. Because they are more soluble in water, mercuric salts are usually more acutely toxic than mercurous salts. Their higher solubility allows them to be more readily absorbed from the gastrointestinal tract. Mercury salts affect primarily the gastrointestinal tract and the kidneys, and can cause severe kidney damage; however, as they cannot cross the blood–brain barrier easily, these salts inflict little neurological damage without continuous or heavy exposure. Mercuric cyanide ($Hg(CN)_2$) is a particularly toxic mercury compound that has been used in murders, as it contains not only mercury but also cyanide, leading to simultaneous cyanide poisoning. The drug n-acetyl penicillamine has been used to treat mercury poisoning with limited success.

Elemental Mercury

Quicksilver (liquid metallic mercury) is poorly absorbed by ingestion and skin contact. Its vapor is the most hazardous form. Animal data indicate less than 0.01% of ingested mercury is absorbed through the intact gastrointestinal tract, though it may not be true for individuals suffering from ileus. Cases of systemic toxicity from accidental swallowing are rare, and attempted suicide via intravenous injection does not appear to result in systemic toxicity, though it still causes damage by physically blocking blood vessels both at the site of injection and the lungs. Though not studied quantitatively, the physical properties of liquid elemental mercury limit its absorption through intact skin and in light of its very low absorption rate from the gastrointestinal tract, skin absorption would not be high. Some mercury vapor is absorbed dermally, but uptake by this route is only about 1% of that by inhalation.

In humans, approximately 80% of inhaled mercury vapor is absorbed via the respiratory tract, where it enters the circulatory system and is distributed throughout the body. Chronic exposure by inhalation, even at low concentrations in the range 0.7–42 $\mu g/m^3$, has been shown in case control studies to cause effects such as tremors, impaired cognitive skills, and sleep disturbance in workers.

Acute inhalation of high concentrations causes a wide variety of cognitive, personality, sensory, and motor disturbances. The most prominent symptoms include tremors (initially affecting the hands and sometimes spreading to other parts of the body), emotional lability (characterized by irritability, excessive shyness, confidence loss, and nervousness), insomnia, memory loss, neuromuscular changes (weakness, muscle atrophy, muscle twitching), headaches, polyneuropathy (paresthesia, stocking-glove sensory loss, hyperactive tendon reflexes, slowed sensory and motor nerve conduction velocities), and performance deficits in tests of cognitive function.

Mechanism

The toxicity of mercury sources can be expected to depend on its nature, i.e., salts vs. organomercury compounds vs. elemental mercury.

One mechanism of mercury toxicity involves its irreversible inhibition of selenoenzymes, such as thioredoxin reductase (IC50 = 9 nM). Although it has many functions, thioredoxin reductase restores vitamins C and E, as well as a number of other important antioxidant molecules, back into their reduced forms, enabling them to counteract oxidative damage. Since the rate of oxygen consumption is particularly high in brain tissues, production of reactive oxygen species (ROS) is accentuated in these vital cells, making them particularly vulnerable to oxidative damage and especially dependent upon the antioxidant protection provided by selenoenzymes. High mercury exposures deplete the amount of cellular selenium available for the biosynthesis of thioredoxin reductase and other selenoenzymes that prevent and reverse oxidative damage, which, if the depletion is severe and long lasting, results in brain cell dysfunctions that can ultimately cause death.

Mercury in its various forms is particularly harmful to fetuses as an environmental toxin in pregnancy, as well as to infants. Women who have been exposed to mercury in substantial excess of dietary selenium intakes during pregnancy are at risk of giving birth to children with serious birth defects. Mercury exposures in excess of dietary selenium intakes in young children can have severe neurological consequences, preventing nerve sheaths from forming properly. Mercury inhibits the formation of myelin.

Diagnosis

Diagnosis of elemental or inorganic mercury poisoning involves determining the history of exposure, physical findings, and an elevated body burden of mercury. Although whole-blood mercury concentrations are typically less than 6 μg/L, diets rich in fish can result in blood mercury concentrations higher than 200 μg/L; it is not that useful to measure these levels for suspected cases of elemental or inorganic poisoning because of mercury's short half-life in the blood. If the exposure is chronic, urine levels can be obtained; 24-hour collections are more reliable than spot collections. It is difficult or impossible to interpret urine samples of patients undergoing chelation therapy, as the therapy itself increases mercury levels in the samples.

Diagnosis of organic mercury poisoning differs in that whole-blood or hair analysis is more reliable than urinary mercury levels.

Prevention

Mercury poisoning can be prevented (or minimized) by eliminating or reducing exposure to mercury and mercury compounds. To that end, many governments and private groups have made efforts to regulate heavily the use of mercury, or to issue advisories about its use. For example, the export from the European Union of mercury and some mercury compounds has been prohibited since the 15th of March, 2010. The variability among regulations and advisories is at times confusing for the lay person as well as scientists.

Country	Regulating agency	Regulated activity	Medium	Type of mercury compound	Type of limit	Limit
US	Occupational Safety and Health Administration	occupational exposure	air	elemental mercury	Ceiling (not to exceed)	0.1 mg/m³
US	Occupational Safety and Health Administration	occupational exposure	air	organic mercury	Ceiling (not to exceed)	0.05 mg/m³
US	Food and Drug Administration	eating	sea food	methylmercury	Maximum allowable concentration	1 ppm (1 mg/L)
US	Environmental Protection Agency	drinking	water	inorganic mercury	Maximum contaminant level	2 ppb (0.002 mg/L)

\The United States Environmental Protection Agency (EPA) issued recommendations in 2004 regarding exposure to mercury in fish and shellfish. The EPA also developed the "Fish Kids" awareness campaign for children and young adults on account of the greater impact of mercury exposure to that population.

Cleaning spilled Mercury

Mercury thermometers and mercury light bulbs are not as common as they used to be, and the amount of mercury they contain is unlikely to be a health concern if handled carefully. However, broken items still require careful cleanup, as mercury can be hard to collect and it is easy to accidentally create a much larger exposure problem.

Treatment

Identifying and removing the source of the mercury is crucial. Decontamination requires removal of clothes, washing skin with soap and water, and flushing the eyes with saline solution as needed.

Chelation Therapy

Chelation therapy for acute inorganic mercury poisoning can be done with DMSA, 2,3-dimercapto-1-propanesulfonic acid (DMPS), D-penicillamine (DPCN), or dimercaprol (BAL). Only DMSA is FDA-approved for use in children for treating mercury poisoning. However, several studies found no clear clinical benefit from DMSA treatment for poisoning due to mercury vapor. No chelator for methylmercury or ethylmercury is approved by the FDA; DMSA is the most frequently used for severe methylmercury poisoning, as it is given orally, has fewer side-effects, and has been found to be superior to BAL, DPCN, and DMPS. α-Lipoic acid (ALA) has been shown to be protective against acute mercury poisoning in several mammalian species when it is given soon after exposure; correct dosage is required, as inappropriate dosages increase toxicity. Although it has been hypothesized that frequent low dosages of ALA may have potential as a mercury chelator, studies in rats have been contradictory.Glutathione and *N*-acetylcysteine (NAC) are recommended by some physicians, but have been shown to increase mercury concentrations in the kidneys and the brain.

Chelation therapy can be hazardous if administered incorrectly. In August 2005, an incorrect form of EDTA (edetate disodium) used for chelation therapy resulted in hypocalcemia, causing cardiac arrest that killed a five-year-old autistic boy.

Other

Experimental findings have demonstrated an interaction between selenium and methylmercury, but epidemiological studies have found little evidence that selenium helps to protect against the adverse effects of methylmercury.

Prognosis

Some of the toxic effects of mercury are partially or wholly reversible, either through specific therapy or through natural elimination of the metal after exposure has been discontinued. Autopsy findings point to a half-life of inorganic mercury in human brains of 27.4 years. Heavy or prolonged exposure can do irreversible damage, in particular in fetuses, infants, and young children. Young's syndrome is believed to be a long-term consequence of early childhood mercury poisoning.

Mercuric chloride may cause cancer as it has caused increases in several types of tumors in rats and mice, while methyl mercury has caused kidney tumors in male rats. The EPA has classified mercuric chloride and methyl mercury as possible human carcinogens (ATSDR, EPA)

Detection in Biological Fluids

Mercury may be measured in blood or urine to confirm a diagnosis of poisoning in hospitalized people or to assist in the forensic investigation in a case of fatal overdosage. Some analytical techniques are capable of distinguishing organic from inorganic forms of the metal. The concentrations in both fluids tend to reach high levels early after exposure to inorganic forms, while lower but very persistent levels are observed following exposure to elemental or organic mercury. Chelation therapy can cause a transient elevation of urine mercury levels.

- The first emperor of unified China, Qin Shi Huang, it is reported, died of ingesting mercury pills that were ironically intended to give him eternal life.
- The phrase *mad as a hatter* is likely a reference to mercury poisoning among milliners (so-called "mad hatter disease), as mercury-based compounds were once used in the manufacture of felt hats in the 18th and 19th century. (The Mad Hatter character of *Alice in Wonderland* was, it is presumed, inspired by an eccentric furniture dealer named Theophilus Carter. Carter was not a victim of mad hatter disease although Lewis Carroll would have been familiar with the phenomenon of dementia that occurred among hatters.)
- In 1810, two British ships, HMS *Triumph* and HMS *Phipps*, salvaged a large load of elemental mercury from a wrecked Spanish vessel near Cadiz, Spain. The

bladders containing the mercury soon ruptured. The element spread about the ships in liquid and vapor forms. The sailors presented with neurologic compromises: tremor, paralysis, and excessive salivation as well as tooth loss, skin problems, and pulmonary complaints. In 1823 William Burnet, MD published a report on the effects of Mercurial vapor. The *Triumph*'s surgeon, Henry Plowman, had concluded that the ailments had arisen from inhaling the mercurialized atmosphere. His treatment was to order the lower deck gun ports to be opened, when it was safe to do so; sleeping on the orlop was forbidden; and no men slept in the lower deck if they were at all symptomatic. Windsails were set to channel fresh air into the lower decks day and night.

- Historically, gold amalgam was widely used in gilding, leading to numerous casualties among the workers. It is estimated that during the construction of Saint Isaac's Cathedral alone, 60 men died from the gilding of the main dome.
- For years, including the early part of his presidency, Abraham Lincoln took a common medicine of his time called "blue mass, which contained significant amounts of mercury.
- On September 5, 1920, silent movie actress Olive Thomas ingested mercury capsules dissolved in an alcoholic solution at the Hotel Ritz in Paris. There is still controversy over whether it was suicide, or whether she consumed the external preparation by mistake. Her husband, Jack Pickford (the brother of Mary Pickford), had syphilis, and the mercury was used as a treatment of the venereal disease at the time. She died a few days later at the American Hospital in Neuilly.
- An early scientific study of mercury poisoning was in 1923–6 by the German inorganic chemist, Alfred Stock, who himself became poisoned, together with his colleagues, by breathing mercury vapor that was being released by his laboratory equipment—diffusion pumps, float valves, and manometers—all of which contained mercury, and also from mercury that had been accidentally spilt and remained in cracks in the linoleum floor covering. He published a number of papers on mercury poisoning, founded a committee in Berlin to study cases of possible mercury poisoning, and introduced the term *micromercurialism*.
- The term *Hunter-Russell syndrome* derives from a study of mercury poisoning among workers in a seed packing factory in Norwich, England in the late 1930s who breathed methylmercury that was being used as a seed disinfectant and preservative.
- Outbreaks of methylmercury poisoning occurred in several places in Japan during the 1950s due to industrial discharges of mercury into rivers and coastal waters. The best-known instances were in Minamata and Niigata. In Minamata alone, more than 600 people died due to what became known as Minamata disease. More than 21,000 people filed claims with the Japanese government, of which almost 3000 became certified as having the disease. In 22 documented cases, pregnant women who consumed contaminated fish showed mild or no symptoms but gave birth to infants with severe developmental disabilities.
- Widespread mercury poisoning occurred in rural Iraq in 1971-1972, when grain

treated with a methylmercury-based fungicide that was intended for planting only was used by the rural population to make bread, causing at least 6530 cases of mercury poisoning and at least 459 deaths (see Basra poison grain disaster).

- On August 14, 1996, Karen Wetterhahn, a chemistry professor working at Dartmouth College, spilled a small amount of dimethylmercury on her latex glove. She began experiencing the symptoms of mercury poisoning five months later and, despite aggressive chelation therapy, died a few months later from brain malfunction due to mercury intoxication.
- In April 2000, Alan Chmurny attempted to kill a former employee, Marta Bradley, by pouring mercury into the ventilation system of her car.
- On March 19, 2008, Tony Winnett, 55, inhaled mercury vapors while trying to extract gold from computer parts (by using liquid mercury to separate gold from the rest of the alloy), and died ten days later. His Oklahoma residence became so contaminated that it had to be gutted.
- In December 2008, actor Jeremy Piven was diagnosed with mercury poisoning possibly resulting from eating sushi twice a day for twenty years or herbal remedies he was also taking.
- In India, a study by the non-profit Centre for Science and Environment has found that in the country's energy capital Singrauli, mercury is slowly entering people's homes, food, water and even blood.

Infantile Acrodynia

Infantile acrodynia (also known as "calomel disease", "erythredemic polyneuropathy", and "pink disease") is a type of mercury poisoning in children characterized by pain and pink discoloration of the hands and feet. The word is derived from the Greek, where άκρο means *end* or *extremity*, and οδυνη means *pain*. Acrodynia resulted primarily from calomel in teething powders and decreased greatly after calomel was excluded from most teething powders in 1954.

Acrodynia is difficult to diagnose, it is most often postulated that the etiology of this syndrome is an idiosyncratic hypersensitivity reaction to mercury because of the lack of correlation with mercury levels, many of the symptoms resemble recognized mercury poisoning.

Medicine

Mercury was once prescribed as a purgative. Many mercury-containing compounds were once used in medicines. eg. see calomel (mercurous chloride), and mercuric chloride

Thiomersal

In 1999, the Centers for Disease Control (CDC) and the American Academy of Pediatrics (AAP) asked vaccine makers to remove the organomercury compound thiomersal (spelled "thimerosal" in the US) from vaccines as quickly as possible, and thiomersal has been phased out of US and European vaccines, except for some preparations of influenza vaccine. The CDC and the AAP followed the precautionary principle, which assumes that there is no harm in exercising caution even if it later turns out to be unwarranted, but their 1999 action sparked confusion and controversy that Thiomersal was the cause of autism.

Since 2000, the thiomersal in child vaccines has been alleged to contribute to autism, and thousands of parents in the United States have pursued legal compensation from a federal fund. A 2004 Institute of Medicine (IOM) committee favored rejecting any causal relationship between thiomersal-containing vaccines and autism. Autism incidence rates increased steadily even after thiomersal was removed from childhood vaccines. Currently there is no accepted scientific evidence that exposure to thiomersal is a factor in causing autism.

Dental amalgam toxicity

Dental amalgam is a possible cause of low-level mercury poisoning due to its use in dental fillings. Discussion on the topic includes debates on whether amalgam should be used, with critics arguing that its toxic effects make it unsafe.

Cosmetics

Some skin whitening products contain the toxic chemical mercury(II) chloride as the active ingredient. When applied, the chemical readily absorbs through the skin into the bloodstream. The use of mercury in cosmetics is illegal in the United States. However, cosmetics containing mercury are often illegally imported. Following a certified case of mercury poisoning resulting from the use of an imported skin whitening product, the United States Food and Drug Administration warned against the use of such products. Symptoms of mercury poisoning have resulted from the use of various mercury-containing cosmetic products. The use of skin whitening products is especially popular amongst Asian women. In Hong Kong in 2002, two products were discovered to contain between 9,000 and 60,000 times the recommended dose.

Fluorescent Lamps

Fluorescent lamps contain mercury which is released when bulbs are broken. Mercury in bulbs is typically present as either elemental mercury liquid, vapor, or both, since the liquid evaporates at ambient temperature. When broken indoors, bulbs may emit sufficient mercury vapor to present health concerns, and the U.S. Environmental Protection Agency recommends evacuating and airing out a room for at least 15 minutes after breaking a fluorescent light bulb. Breakage of multiple bulbs presents a greater concern. A 1987 report described a 23-month-old toddler who suffered anorexia, weight loss, irritability, profuse sweating, and peeling and redness of fingers and toes. This case of acrodynia was traced to exposure of mercury from a carton of 8-foot fluorescent light bulbs that had broken in a potting shed adjacent to the main nursery. The glass was cleaned up and discarded, but the child often used the area for play.

Assassination

Mercury has been used at various times to assassinate people. In 2008, Russian lawyer Karinna Moskalenko claimed to have been poisoned by mercury left in her car, while in 2010 journalists Viktor Kalashnikov and Marina Kalashnikova accused Russia's FSB of trying to poison them.

LEAD POISONING

Lead poisoning is a type of metal poisoning caused by lead in the body. The brain is the most sensitive. Symptoms may include abdominal pain, constipation, headaches, irritability, memory problems, inability to have children, and tingling in the hands and feet. It causes almost 10% of intellectual disability of otherwise unknown cause and can result in behavioral problems. Some of the effects are permanent. In severe cases anemia, seizures, coma, or death may occur.

Exposure to lead can occur by contaminated air, water, dust, food, or consumer products. Children are at greater risk as they are more likely to put objects in their mouth such as those that contain lead paint and absorb a greater proportion of the lead that they eat. Exposure at work is a common cause of lead poisoning in adults with certain occupations at particular risk. Diagnosis is typically by measurement of the blood lead level.The Centers for Disease Control (US) has set the upper limit for blood lead for adults at 10 µg/dl (10 µg/100 g) and for children at 5 µg/dl.Elevated lead may also be detected by changes in red blood cells or dense lines in the bones of children as seen on X-ray.

Lead poisoning is preventable. This includes by individual efforts such as removing lead-containing items from the home, workplace efforts such as improved ventilation and monitoring, and nationwide policies such as laws that ban lead in products such as paint and gasoline, reduce allowable levels in water or soil, and provide for cleanup of contaminated soil. The major treatments are removal of the source of lead and the use of medications that bind lead so it can be eliminated from the body, known as chelation therapy. Chelation therapy in children is recommended when blood levels are greater than 40-45 ug/dl. Medications used include dimercaprol, edetate calcium disodium, and succimer.

In 2013, lead is believed to have resulted in 853,000 deaths. It occurs most commonly in the developing world. Those who are poor are at greater risk. Lead is believed to result in 0.6% of the world's disease burden. People have been mining and using lead for thousands of years. Descriptions of lead poisoning date to at least 2000 BC, while efforts to limit lead's use date back to at least the 1500s. Concerns for low levels of exposure begin in the 1970s with there being no safe threshold for lead exposure.

Classification

Classically, "lead poisoning" or "lead intoxication" has been defined as exposure to high levels of lead typically associated with severe health effects. Poisoning is a pattern of symptoms that occur with toxic effects from mid to high levels of exposure; toxicity is a wider spectrum of effects, including subclinical ones (those that do not cause symptoms).

However, professionals often use “lead poisoning” and “lead toxicity” interchangeably, and official sources do not always restrict the use of “lead poisoning” to refer only to symptomatic effects of lead.

The amount of lead in the blood and tissues, as well as the time course of exposure, determine toxicity. Lead poisoning may be acute (from intense exposure of short duration) or chronic (from repeat low-level exposure over a prolonged period), but the latter is much more common. Diagnosis and treatment of lead exposure are based on blood lead level (the amount of lead in the blood), measured in micrograms of lead per deciliter of blood (μg/dL). Urine lead levels may be used as well, though less commonly. In cases of chronic exposure lead often sequesters in the highest concentrations first in the bones, then in the kidneys. If a provider is performing a provocative excretion test, or “chelation challenge”, a measurement obtained from urine rather than blood is likely to provide a more accurate representation of total lead burden to a skilled interpreter.

The US Centers for Disease Control and Prevention and the World Health Organization state that a blood lead level of 10 μg/dL or above is a cause for concern; however, lead may impair development and have harmful health effects even at lower levels, and there is no known safe exposure level.Authorities such as the American Academy of Pediatrics define lead poisoning as blood lead levels higher than 10 μg/dL.

Lead forms a variety of compounds and exists in the environment in various forms. Features of poisoning differ depending on whether the agent is an organic compound (one that contains carbon), or an inorganic one. Organic lead poisoning is now very rare, because countries across the world have phased out the use of organic lead compounds as gasoline additives, but such compounds are still used in industrial settings. Organic lead compounds, which cross the skin and respiratory tract easily, affect the central nervous system predominantly.

Signs and Symptoms

Lead poisoning can cause a variety of symptoms and signs which vary depending on the individual and the duration of lead exposure. Symptoms are nonspecific and may be subtle, and someone with elevated lead levels may have no symptoms.Symptoms usually develop over weeks to months as lead builds up in the body during a chronic exposure, but acute symptoms from brief, intense exposures also occur. Symptoms from exposure to organic lead, which is probably more toxic than inorganic lead due to its lipid solubility, occur rapidly.Poisoning by organic lead compounds has symptoms predominantly in the central nervous system, such as insomnia, delirium, cognitive deficits, tremor, hallucinations, and convulsions.

Symptoms may be different in adults and children; the main symptoms in adults are headache, abdominal pain, memory loss, kidney failure, male reproductive problems, and weakness, pain, or tingling in the extremities.

Early symptoms of lead poisoning in adults are commonly nonspecific and include depression, loss of appetite, intermittent abdominal pain, nausea, diarrhea, constipation, and muscle pain. Other early signs in adults include malaise, fatigue, decreased libido, and problems with sleep. An unusual taste in the mouth and personality changes are also early signs.

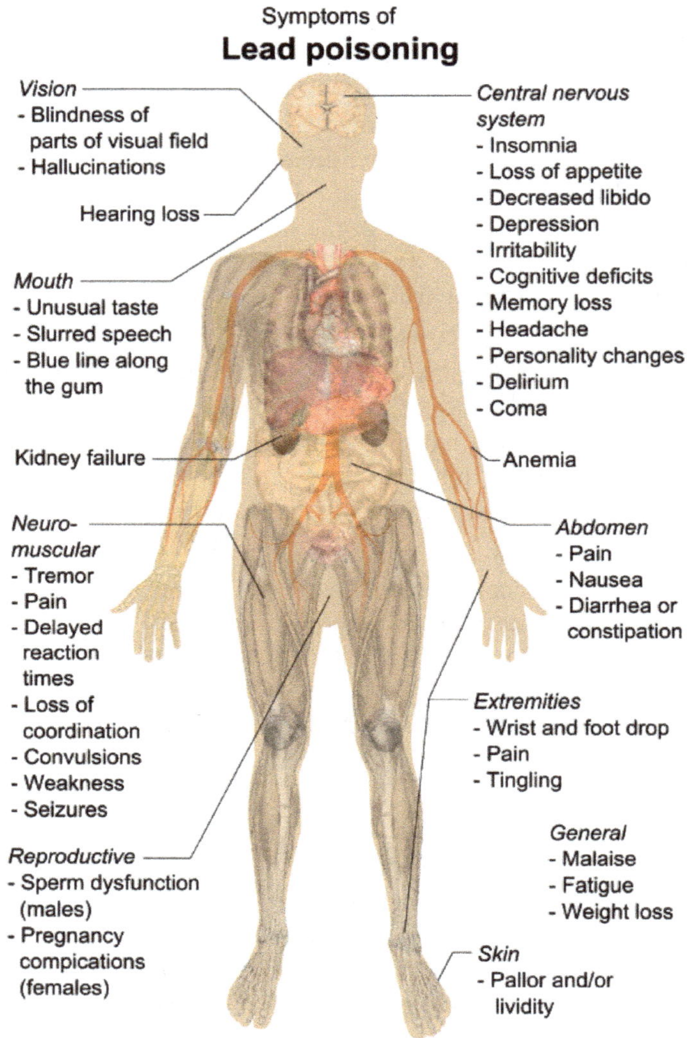

Symptoms of lead poisoning.

In adults, symptoms can occur at levels above 40 μg/dL, but are more likely to occur only above 50–60 μg/dL. Symptoms begin to appear in children generally at around 60 μg/dL. However, the lead levels at which symptoms appear vary widely depending on unknown characteristics of each individual. At blood lead levels between 25 and 60 μg/dL, neuropsychiatric effects such as delayed reaction times, irritability, and difficulty concentrating, as well as slowed motor nerve conduction and headache can occur. Anemia may appear at blood lead levels higher than 50 μg/dL. In adults, abdominal colic, involving paroxysms of pain, may appear at blood lead levels greater than 80 μg/dL.Signs that occur in adults at blood lead levels exceeding 100 μg/dL include wrist drop and foot drop, and signs of encephalopathy (a condition characterized by brain swelling), such as those that accompany increased pressure within the skull, delirium, coma, seizures, and headache. In children, signs of encephalopathy such as bizarre behavior, discoordination, and apathy occur at lead levels exceeding 70 μg/dL. For both adults and children, it is rare to be asymptomatic if blood lead levels exceed 100 μg/dL.

Acute Poisoning

In acute poisoning, typical neurological signs are pain, muscle weakness, numbness and tingling, and, rarely, symptoms associated with inflammation of the brain. Abdominal pain, nausea, vomiting, diarrhea, and constipation are other acute symptoms. Lead's effects on the mouth include astringency and a metallic taste. Gastrointestinal problems, such as constipation, diarrhea, poor appetite, or weight loss, are common in acute poisoning. Absorption of large amounts of lead over a short time can cause shock (insufficient fluid in the circulatory system) due to loss of water from the gastrointestinal tract. Hemolysis (the rupture of red blood cells) due to acute poisoning can cause anemia and hemoglobin in the urine. Damage to kidneys can cause changes in urination such as decreased urine output. People who survive acute poisoning often go on to display symptoms of chronic poisoning.

Chronic Poisoning

Chronic poisoning usually presents with symptoms affecting multiple systems, but is associated with three main types of symptoms: gastrointestinal, neuromuscular, and neurological. Central nervous system and neuromuscular symptoms usually result from intense exposure, while gastrointestinal symptoms usually result from exposure over longer periods. Signs of chronic exposure include loss of short-term memory or concentration, depression, nausea, abdominal pain, loss of coordination, and numbness and tingling in the extremities. Fatigue, problems with sleep, headaches, stupor, slurred speech, and anemia are also found in chronic lead poisoning. A "lead hue" of the skin with pallor and/or lividity is another feature. A blue line along the gum with bluish black edging to the teeth, known as a Burton line, is another indication of chronic lead poisoning. Children with chronic poisoning may refuse to play or may have hyperkinetic or aggressive behavior disorders. Visual disturbance may present with gradually progressing blurred vision as a result of central scotoma, caused by toxic optic neuritis.

Effects on Children

A fetus developing in the womb of a woman who has elevated blood lead level is susceptible to lead poisoning by intrauterine exposure, and is at greater risk of being born prematurely or with a low birth weight.

Children are more at risk for lead poisoning because their smaller bodies are in a continuous state of growth and development. Lead is absorbed at a faster rate compared to adults, which causes more physical harm than to older people. Furthermore, children, especially as they are learning to crawl and walk, are constantly on the floor and therefore more prone to ingesting and inhaling dust that is contaminated with lead.

The classic signs and symptoms in children are loss of appetite, abdominal pain, vomiting, weight loss, constipation, anemia, kidney failure, irritability, lethargy, learning disabilities, and behavioral problems.Slow development of normal childhood behaviors, such as talking and use of words, and permanent intellectual disability are both commonly seen. Although less common, it is possible for fingernails to develop leukonychia striata if exposed to abnormally high lead concentrations.

Complications

Lead affects every one of the body's organ systems, especially the nervous system, but also the bones and teeth, the kidneys, and the cardiovascular, immune, and reproductive systems. Hearing loss and tooth decay have been linked to lead exposure, as have cataracts. Intrauterine and neonatal lead exposure promote tooth decay. Aside from the developmental effects unique to young children, the health effects experienced by adults are similar to those in children, although the thresholds are generally higher.

Kidneys

Kidney damage occurs with exposure to high levels of lead, and evidence suggests that lower levels can damage kidneys as well. The toxic effect of lead causes nephropathy and may cause Fanconi syndrome, in which the proximal tubular function of the kidney is impaired. Long-term exposure at levels lower than those that cause lead nephropathy have also been reported as nephrotoxic in patients from developed countries that had chronic kidney disease or were at risk because of hypertension or diabetes mellitus. Lead poisoning inhibits excretion of the waste product urate and causes a predisposition for gout, in which urate builds up. This condition is known as *saturnine gout*.

Cardiovascular System

Evidence suggests lead exposure is associated with high blood pressure, and studies have also found connections between lead exposure and coronary heart disease, heart rate variability, and death from stroke, but this evidence is more limited. People who have been exposed to higher concentrations of lead may be at a higher risk for cardiac autonomic dysfunction on days when ozone and fine particles are higher.

Reproductive System

Lead affects both the male and female reproductive systems. In men, when blood lead levels exceed 40 μg/dL, sperm count is reduced and changes occur in volume of sperm, their motility, and their morphology. A pregnant woman's elevated blood lead level can lead to miscarriage, prematurity, low birth weight, and problems with development during childhood. Lead is able to pass through the placenta and into breast milk, and blood lead levels in mothers and infants are usually similar. A fetus may be poisoned *in utero* if lead from the mother's bones is subsequently mobilized by the changes in metabolism due to pregnancy; increased calcium intake in pregnancy may help mitigate this phenomenon.

Nervous System

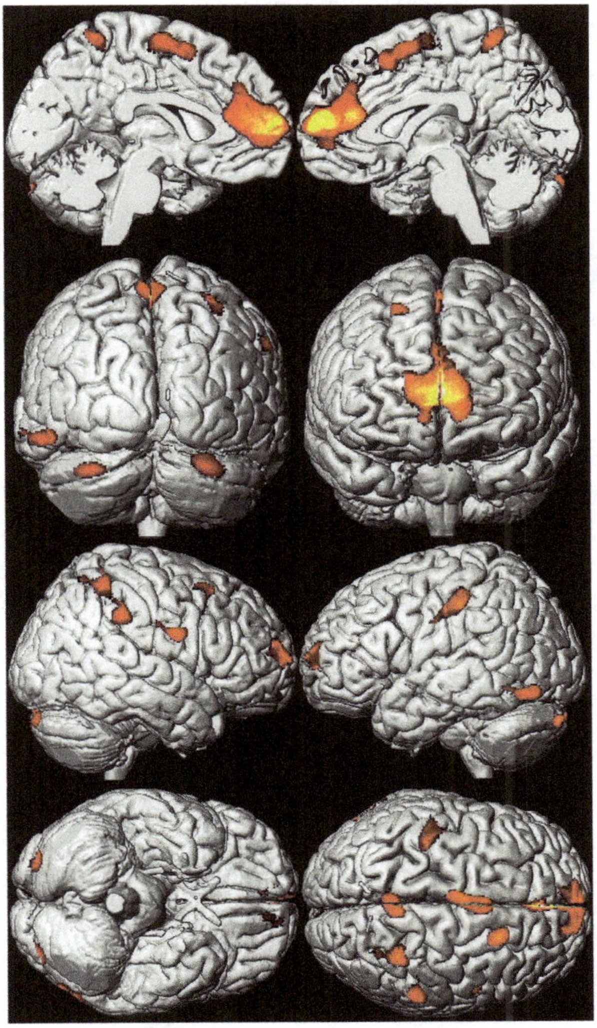

The brains of adults who were exposed to lead as children show decreased volume, especially in the prefrontal cortex, on MRI. Areas of volume loss are shown in color over a template of a normal brain.

Lead affects the peripheral nervous system (especially motor nerves) and the central nervous system. Peripheral nervous system effects are more prominent in adults and central nervous system effects are more prominent in children. Lead causes the axons of nerve cells to degenerate and lose their myelin coats.

Lead exposure in young children has been linked to learning disabilities, and children with blood lead concentrations greater than 10 μg/dL are in danger of developmental disabilities. Increased blood lead level in children has been correlated with decreases in intelligence, nonverbal reasoning, short-term memory, attention, reading and arithmetic ability, fine motor skills, emotional regulation, and social engagement.The effect of lead on children's cognitive abilities takes place at very low levels. There is apparently no lower threshold to the dose-response relationship (unlike other heavy metals such as mercury). Reduced academic performance has been associated with lead exposure even at blood lead levels lower than 5 μg/dL. Blood lead levels below 10 μg/dL have been reported to be associated with lower IQ and behavior problems such as aggression, in proportion with blood lead levels.Between the blood lead levels of 5 and 35 μg/dL, an IQ decrease of 2–4 points for each μg/dL increase is reported in children. However, studies that show associations between low-level lead exposure and health effects in children may be affected by confounding and overestimate the effects of low-level lead exposure.

High blood lead levels in adults are also associated with decreases in cognitive performance and with psychiatric symptoms such as depression and anxiety. It was found in a large group of current and former inorganic lead workers in Korea that blood lead levels in the range of 20–50 μg/dL were correlated with neuro-cognitive defects. Increases in blood lead levels from about 50 to about 100 μg/dL in adults have been found to be associated with persistent, and possibly permanent, impairment of central nervous system function.

Lead exposure in children is also correlated with neuropsychiatric disorders such as attention deficit hyperactivity disorder and anti-social behaviour. Elevated lead levels in children are correlated with higher scores on aggression and delinquency measures. A correlation has also been found between prenatal and early childhood lead exposure and violent crime in adulthood. Countries with the highest air lead levels have also been found to have the highest murder rates, after adjusting for confounding factors. A May 2000 study by economic consultant Rick Nevin theorizes that lead exposure explains 65% to 90% of the variation in violent crime rates in the US. A 2007 paper by the same author claims to show a strong association between preschool blood lead and subsequent crime rate trends over several decades across nine countries. It is believed that the U.S. ban on lead paint in buildings in the late 1970s, as well as the phaseout of leaded gasoline in the 1970s and 1980s, partially helped contribute to the decline of violent crime in the United States since the early 1990s.

Exposure Routes

Lead is a common environmental pollutant. Causes of environmental contamination include industrial use of lead, such as is found in facilities that process lead-acid batteries or produce lead wire or pipes, and metal recycling and foundries. Children living near facilities that process lead, such as lead smelters, have been found to have unusually high blood lead levels. In August 2009, parents rioted in China after lead poisoning was found in nearly 2000 children living near zinc and manganese smelters. Lead exposure can occur from contact with lead in air, household dust, soil, water, and commercial products.

Leaded gasoline has also been linked to increases in lead pollution.Some research has suggested a link between leaded gasoline and crime rates.

Occupational Exposure

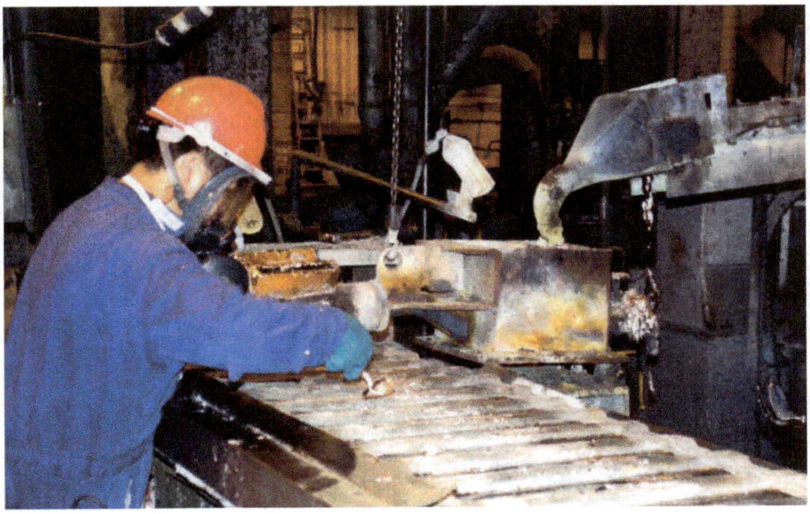

Battery recycling workers are at risk for lead exposure. This worker ladles molten lead into billets in a lead-acid battery recovery facility.

In adults, occupational exposure is the main cause of lead poisoning. People can be exposed when working in facilities that produce a variety of lead-containing products; these include radiation shields, ammunition, certain surgical equipment, developing dental x-ray films prior to digital x-rays (each film packet had a lead liner to prevent the radiation from going through), fetal monitors, plumbing, circuit boards, jet engines, and ceramic glazes. In addition, lead miners and smelters, plumbers and fitters, auto mechanics, glass manufacturers, construction workers, battery manufacturers and recyclers, firing range instructors, and plastic manufacturers are at risk for lead exposure. Other occupations that present lead exposure risks include welding, manufacture of rubber, printing, zinc and copper smelting, processing of ore, combustion of solid waste, and production of paints and pigments. Parents who are exposed to lead in the workplace can bring lead dust home on clothes or skin and expose their children.

Food

Lead may be found in food when food is grown in soil that is high in lead, airborne lead contaminates the crops, animals eat lead in their diet, or lead enters the food either from what it was stored or cooked in.

Paint

Some lead compounds are colorful and are used widely in paints, and lead paint is a major route of lead exposure in children. A study conducted in 1998–2000 found that 38 million housing units in the US had lead-based paint, down from a 1990 estimate of 64 million. Deteriorating lead paint can produce dangerous lead levels in household dust and soil. Deteriorating lead paint and lead-containing household dust are the main causes of chronic lead poisoning. The lead breaks down into the dust and since children are more prone to crawling on the floor, it is easily ingested. Many young children display pica, eating things that are not food. Even a small amount of a lead-containing product such as a paint chip or a sip of glaze can contain tens or hundreds of milligrams of lead. Eating chips of lead paint presents a particular hazard to children, generally producing more severe poisoning than occurs from dust. Because removing lead paint from dwellings, e.g. by sanding or torching creates lead-containing dust and fumes, it is generally safer to seal the lead paint under new paint (excepting moveable windows and doors, which create paint dust when operated). Alternately, special precautions must be taken if the lead paint is to be removed. In oil painting it was once common for colours such as yellow or white to be made with lead carbonate. Lead white oil colour was the main white of oil painters until superseded by compounds containing zinc or titanium in the mid-20th century. It is speculated that the painter Caravaggio and possibly Francisco Goya and Vincent Van Gogh had lead poisoning due to overexposure or carelessness when handling this colour.

Soil

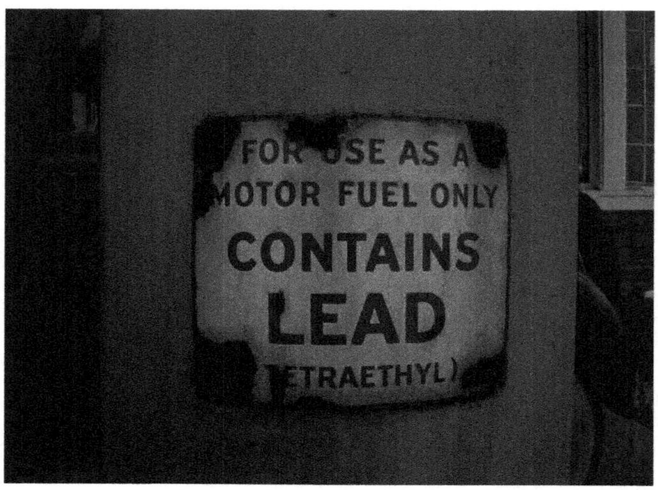

A lead warning on a fuel pump. Tetraethyllead, which used to be added to automotive gasoline (and still is added to some aviation gasolines), contributed to soil contamination.

Residual lead in soil contributes to lead exposure in urban areas. It has been thought that the more polluted an area is with various contaminants, the more likely it is to contain lead. However, this is not always the case, as there are several other reasons for lead contamination in soil. Lead content in soil may be caused by broken-down lead paint, residues from lead-containing gasoline, used engine oil, or pesticides used in the past, contaminated landfills, or from nearby industries such as foundries or smelters. Although leaded soil is less of a problem in countries that no longer have leaded gasoline, it remains prevalent, raising concerns about the safety of urban agriculture; eating food grown in contaminated soil can present a lead hazard.

Water

Lead from the atmosphere or soil can end up in groundwater and surface water. It is also potentially in drinking water, e.g. from plumbing and fixtures that are either made of lead or have lead solder.Since acidic water breaks down lead in plumbing more readily, chemicals can be added to municipal water to increase the pH and thus reduce the corrosivity of the public water supply. Chloramines, which were adopted as a substitute for chlorine disinfectants due to fewer health concerns, increase corrositivity. In the US, 14–20% of total lead exposure is attributed to drinking water. In 2004, a team of seven reporters from *The Washington Post* discovered high levels of lead in the drinking water in Washington, D.C. and won an award for investigative reporting for a series of articles about this contamination. In the Flint water crisis, a switch to a more corrosive municipal water source elevated lead levels in drinking water in domestic tap water.

In Australia, collecting rainwater from roof runoff used as potable water may contain lead if there are lead contaminants on the roof or in the storage tank. The Australian Drinking Water Guidelines allow a maximum of .01 mg/L lead in water.

Lead-Containing Products

Lead can be found in products such as kohl, an ancient cosmetic from the Middle East, South Asia, and parts of Africa that has many names; and from some toys. In 2007, millions of toys made in China were recalled from multiple countries owing to safety hazards including lead paint. Vinyl mini-blinds, found especially in older housing, may contain lead. Lead is commonly incorporated into herbal remedies such as Indian Ayurvedic preparations and remedies of Chinese origin. There are also risks of elevated blood lead levels caused by folk remedies like *azarcon* and *greta*, which each contain about 95% lead.

Ingestion of metallic lead, such as small lead fishing lures, increases blood lead levels and can be fatal. Ingestion of lead-contaminated food is also a threat. Ceramic glaze often contains lead, and dishes that have been improperly fired can leach the metal into food, potentially causing severe poisoning. In some places, the solder in cans used for food contains lead. When manufacturing medical instruments and hardware, solder containing lead may be present. People who eat animals hunted with lead bullets may be at risk for lead exposure. Bullets lodged in the body rarely cause significant levels of lead, but bullets lodged in the joints are the exception, as they deteriorate and release lead into the body over time.

In May 2015, Indian food safety regulators in the state of Uttar Pradesh found that samples of Maggi 2 Minute Noodles contained lead up to 17 times beyond permissible limits. On 3 June 2015, New Delhi Government banned the sale of Maggi noodles in New Delhi stores for 15 days because it was found to contain lead beyond the permissible limit. The Gujarat FDA on June 4, 2015 banned the noodles for 30 days after 27 out of 39 samples were detected with objectionable levels of metallic lead, among other things. Some India's biggest retailers like Future Group, Big Bazaar, Easyday and Nilgiris have imposed a nationwide ban on Maggi noodles. Many other states too have banned Maggi noodles.

Bullets

Contact with ammunition is a source of lead exposure. As of 2013, lead-based ammunition production is the second largest annual use of lead in the US, accounting for over 60,000 metric tons consumed in 2012, second only to the manufacture of storage batteries. The Environmental Protection Agency (EPA) does not regulate lead, as a matter of law. Lead birdshot is banned in some areas, but this is primarily for the benefit of the birds and their predators, rather than humans. Non-lead alternatives include steel, tungsten-nickel-iron, bismuth-tin, and tungsten-polymer.

Because game animals can be shot using lead bullets, the potential for lead ingestion from game meat consumption has been studied clinically and epidemiologically. In a recent study conducted by the CDC, a cohort from North Dakota was enrolled and asked to self-report historical consumption of game meat, and participation in other activities that could cause lead exposure. The study found that participants' age, sex, housing age, current hobbies with potential for lead exposure, and game consumption were all associated with blood lead level (PbB).

This study has been cited by popular media as simple evidence that hunting increases exposure to lead poisoning, prompting the University of Illinois Extension to release a statement that there is no such risk. Concerning the CDC report, the authors' conclusion in a related Epi-AID Trip Report notes the small increase associated with game consumption in the study, and urges interpretation with respect to environmental context:

While this study suggests that consumption of wild game meat can adversely affect PbB, no participant had PbB higher than the CDC recommended threshold of 10μg/dl—the level at which CDC recommends case management; and the geometric mean PbB among this study population (1.17μg/dl) was lower than the overall population geometric mean PbB in the United States (1.60 μg/dl). The clinical significance of low PbB in this sample population and the small quantitative increase of 0.30μg/dl in PbB associated with wild game consumption should be interpreted in the context of naturally occurring PbB.

Copper-jacketed, lead-based bullets are more economical to produce and use than lead or any other material. Alternative materials are available such as steel, copper, and tungsten, but alternatives are universally less effective and/or more expensive. However, the biggest impediment to using the vast majority of alternatives relates to current laws in the United States pertaining to armor-piercing rounds. Laws and regulations relating to armor-piercing ammunition expressly prohibit the use of brass, bronze, steel, tungsten, and nearly every metallic alternative in any bullet that can be shot by a handgun, which at this time is nearly every caliber smaller than 50BMG (including the popular .223 Remington, .308 Winchester and .30-06 to name just a few). Some lead-based bullets are resistant to fragmentation, offering hunters the ability to clean game animals with negligible risk of including lead fragments in prepared meat. Other bullets are prone to fragmentation and exacerbate the risk of lead ingestion from prepared meat. In practice, use of a non-fragmenting bullet and proper cleaning of the game animal's wound can eliminate the risk of lead ingestion from eating game; however, isolating such practice to experimentally determine its association with blood lead levels in study is difficult. Bismuth is an element used as a lead-replacement for shotgun pellets used in waterfowl hunting although shotshells made from bismuth are nearly ten times the cost of lead.

Pathophysiology

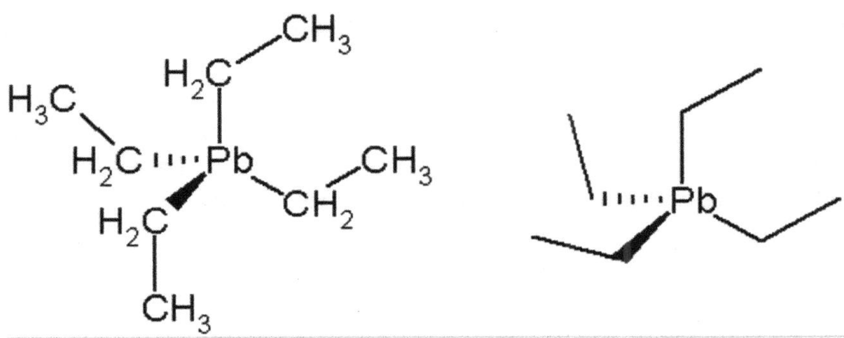

Tetraethyllead, still used as an additive in some fuels, can be absorbed through the skin.

Exposure occurs through inhalation, ingestion or occasionally skin contact. Lead may be taken in through direct contact with mouth, nose, and eyes (mucous membranes), and through breaks in the skin. Tetraethyllead, which was a gasoline additive and is still used in fuels such as aviation fuel, passes through the skin; however inorganic lead found in paint, food, and most lead-containing consumer products is only minimally absorbed through the skin. The main sources of absorption of inorganic lead are from ingestion and inhalation. In adults, about 35–40% of inhaled lead dust is deposited in the lungs, and about 95% of that goes into the bloodstream.Of ingested inorganic lead, about 15% is absorbed, but this percentage is higher in children, pregnant women, and people with deficiencies of calcium, zinc, or iron. Infants may absorb about 50% of ingested lead, but little is known about absorption rates in children.

The main body compartments that store lead are the blood, soft tissues, and bone; the half-life of lead in these tissues is measured in weeks for blood, months for soft tissues, and years for bone. Lead in the bones, teeth, hair, and nails is bound tightly and not available to other tissues, and is generally thought not to be harmful. In adults, 94% of absorbed lead is deposited in the bones and teeth, but children only store 70% in this manner, a fact which may partially account for the more serious health effects on children. The estimated half-life of lead in bone is 20 to 30 years, and bone can introduce lead into the bloodstream long after the initial exposure is gone. The half-life of lead in the blood in men is about 40 days, but it may be longer in children and pregnant women, whose bones are undergoing remodeling, which allows the lead to be continuously re-introduced into the bloodstream. Also, if lead exposure takes place over years, clearance is much slower, partly due to the re-release of lead from bone. Many other tissues store lead, but those with the highest concentrations (other than blood, bone, and teeth) are the brain, spleen, kidneys, liver, and lungs. Lead is removed from the body very slowly, mainly through urine. Smaller amounts of lead are also eliminated through the feces, and very small amounts in hair, nails, and sweat.

Lead has no known physiologically relevant role in the body, and its harmful effects are myriad. Lead and other heavy metals create reactive radicals which damage cell structures including DNA and cell membranes. Lead also interferes with DNA transcription, enzymes that help in the synthesis of vitamin D, and enzymes that maintain the integrity of the cell membrane. Anemia may result when the cell membranes of red blood cells become more fragile as the result of damage to their membranes.Lead interferes with metabolism of bones and teeth and alters the permeability of blood vessels and collagen synthesis. Lead may also be harmful to the developing immune system, causing production of excessive inflammatory proteins; this mechanism may mean that lead exposure is a risk factor for asthma in children. Lead exposure has also been associated with a decrease in activity of immune cells such as polymorphonuclear leukocytes. Lead also interferes with the normal metabolism of calcium in cells and causes it to build up within them.

Enzymes

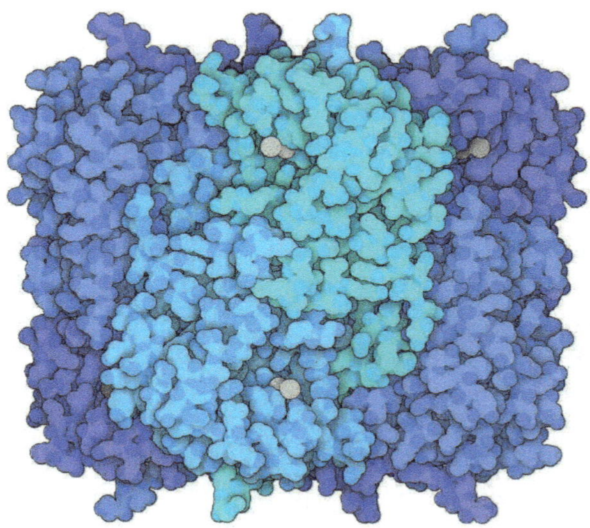

ALAD enzyme with lead bound (PDB: 1QNV).

The primary cause of lead's toxicity is its interference with a variety of enzymes because it binds to sulfhydryl groups found on many enzymes. Part of lead's toxicity results from its ability to mimic other metals that take part in biological processes, which act as cofactors in many enzymatic reactions, displacing them at the enzymes on which they act. Lead is able to bind to and interact with many of the same enzymes as these metals but, due to its differing chemistry, does not properly function as a cofactor, thus interfering with the enzyme's ability to catalyze its normal reaction or reactions. Among the essential metals with which lead interacts are calcium, iron, and zinc.

The lead ion has a lone pair in its electronic structure, which can result in a distortion in the coordination of ligands, and in 2007 was hypothesized to be important in lead poisoning's effects on enzymes (see Lone pair § Unusual lone pairs).

One of the main causes for the pathology of lead is that it interferes with the activity of an essential enzyme called delta-aminolevulinic acid dehydratase, or ALAD (see image of the enzyme structure), which is important in the biosynthesis of heme, the cofactor found in hemoglobin. Lead also inhibits the enzyme ferrochelatase, another enzyme involved in the formation of heme. Ferrochelatase catalyzes the joining of protoporphyrin and Fe^{2+} to form heme. Lead's interference with heme synthesis results in production of zinc protoporphyrin and the development of anemia. Another effect of lead's interference with heme synthesis is the buildup of heme precursors, such as aminolevulinic acid, which may be directly or indirectly harmful to neurons.

Neurons

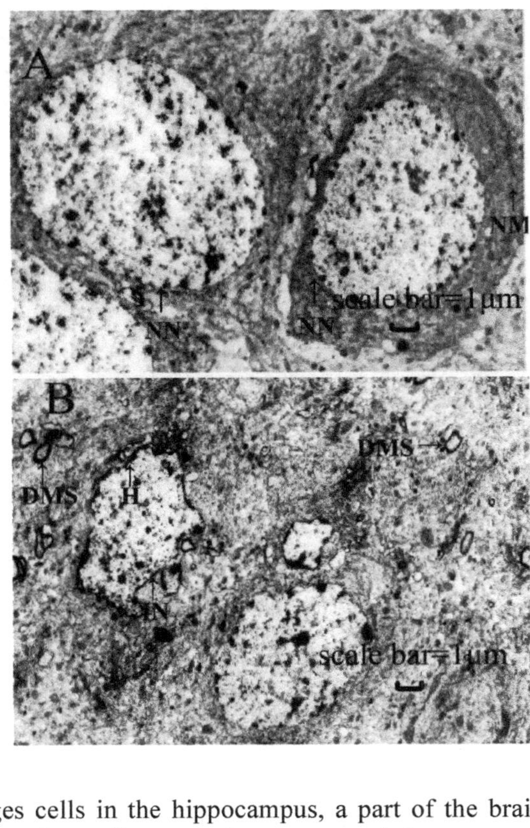

Lead exposure damages cells in the hippocampus, a part of the brain involved in memory. Hippocampi of lead-exposed rats (bottom) show structural damage such as irregular nuclei (IN) and denaturation of myelin (DNS) compared to controls (top).

The brain is the organ most sensitive to lead exposure. Lead is able to pass through the endothelial cells at the blood brain barrier because it can substitute for calcium ions and be uptaken by calcium-ATPase pumps. Lead poisoning interferes with the normal development of a child's brain and nervous system; therefore children are at greater risk of lead neurotoxicity than adults are. In a child's developing brain, lead interferes with synapse formation in the cerebral cortex, neurochemical development (including that of neurotransmitters), and organization of ion channels. It causes loss of neurons' myelin sheaths, reduces numbers of neurons, interferes with neurotransmission, and decreases neuronal growth.

Lead interferes with the release of neurotransmitters, chemicals used by neurons to send signals to other cells. It interferes with the release of glutamate, a neurotransmitter important in many functions including learning, by blocking NMDA receptors. The targeting of NMDA receptors is thought to be one of the main causes for lead's toxicity to neurons. A Johns Hopkins University report found that in addition to inhibiting the NMDA receptor, lead exposure decreased the level of expression of the gene for the receptor in part of the brain. In addition, lead has been found in animal studies to cause programmed cell death in brain cells.

Diagnosis

Diagnosis includes determining the clinical signs and the medical history, with inquiry into possible routes of exposure. Clinical toxicologists, medical specialists in the area of poisoning, may be involved in diagnosis and treatment. The main tool in diagnosing and assessing the severity of lead poisoning is laboratory analysis of the blood lead level (BLL).

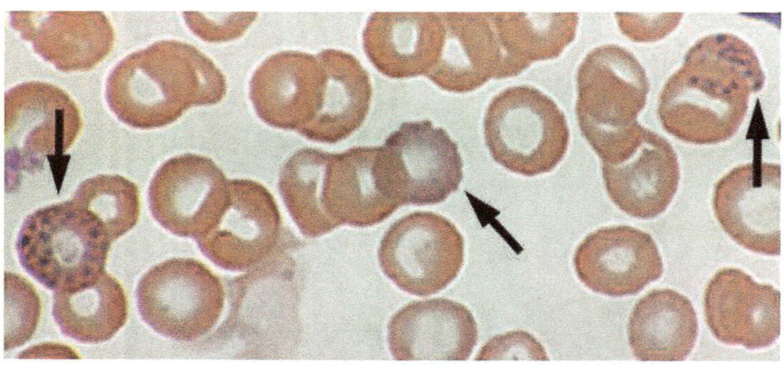

Basophilic stippling (arrows) of red blood cells in a 53-year-old who had elevated blood lead levels due to drinking repeatedly from glasses decorated with lead paint.

Blood film examination may reveal basophilic stippling of red blood cells (dots in red blood cells visible through a microscope), as well as the changes normally associated with iron-deficiency anemia (microcytosis and hypochromasia). However, basophilic stippling is also seen in unrelated conditions, such as megaloblastic anemia caused by vitamin B12 (colbalamin) and folate deficiencies.

Exposure to lead also can be evaluated by measuring erythrocyte protoporphyrin (EP) in blood samples. EP is a part of red blood cells known to increase when the amount of lead in the blood is high, with a delay of a few weeks. Thus EP levels in conjunction with blood lead levels can suggest the time period of exposure; if blood lead levels are high but EP is still normal, this finding suggests exposure was recent. However, the EP level alone is not sensitive enough to identify elevated blood lead levels below about 35 μg/dL. Due to this higher threshold for detection and the fact that EP levels also increase in iron deficiency, use of this method for detecting lead exposure has decreased.

Blood lead levels are an indicator mainly of recent or current lead exposure, not of total body burden.Lead in bones can be measured noninvasively by X-ray fluorescence; this may be the best measure of cumulative exposure and total body burden. However this method is not widely available and is mainly used for research rather than routine diagnosis. Another radiographic sign of elevated lead levels is the presence of radiodense lines called lead lines at the metaphysis in the long bones of growing children, especially around the knees. These lead lines, caused by increased calcification due to disrupted metabolism in the growing bones, become wider as the duration of lead exposure increases. X-rays may also reveal lead-containing foreign materials such as paint chips in the gastrointestinal tract.

Fecal lead content that is measured over the course of a few days may also be an accurate way to estimate the overall amount of childhood lead intake. This form of measurement may serve as a useful way to see the extent of oral lead exposure from all the diet and environmental sources of lead.

Lead poisoning shares symptoms with other conditions and may be easily missed. Conditions that present similarly and must be ruled out in diagnosing lead poisoning include carpal tunnel syndrome, Guillain–Barré syndrome, renal colic, appendicitis, encephalitis in adults, and viral gastroenteritis in children. Other differential diagnoses in children include constipation, abdominal colic, iron deficiency, subdural hematoma, neoplasms of the central nervous system, emotional and behavior disorders, and intellectual disability.

Reference Levels

The current reference range for acceptable blood lead concentrations in healthy persons without excessive exposure to environmental sources of lead is less than 5 μg/dL for children. It was less than 25 μg/dL for adults. Previous to 2012 the value for children was 10 (μg/dl). The current biological exposure index (a level that should not be exceeded) for lead-exposed workers in the U.S. is 30 μg/dL in a random blood specimen.

The National Institute for Occupational Safety and Health (CDC/NIOSH) reference blood lead level in adults is 10 μg/dL The U.S. national BLL geometric mean among adults was 1.2 μg/dL in 2009–2010.

Blood lead concentrations in poisoning victims have ranged from 30->80 μg/dL in children exposed to lead paint in older houses, 77–104 μg/dL in persons working with pottery glazes, 90–137 μg/dL in individuals consuming contaminated herbal medicines, 109–139 μg/dL in indoor shooting range instructors and as high as 330 μg/dL in those drinking fruit juices from glazed earthenware containers.

Prevention

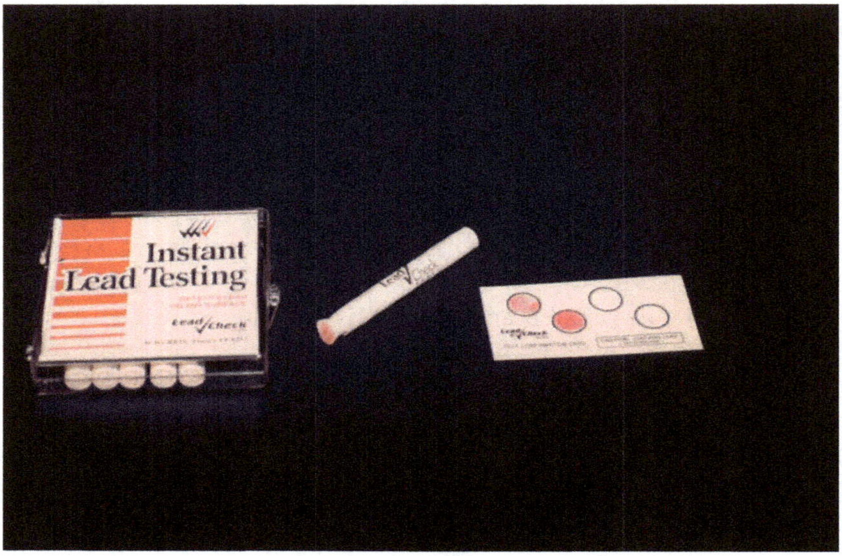

Testing kits are commercially available for detecting lead. These swabs, when wiped on a surface, turn red in the presence of lead.

In most cases, lead poisoning is preventable by avoiding exposure to lead. Prevention strategies can be divided into individual (measures taken by a family), preventive medicine (identifying and intervening with high-risk individuals), and public health (reducing risk on a population level).

Recommended steps by individuals to reduce the blood lead levels of children include increasing their frequency of hand washing and their intake of calcium and iron, discouraging them from putting their hands to their mouths, vacuuming frequently, and eliminating the presence of lead-containing objects such as blinds and jewellery in the house. In houses with lead pipes or plumbing solder, these can be replaced. Less permanent but cheaper methods include running water in the morning to flush out the most contaminated water, or adjusting the water's chemistry to prevent corrosion of pipes. Lead testing kits are commercially available for detecting the presence of lead in the household. As hot water is more likely than cold water to contain higher amounts of lead, use only cold water from the tap for drinking, cooking, and for making baby formula. Since most of the lead in household water usually comes from plumbing in the house and not from the local water supply, using cold water can avoid lead exposure. Measures such as dust control and household education do not appear to be effective in changing children's blood levels.

Screening is an important method in preventive medicine strategies. Screening programs exist to test the blood of children at high risk for lead exposure, such as those who live near lead-related industries.

Prevention measures also exist on national and municipal levels. Recommendations by health professionals for lowering childhood exposures include banning the use of lead where it is not essential and strengthening regulations that limit the amount of lead in soil, water, air, household dust, and products. Regulations exist to limit the amount of lead in paint; for example, a 1978 law in the US restricted the lead in paint for residences, furniture, and toys to 0.06% or less. In October 2008, the US Environmental Protection Agency reduced the allowable lead level by a factor of ten to 0.15 micrograms per cubic meter of air, giving states five years to comply with the standards. The European Union's Restriction of Hazardous Substances Directive limits amounts of lead and other toxic substances in electronics and electrical equipment. In some places, remediation programs exist to reduce the presence of lead when it is found to be high, for example in drinking water. As a more radical solution, entire towns located near former lead mines have been "closed" by the government, and the population resettled elsewhere, as was the case with Picher, Oklahoma in 2009.

Treatment

CDC management guidelines for children with elevated blood levels	
Blood lead level (μg/dL)	**Treatment**
10–14	Education, repeat screening
15–19	Repeat screening, case management to abate sources
20–44	Medical evaluation, case management
45–69	Medical evaluation, chelation, case management
>69	Hospitalization, immediate chelation, case management

The mainstays of treatment are removal from the source of lead and, for people who have significantly high blood lead levels or who have symptoms of poisoning, chelation therapy. Treatment of iron, calcium, and zinc deficiencies, which are associated with increased lead absorption, is another part of treatment for lead poisoning. When lead-containing materials are present in the gastrointestinal tract (as evidenced by abdominal X-rays), whole bowel irrigation, cathartics, endoscopy, or even surgical removal may be used to eliminate it from the gut and prevent further exposure. Lead-containing bullets and shrapnel may also present a threat of further exposure and may need to be surgically removed if they are in or near fluid-filled or synovial spaces. If lead encephalopathy is present, anticonvulsants may be given to control seizures, and treatments to control swelling of the brain include corticosteroids and mannitol. Treatment of organic lead poisoning involves removing the lead compound from the skin, preventing further exposure, treating seizures, and possibly chelation therapy for people with high blood lead concentrations.

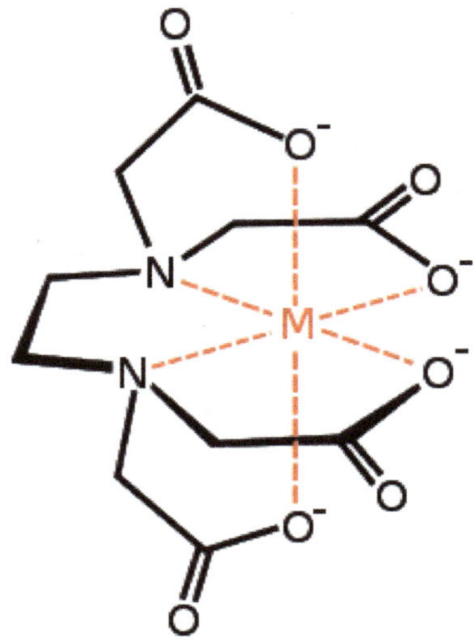

EDTA, a chelating agent, binds a heavy metal, sequestering it.

A chelating agent is a molecule with at least two negatively charged groups that allow it to form complexes with metal ions with multiple positive charges, such as lead. The chelate that is thus formed is nontoxic and can be excreted in the urine, initially at up to 50 times the normal rate. The chelating agents used for treatment of lead poisoning are edetate disodium calcium ($CaNa_2EDTA$), dimercaprol (BAL), which are injected, and succimer and d-penicillamine, which are administered orally. Chelation therapy is used in cases of acute lead poisoning, severe poisoning, and encephalopathy, and is considered for people with blood lead levels above 25 μg/dL. While the use of chelation for people with symptoms of lead poisoning is widely supported, use in asymptomatic people with high blood lead levels is more controversial. Chelation therapy is of limited value for cases of chronic exposure to low levels of lead. Chelation therapy is usually stopped when symptoms resolve or when blood lead levels return to premorbid levels. When lead exposure has taken place over a long period, blood lead levels may rise after chelation is stopped because lead is leached into blood from stores in the bone; thus repeated treatments are often necessary.

People receiving dimercaprol need to be assessed for peanut allergies since the commercial formulation contains peanut oil. Calcium EDTA is also effective if administered four hours after the administration of dimercaprol. Administering dimercaprol, DMSA (Succimer), or DMPS prior to calcium EDTA is necessary to prevent the redistribution of lead into the central nervous system. Dimercaprol used alone may also redistribute lead to the brain and testes. An adverse side effect of calcium EDTA is renal toxicity. Succimer (DMSA) is the preferred agent in mild to moderate lead poisoning cases. This may be the case in instances where children have a blood lead level >25μg/dL. The most reported adverse side effect for succimer is gastrointestinal disturbances. It is also important to note that chelation therapy only lowers blood lead levels and may not prevent the lead-induced cognitive problems associated with lower lead levels in tissue. This may be because of the inability of these agents to remove sufficient amounts of lead from tissue or inability to reverse preexisting damage. Chelating agents can have adverse effects; for example, chelation therapy can lower the body's levels of necessary nutrients like zinc. Chelating agents taken orally can increase the body's absorption of lead through the intestine.

Chelation challenge, also known as provocation testing, is used to indicate an elevated and mobilizable body burden of heavy metals including lead. This testing involves collecting urine before and after administering a one-off dose of chelating agent to mobilize heavy metals into the urine. Then urine is analyzed by a laboratory for levels of heavy metals; from this analysis overall body burden is inferred. Chelation challenge mainly measures the burden of lead in soft tissues, though whether it accurately reflects long-term exposure or the amount of lead stored in bone remains controversial. Although the technique has been used to determine whether chelation therapy is indicated and to diagnose heavy metal exposure, some evidence does not support these uses as blood levels after chelation are not comparable to the reference range typically used to diagnose heavy metal poisoning. The single chelation dose could also redistribute the heavy metals to more sensitive areas such as central nervous system tissue.

Epidemiology

Since lead has been used widely for centuries, the effects of exposure are worldwide. Environmental lead is ubiquitous, and everyone has some measurable blood lead level. Atmospheric lead pollution increased dramatically beginning in the 1950s as a result of the widespread use of leaded gasoline. Lead is one of the largest environmental medicine problems in terms of numbers of people exposed and the public health toll it takes. Lead exposure accounts for about 0.2% of all deaths and 0.6% of disability adjusted life years globally.

Although regulation reducing lead in products has greatly reduced exposure in the developed world since the 1970s, lead is still allowed in products in many developing countries. In all countries that have banned leaded gasoline, average blood lead levels have fallen sharply. However, some developing countries still allow leaded gasoline, which is the primary source of lead exposure in most developing countries. Beyond exposure from gasoline, the frequent use of pesticides in developing countries adds a risk of lead exposure and subsequent poisoning. Poor children in developing countries are at especially high risk for lead poisoning. Of North American children, 7% have blood lead levels above 10 μg/dL, whereas among Central and South American children, the percentage is 33 to 34%. About one fifth of the world's disease burden from lead poisoning occurs in the Western Pacific, and another fifth is in Southeast Asia.

In developed countries, people with low levels of education living in poorer areas are most at risk for elevated lead. In the US, the groups most at risk for lead exposure are the impoverished, city-dwellers, and immigrants. African-American children and those living in old housing have also been found to be at elevated risk for high blood lead levels in the US. Low-income people often live in old housing with lead paint, which may begin to peel, exposing residents to high levels of lead-containing dust.

Risk factors for elevated lead exposure include alcohol consumption and smoking (possibly because of contamination of tobacco leaves with lead-containing pesticides). Adults with certain risk factors might be more susceptible to toxicity; these include calcium and iron deficiencies, old age, disease of organs targeted by lead (e.g. the brain, the kidneys), and possibly genetic susceptibility. Differences in vulnerability to lead-induced neurological damage between males and females have also been found, but some studies have found males to be at greater risk, while others have found females to be.

In adults, blood lead levels steadily increase with increasing age. In adults of all ages, men have higher blood lead levels than women do. Children are more sensitive to elevated blood lead levels than adults are. Children may also have a higher intake of lead than adults; they breathe faster and may be more likely to have contact with and ingest soil. Children of ages one to three tend to have the highest blood lead levels, possibly because at that age they begin to walk and explore their environment, and they use their mouths in their exploration. Blood levels usually peak at about 18–24 months old. In many countries including the US, household paint and dust are the major route of exposure in children.

Notable Cases

Cases of mass lead poisoning can occur, primarily in underdeveloped countries.

15,000 people are being relocated from Jiyuan in central Henan province to other locations after 1000 children living around China's largest smelter plant (owned and operated by Yuguang Gold and Lead) were found to have excess lead in their blood. The total cost of this project is estimated to around 1 billion yuan ($150 million). 70% of the cost will be paid by local government and the smelter company, while the rest will be paid by the residents themselves. The government has suspended production at 32 of 35 lead plants. The affected area includes people from 10 different villages.

The Zamfara State lead poisoning epidemic occurred in Nigeria in 2010. As of October 5, 2010 at least 400 children have died from the effects of lead poisoning.

Prognosis

Reversibility

Outcome is related to the extent and duration of lead exposure. Effects of lead on the physiology of the kidneys and blood are generally reversible; its effects on the central nervous system are not. While peripheral effects in adults often go away when lead exposure ceases, evidence suggests that most of lead's effects on a child's central nervous system are irreversible. Children with lead poisoning may thus have adverse health, cognitive, and behavioral effects that follow them into adulthood.

Encephalopathy

Lead encephalopathy is a medical emergency and causes permanent brain damage in 70–80% of children affected by it, even those that receive the best treatment. The mortality rate for people who develop cerebral involvement is about 25%, and of those who survive who had lead encephalopathy symptoms by the time chelation therapy was begun, about 40% have permanent neurological problems such as cerebral palsy.

Long-term

Exposure to lead may also decrease lifespan and have health effects in the long term. Death rates from a variety of causes have been found to be higher in people with elevated blood lead levels; these include cancer, stroke, and heart disease, and general death rates from all causes. Lead is considered a possible human carcinogen based on evidence from animal studies. Evidence also suggests that age-related mental decline and psychiatric symptoms are correlated with lead exposure. Cumulative exposure over a prolonged period may have a more important effect on some aspects of health than recent exposure. Some health effects, such as high blood pressure, are only significant risks when lead exposure is prolonged (over about one year).

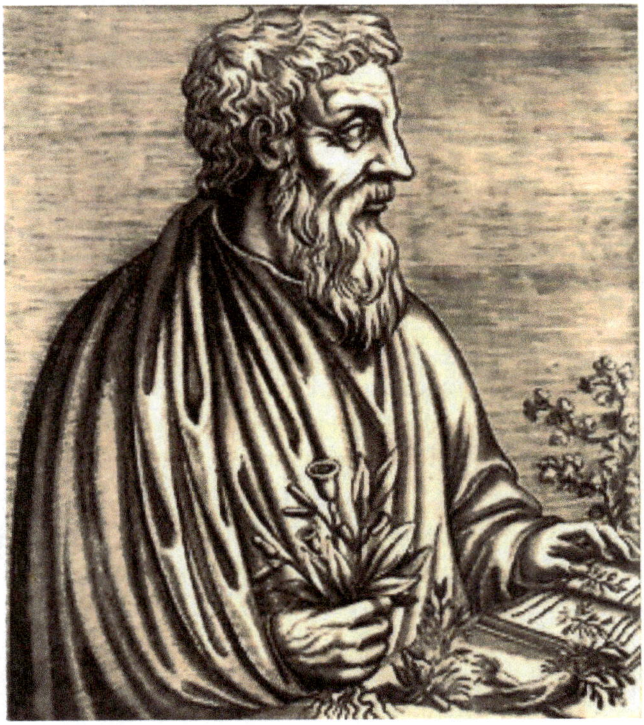

Dioscorides noted lead's effect on the mind in the first century A.D.

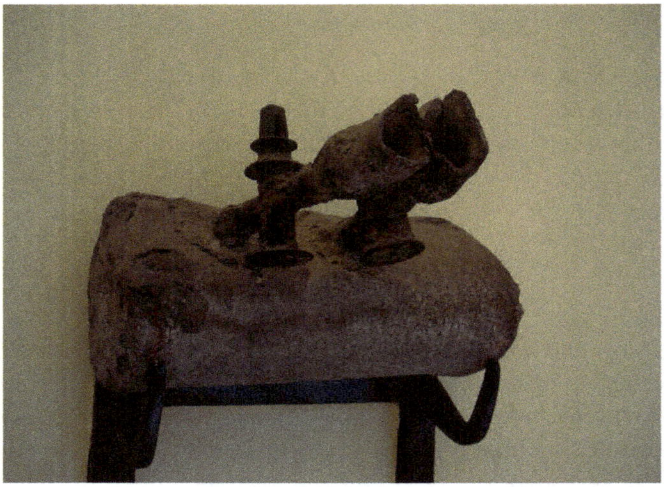

Roman lead water pipes with taps.

Lead poisoning was among the first known and most widely studied work and environmental hazards. One of the first metals to be smelted and used, lead is thought to have been discovered and first mined in Anatolia around 6500 BCE. Its density, workability, and corrosion resistance were among the metal's attractions.

In the 2nd century BCE the Greek botanist Nicander described the colic and paralysis seen in lead-poisoned people. Dioscorides, a Greek physician who lived in the 1st century CE, wrote that lead makes the mind give way.

Lead was used extensively in Roman aqueducts from about 500 BCE to 300 CE Julius Caesar's engineer, Vitruvius, reported, water is much more wholesome from earthenware pipes than from lead pipes. For it seems to be made injurious by lead, because white lead is produced by it, and this is said to be harmful to the human body." Gout, prevalent in affluent Rome, is thought to be the result of lead, or leaded eating and drinking vessels. Sugar of lead (lead(II) acetate) was used to sweeten wine, and the gout that resulted from this was known as saturnine gout. It is even hypothesized that lead poisoning may have contributed to the decline of the Roman Empire, a hypothesis thoroughly disputed:

The great disadvantage of lead has always been that it is poisonous. This was fully recognised by the ancients, and Vitruvius specifically warns against its use. Because it was nevertheless used in profusion for carrying drinking water, the conclusion has often been drawn that the Romans must therefore have suffered from lead poisoning; sometimes conclusions are carried even further and it is inferred that this caused infertility and other unwelcome conditions, and that lead plumbing was largely responsible for the decline and fall of Rome.

Two things make this otherwise attractive hypothesis impossible. First, the calcium carbonate deposit that formed so thickly inside the aqueduct channels also formed inside the pipes, effectively insulating the water from the lead, so that the two never touched. Second, because the Romans had so few taps and the water was constantly running, it was never inside the pipes for more than a few minutes, and certainly not long enough to become contaminated. However, recent research supports the idea that the lead found in the water came from the supply pipes, rather than another source of contamination. It was not unknown for locals to punch holes in the pipes to draw water off, increasing the number of people exposed to the lead.

Thirty years ago, Jerome Nriagu argued in a milestone paper that Roman civilization collapsed as a result of lead poisoning. Clair Patterson, the scientist who convinced governments to ban lead from gasoline, enthusiastically endorsed this idea, which nevertheless triggered a volley of publications aimed at refuting it. Although today lead is no longer seen as the prime culprit of Rome's demise, its status in the system of water distribution by lead pipes (fistulæ) still stands as a major public health issue. By measuring Pb isotope compositions of sediments from the Tiber River and the Trajanic Harbor, the present work shows that "tap water" from ancient Rome had 100 times more lead than local spring waters.

Romans also consumed lead through the consumption of defrutum, carenum, and sapa, musts made by boiling down fruit in lead cookware. Defrutum and its relatives were used in ancient Roman cuisine and cosmetics, including as a food preservative. The use of leaden cookware, though popular, was not the general standard and copper cookware was used far more generally. There is also no indication how often sapa was added or in what quantity.

The consumption of sapa as having a role in the fall of the Roman Empire was used in a theory proposed by geochemist Jerome Nriagu to state that lead poisoning contributed to the decline of the Roman Empire. In 1984, John Scarborough, a pharmacologist and classicist, criticized the conclusions drawn by Nriagu's book as so full of false evidence, miscitations, typographical errors, and a blatant flippancy regarding primary sources that the reader cannot trust the basic arguments.

After antiquity, mention of lead poisoning was absent from medical literature until the end of the Middle Ages. In 1656 the German physician Samuel Stockhausen recognized dust and fumes containing lead compounds as the cause of disease, called since ancient Roman times *morbi metallici*, that were known to afflict miners, smelter workers, potters, and others whose work exposed them to the metal.

The painter Caravaggio might have died of lead poisoning. Bones with high lead levels were recently found in a grave thought likely to be his. Paints used at the time contained high amounts of lead salts. Caravaggio is known to have exhibited violent behavior, as caused by lead poisoning.

In 17th-century Germany, the physician Eberhard Gockel discovered lead-contaminated wine to be the cause of an epidemic of colic. He had noticed that monks who did not drink wine were healthy, while wine drinkers developed colic, and traced the cause to sugar of lead, made by simmering litharge with vinegar. As a result, Eberhard Ludwig, Duke of Württemberg issued an edict in 1696 banning the adulteration of wines with litharge.

In the 18th century lead poisoning was fairly frequent on account of the widespread drinking of rum, which was made in stills with a lead component (the "worm"). It was a significant cause of mortality amongst slaves and sailors in the colonial West Indies. Lead poisoning from rum was also noted in Boston. Benjamin Franklin suspected lead to be a risk in 1786. Also in the 18th century, "Devonshire colic was the name given to the symptoms suffered by people of Devon who drank cider made in presses that were lined with lead. Lead was added to cheap wine illegally in the 18th and early 19th centuries as a sweetener. The composer Beethoven, a heavy wine drinker, suffered elevated lead levels (as later detected in his hair) possibly due to this; the cause of his death is controversial, but lead poisoning is a contender as a factor.

With the Industrial Revolution in the 19th century, lead poisoning became common in the work setting.The introduction of lead paint for residential use in the 19th century increased childhood exposure to lead; for millennia before this, most lead exposure had been occupational. An important step in the understanding of childhood lead poisoning occurred when toxicity in children from lead paint was recognized in Australia in 1897. France, Belgium, and Austria banned white lead interior paints in 1909; the League of Nations followed suit in 1922. However, in the United States, laws banning lead house paint were not passed until 1971, and it was phased out and not fully banned until 1978.

The 20th century saw an increase in worldwide lead exposure levels due to the increased widespread use of the metal. Beginning in the 1920s, lead was added to gasoline to improve its combustion; lead from this exhaust persists today in soil and dust in buildings. Blood lead levels worldwide have been declining sharply since the 1980s, when leaded gasoline began to be phased out. In those countries that have banned lead in solder for food and drink cans and have banned leaded gasoline additives, blood lead levels have fallen sharply since the mid-1980s.

The levels found today in most people are orders of magnitude greater than those of pre-industrial society. Due to reductions of lead in products and the workplace, acute lead poisoning is rare in most countries today, but low level lead exposure is still common. It was not until the second half of the 20th century that subclinical lead exposure became understood to be a problem. During the end of the 20th century, the blood lead levels deemed acceptable steadily declined. Blood lead levels once considered safe are now considered hazardous, with no known safe threshold.

In the late 1950s through the 1970s Herbert Needleman and Clair Cameron Patterson did research trying to prove lead's toxicity to humans. In the 1980s Needleman was falsely accused of scientific misconduct by the lead industry associates.

In 2002 Tommy Thompson, secretary of Health and Human Services appointed at least two persons with conflicts of interest to the CDC's Lead Advisory Committee.

In 2014 a case by the state of California against a number of companies decided against Sherwin-Williams, NL Industries and ConAgra and ordered them to pay $1.15 billion. The case is currently under appeal.

Studies have found a weak link between lead from leaded gasoline and crime rates.

Other Species

Humans are not alone in suffering from lead's effects; plants and animals are also affected by lead toxicity to varying degrees depending on species. Animals experience many of the same effects of lead exposure as humans do, such as abdominal pain, peripheral neuropathy, and behavioral changes such as increased aggression. Much of what is known about human lead toxicity and its effects is derived from animal studies. Animals are used to test the effects of treatments, such as chelating agents, and to provide information on the pathophysiology of lead, such as how it is absorbed and distributed in the body.

Farm animals such as cows and horses as well as pet animals are also susceptible to the effects of lead toxicity. Sources of lead exposure in pets can be the same as those that present health threats to humans sharing the environment, such as paint and blinds, and there is sometimes lead in toys made for pets. Lead poisoning in a pet dog may indicate that children in the same household are at increased risk for elevated lead levels.

Wildlife

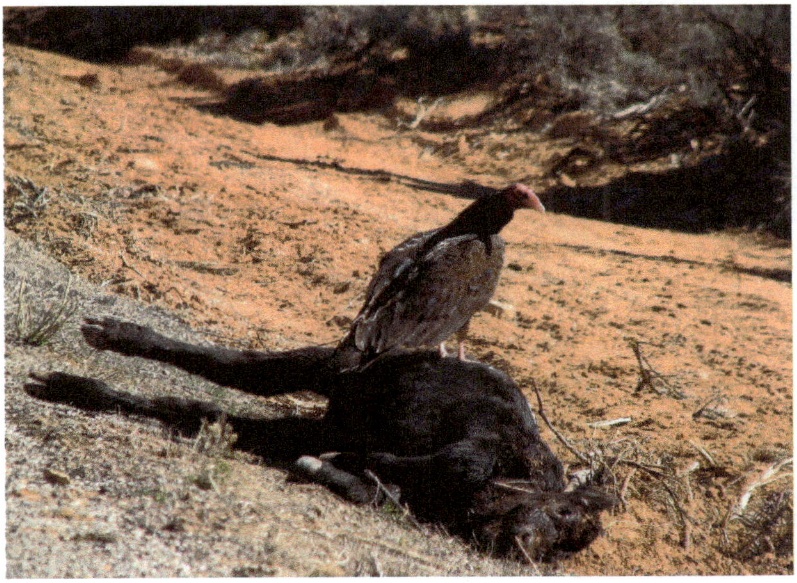

Turkey vultures, *Cathartes aura* (shown), and California condors can be poisoned when they eat carcasses of animals shot with lead pellets.

Lead, one of the leading causes of toxicity in waterfowl, has been known to cause die-offs of wild bird populations. When hunters use lead shot, waterfowl such as ducks can ingest the spent pellets later and be poisoned; predators that eat these birds are also at risk. Lead shot-related waterfowl poisonings were first documented in the US in the 1880s. By 1919, the spent lead pellets from waterfowl hunting was positively identified as the source of waterfowl deaths. Lead shot has been banned for hunting waterfowl in several countries, including the US in 1991 and Canada in 1997.Other threats to wildlife include lead paint, sediment from lead mines and smelters, and lead weights from fishing lines.Lead in some fishing gear has been banned in several countries.

The critically endangered California condor has also been affected by lead poisoning. As scavengers, condors eat carcasses of game that have been shot but not retrieved, and with them the fragments from lead bullets; this increases their lead levels. Among condors around the Grand Canyon, lead poisoning due to eating lead shot is the most frequently diagnosed cause of death. In an effort to protect this species, in areas designated as the California condor's range the use of projectiles containing lead has been banned to hunt deer, feral pigs, elk, pronghorn antelope, coyotes, ground squirrels, and other non-game wildlife. Also, conservation programs exist which routinely capture condors, check their blood lead levels, and treat cases of poisoning.

COPPER TOXICITY

Copper toxicity, also called **copperiedus**, refers to the consequences of an excess of copper in the body. Copperiedus can occur from eating acid foods cooked in uncoated copper cookware, or from exposure to excess copper in drinking water or other environmental sources.

Representation in ICD-9-CM, ICD-10-CM and SNOMED-CT

ICD-9-CM 985.8 *Toxic effect of other specified metals*

ICD-9-CM code **985.8** *Toxic effect of other specified metals* includes acute & chronic copper poisoning (or other toxic effect) whether intentional, accidental, industrial etc.

- In addition, it includes poisoning and toxic effects of other metals including tin, selenium nickel, iron, heavy metals, thallium, silver, lithium, cobalt, aluminum and bismuth. Some poisonings, e.g. zinc phosphide, would/could also be included as well as under 989.4 Poisoning due to other pesticides, etc.
- Excluded are toxic effects of mercury, arsenic, manganese, beryllium, antimony, cadmium, and chromium.

ICD-10-CM

Header text code	term
T56.4X1D	Toxic effect of copper and its compounds, accidental (unintentional), subsequent encounter
T56.4X1S	Toxic effect of copper and its compounds, accidental (unintentional), sequela
T56.4X2D	Toxic effect of copper and its compounds, intentional self-harm, subsequent encounter
T56.4X2S	Toxic effect of copper and its compounds, intentional self-harm, sequela
T56.4X3D	Toxic effect of copper and its compounds, assault, subsequent encounter
T56.4X3S	Toxic effect of copper and its compounds, assault, sequela
T56.4X4D	Toxic effect of copper and its compounds, undetermined, subsequent encounter
T56.4X4S	Toxic effect of copper and its compounds, undetermined, sequela

SNOMED-CT 46655005 *Copper poisoning (disorder)*

concept id	term
46655005	Copper
43098002	Copper fever
49443005	Phytogenous chronic copper poisoning
50288007	Chronic copper poisoning
73475009	Hepatogenous chronic copper poisoning
875001	Chalcosis of eye
90632001	Acute copper poisoning

Toxicity

Copper in the blood and blood stream exists in two forms: bound to ceruloplasmin (85–95%), and the rest "free", loosely bound to albumin and small molecules. Free copper normally reduces oxidative stress, as it is involved in the metabolic elimination of reactive oxygen species, such as with the superoxide radical through Cu-Zn dependent superoxide dismutase. Excessive free copper impairs zinc homeostasis, and vice versa, which in turn impairs antioxidant enzyme function, increasing oxidative stress. Chronically elevated levels of copper intake produces zinc deficiency.

Nutritionally, there is a distinct difference between organic and inorganic copper, according to whether the copper ion is bound to an organic ligand. Organic copper, like that found in food, is a beneficial micronutrient needed for good health. Inorganic metallic copper, like that found in electrical wire, plumbing pipes, brass fittings, redox water filters, sheet metal, cooking utensils, jewelry and pennies, is a neurotoxic heavy metal linked to physical and psychiatric symptoms on par with mercury and lead.

Symptoms and Presentation

Acute symptoms of copper poisoning by ingestion include vomiting, hematemesis (vomiting of blood), hypotension (low blood pressure), melena (black "tarry" feces), coma, jaundice (yellowish pigmentation of the skin), and gastrointestinal distress. Individuals with glucose-6-phosphate deficiency may be at increased risk of hematologic effects of copper. Hemolytic anemia resulting from the treatment of burns with copper compounds is infrequent.

Chronic (long-term) effects of copper exposure can damage the liver and kidneys. Mammals have efficient mechanisms to regulate copper stores such that they are generally protected from excess dietary copper levels.

Those same protection mechanisms can cause milder symptoms, which are often misdiagnosed as psychiatric disorders. There is a lot of research going on regarding the function of the Cu/Zn ratio in many conditions, neurological, endocrinological and psychological. The diagnostic difficulties arise from the fact that many of the substances that protect us from excess copper perform important functions in our neurological and endocrine systems. When they are used to bind copper in the plasma, to prevent it from being absorbed in the tissues, their own function may go unfulfilled. Such symptoms often include mood swings, irritability, depression, fatigue, excitation, difficulty focusing, feeling out of control, etc. To further complicate diagnosis, some symptoms of excess copper are similar to those of a copper deficit.

The U.S. Environmental Protection Agency's Maximum Contaminant Level (MCL) in drinking water is 1.3 milligrams per liter. The MCL for copper is based on the expectation that a lifetime of consuming copper in water at this level is without adverse effect (gastrointestinal). The US EPA lists copper as a micronutrient and a toxin. Toxicity in mammals includes a wide range of animals and effects such as liver cirrhosis, necrosis in kidneys and the brain, gastrointestinal distress, lesions, low blood pressure, and fetal mortality. The Occupational Safety and Health Administration (OSHA) has set a limit of 0.1 mg/m^3 for copper fumes (vapor generated from heating copper) and 1 mg/m^3 for copper dusts (fine metallic copper particles) and mists (aerosol of soluble copper) in workroom air during an eight-hour work shift, 40-hour work week. Toxicity to other species of plants and animals is noted to varying levels.

EPA Cancer Data

The EPA lists no evidence for human cancer incidence connected with copper, and lists animal evidence linking copper to cancer as "inadequate". Two studies in mice have shown no increased incidence of cancer. One of these used regular injections of copper compounds, including cupric oxide. One study of two strains of mice fed copper compounds found a varying increased incidence of reticulum cell sarcoma in males of one strain, but not the other (there was a slightly increased incidence in females of both strains). These results have not been repeated.

Treatment

In cases of suspected copper poisoning, penicillamine is the drug of choice, and dimercaprol, a heavy metal chelating agent, is often administered. Vinegar is not recommended to be given, as it assists in solubilizing insoluble copper salts. The inflammatory symptoms are to be treated on general principles, as are the nervous ones.

There is some evidence that alpha-lipoic acid (ALA) may work as a milder chelator of tissue-bound copper. Alpha lipoic acid is also being researched for chelating other heavy metals, such as mercury.

Cookware

Cookware in which copper is the main structural element (as opposed to copper clad, copper sandwiched or copper colored) is sometimes manufactured without a lining when intended to be used for any of a number of specific culinary tasks, such as preparing preserves or meringues. Otherwise, copper cookware is lined with a non-reactive metal to prevent contact between acidic foods and the structural copper element of the cookware.

Excepting for acute or chronic conditions, exposure to copper in cooking is generally considered harmless. Following Paracelsus, dosage makes the poison; as this pertains to copper a defense mechanism has apparently evolved as a consequence of which toxicity in man is very unusual.

Acute exposure and attendant copper toxicity is possible when cooking or storing highly acidic foods in unlined copper vessels for extended periods, or by exposing foodstuffs to reactive copper salts (copper corrosion, or verdigris). Continuous, small (chronic) exposures of acidic foods to copper may also result in toxicity in cases where either surface area interaction potentials are significant, pH is exceptionally low and concentrated (in the case of cooking with, for example, vinegar or wine), or both, and insufficient time elapses between exposures for normal homeostatic elimination of excess copper.

Exceptions to the above may be observed in the case of jam, jelly and preserve -making, wherein unlined copper vessels are used to cook (not to store) acidic preparations, in this case of fruit. Methods of jamming and preserving specify sugar as chemically necessary to the preserving (antibacterial) action, which has the additional effect of mediating (buffering) the interaction of fruit acid with copper,permitting the use of the metal for its efficient thermal transfer properties.

Non-Sparking Tools

OSHA has set safety standards for grinding and sharpening copper and copper alloy tools, which are often used in nonsparking applications. These standards are recorded in the Code of Federal Regulations 29 CFR 1910.134 and 1910.1000.

Note: The most important nonsparking copper alloy is beryllium copper, and can lead to beryllium poisoning.

Drinking Water

With an LD_{50} of 30 mg/kg in rats, "gram quantities" of copper sulfate are potentially lethal in humans.The suggested safe level of copper in drinking water for humans varies depending on the source, but tends to be pegged at 2.0 mg/l.

Birth Control

Estrogen birth control pills may increase the amount of copper in humans, but was not shown to increase absorption. Copper Intrauterine devices (IUDs) have been questioned anecdotally, with people claiming copper toxicity, but there is currently no scientific evidence to substantiate this claim. Estrogen increases the absorption of copper, making women more likely to carry excess copper even when no birth control is used.

The amount of estrogen (or copper) contained in these modern forms of contraception are generally considered safe, and the former restrictions for estrogen use (not to be used by women older than 40, 35 for smokers) were lifted in 1989.

There are conditions in which an individual's copper metabolism is compromised to such an extent that birth control may cause an issue with copper accumulation. They include toxicity or just increased copper from other sources, as well as the increased copper level of the individual's mother via the placenta before birth. The two hormones commonly used in birth control, estrogen and progestin, protect from each other's complications, so a combination method may work best. At least when existing imbalances have been treated.

Pathophysiology

A significant portion of the toxicity of copper comes from its ability to accept and donate single electrons as it changes oxidation state. This catalyzes the production of very reactive radical ions, such as hydroxyl radical in a manner similar to Fenton chemistry. This catalytic activity of copper is used by the enzymes with which it is associated, thus is only toxic when unsequestered and unmediated. This increase in unmediated reactive radicals is generally termed oxidative stress, and is an active area of research in a variety of diseases where copper may play an important but more subtle role than in acute toxicity.

Some of the effects of aging may be associated with excess copper.

Indian Childhood Cirrhosis

One manifestation of copper toxicity, cirrhosis of the liver in children (Indian childhood cirrhosis), has been linked to boiling milk in copper cookware. The Merck Manual states recent studies suggest that a genetic defect is associated with this particular cirrhosis.

Wilson's Disease

An inherited condition called Wilson's disease causes the body to retain copper, since it is not excreted by the liver into the bile. This disease, if untreated, can lead to brain and liver damage, and bis-choline tetrathiomolybdate is under investigation as a therapy against Wilson's disease.

Alzheimer's Disease

Elevated free copper levels exist in Alzheimer's disease, which has been hypothesized to be linked to inorganic copper consumption. Copper and zinc are known to bind to amyloid beta proteins in Alzheimer's disease. This bound form is thought to mediate the production of reactive oxygen species in the brain.

Aquatic Life

Too much copper in water may damage marine and freshwater organisms such as fish and molluscs.Fish species vary in their sensitivity to copper, with the LD50 for 96-h exposure to copper sulphate reported to be in the order of 58 mg per litre for Tilapia (*Oreochromis niloticus*) and 70 mg per litre for catfish (*Clarias gariepinus*) The chronic effect of sublethal concentrations of copper on fish and other creatures is damage to gills, liver, kidneys and the nervous system. It also interferes with the sense of smell in fish, thus preventing them from choosing good mates or finding their way to mating areas.

Copper-based paint is a common marine antifouling agent. In the United States, copper-based paint replaced tributyltin, which was banned due to its toxicity, as a way for boats to control organic growth on their hulls. In 2011, Washington state became the first U.S. state to ban the use of copper-based paint for boating, although it only applied to recreational boats. California has also pursued initiatives to reduce the effect of copper leaching, with the U.S. EPA pursuing research.

Bacteria

Copper and copper alloys such as brass have been found to be toxic to bacteria via the oligodynamic effect. The exact mechanism of action is unknown, but common to other heavy metals. Viruses are less susceptible to this effect than bacteria. Associated applications include the use of brass doorknobs in hospitals, which have been found to self-disinfect after eight hours, and mineral sanitizers, in which copper can act as an algicide. Overuse of copper sulfate as an algicide has been speculated to have caused a copper poisoning epidemic on Great Palm Island in 1979.

ARSENIC POISONING

Arsenic poisoning is a medical condition that occurs due to elevated levels of arsenic in the body. If exposure occurs over a brief period of time symptoms may include vomiting, abdominal pain, encephalopathy, and watery diarrhea that contains blood. Long-term exposure can result in thickening of the skin, darker skin, abdominal pain, diarrhea, heart disease, numbness, and cancer.

The most common reason for long-term exposure is contaminated drinking water. Groundwater most often becomes contaminated naturally; however, contamination may also occur from mining or agriculture. Recommended levels in water are less than 10–50 ug/l (10–50 parts per billion). Other routes of exposure include toxic waste sites and traditional medicines. Most cases of poisoning are accidental. Arsenic acts via changing the functioning of around 200 enzymes. Diagnosis is by testing the urine, blood, or hair.

Prevention is by using water that does not contain high levels of arsenic. This may be achieved by the use of special filters or using rainwater. There is not good evidence to support specific treatments for long-term poisoning. For acute poisonings treating dehydration is important. Dimercaptosuccinic acid (DMSA) or dimercaptopropane sulfonate (DMPS) may be used while dimercaprol (BAL) is not recommended. Hemodialysis may also be used.

Through drinking water, more than 200 million people globally are exposed to higher than safe levels of arsenic. The areas most affected are Bangladesh and West Bengal. Acute poisoning is uncommon.The toxicity of arsenic has been described as far back as 1500 BC in the Ebers papyrus.

Signs and Symptoms

Symptoms of arsenic poisoning begin with headaches, confusion, severe diarrhea, and drowsiness. As the poisoning develops, convulsions and changes in fingernail pigmentation called leukonychia striata (Mees's lines, or Aldrich-Mees's lines) may occur. When the poisoning becomes acute, symptoms may include diarrhea, vomiting, vomiting blood, blood in the urine, cramping muscles, hair loss, stomach pain, and more convulsions. The organs of the body that are usually affected by arsenic poisoning are the lungs, skin, kidneys, and liver. The final result of arsenic poisoning is coma and death.

Arsenic is related to heart disease (hypertension-related cardiovascular disease), cancer, stroke(cerebrovascular diseases), chronic lower respiratory diseases, and diabetes.

Chronic exposure to arsenic is related to vitamin A deficiency, which is related to heart disease and night blindness.

Inorganic arsenites (arsenic(III)) in drinking water have a much higher acute toxicity than organic arsenates (arsenic(V)). The acute minimal lethal dose of arsenic in adults is estimated to be 70 to 200 mg or 1 mg/kg/day.

Cancer

Arsenic increases the risk of cancer. Exposure is related to skin, lung, liver, and kidney cancer among others.

Its comutagenic effects may be explained by interference with base and nucleotide excision repair, eventually through interaction with zinc finger structures. Dimethylarsinic acid, DMA(V), caused DNA single stand breaks resulting from inhibition of repair enzymes at levels of 5 to 100 mM in human epithelial type II cells.

MMA(III) and DMA(III) were also shown to be directly genotoxic by effectuating scissions in supercoiled ΦX174 DNA. Increased arsenic exposure is associated with an increased frequency of chromosomal aberrations, micronuclei and sister-chromatid exchanges. An explanation for chromosomal aberrations is the sensitivity of the protein tubulin and the mitotic spindle to arsenic. Histological observations confirm effects on cellular integrity, shape and locomotion.

DMA(III) is able to form reactive oxygen species (ROS) by reaction with molecular oxygen. Resulting metabolites are the dimethylarsenic radical and the dimethylarsenic peroxyl radical. Both DMA(III) and DMA(V) were shown to release iron from horse spleen as well as from human liver ferritin if ascorbic acid was administered simultaneously. Thus, formation of ROS can be promoted. Moreover, arsenic could cause oxidative stress by depleting the cell's antioxidants, especially the ones containing thiol groups. The accumulation of ROS like the cited above and hydroxyl radicals, superoxide radicals and hydrogen peroxides causes aberrant gene expression at low concentrations and lesions of lipids, proteins and DNA in higher concentrations which eventually lead to cellular death. In a rat animal model, urine levels of 8-hydroxy-2'-desoxyguanosine (as a biomarker of ROS DNA damage) were measured after treatment with DMA(V). In comparison to control levels, they turned out to be significantly increased. This theory is further supported by a cross-sectional study which found elevated mean serum lipid peroxides (LPO) in the As exposed individuals which correlated with blood levels of inorganic arsenic and methylated metabolites and inversely correlated with nonprotein sulfhydryl (NPSH) levels in whole blood. Another study found an association of As levels in whole blood with the level of reactive oxidants in plasma and an inverse relationship with plasma antioxidants. A finding of the latter study indicates that methylation might in fact be a detoxification pathway with regard to oxidative stress: the results showed that the lower the As methylation capacity was, the lower the level of plasma antioxidant capacity. As reviewed by Kitchin (2001), the oxidative stress theory provides an explanation for the preferred tumor sites connected with arsenic exposure. Considering that a high partial pressure of oxygen is present in lungs and DMA(III) is excreted in gaseous state via the lungs this seems to be a plausible mechanism for special vulnerability. The fact that DMA is produced by methylation in the liver, excreted via the kidneys and latter on stored in the bladder accounts for the other tumor localizations.

Regarding DNA methylation, some studies suggest interaction of As with methyltransferases which leads to an inactivation of tumor suppressor genes through hypermethylation, others state that hypomethylation might occur due to a lack of SAM resulting in aberrant gene activation. An experiment by Zhong et al. (2001) with arsenite-exposed human lung A549, kidney UOK123, UOK109 and UOK121 cells isolated eight different DNA fragments by methylation-sensitive arbitrarily primed PCR. It turned out that six of the fragments were hyper- and two of them were hypomethylated.Higher levels of DNA methltransferase mRNA and enzyme activity were found.

Kitchin (2001) proposed a model of altered growth factors which lead to cell proliferation and thus to carcinogenesis. From observations, it is known that chronic low-dose arsenic poisoning can lead to increased tolerance to its acute toxicity. MRP1-overexpressing lung tumor GLC4/Sb30 cells poorly accumulate arsenite and arsenate. This is mediated through MRP-1 dependent efflux. The efflux requires GSH, but no As-GSH complex formation.

Although many mechanisms have been proposed, no definite model can be given for the mechanisms of chronic arsenic poisoning. The prevailing events of toxicity and carcinogenicity might be quite tissue-specific. Current consensus on the mode of carcinogenesis is that it acts primarily as a tumor promoter. Its co-carcinogenicity has been demonstrated in several models. However, the finding of several studies that chronically arsenic-exposed Andean populations (as most extremely exposed to UV-light) do not develop skin cancer with chronic arsenic exposure, is puzzling.

Causes

Organic arsenic is less harmful than inorganic arsenic. Seafood is a common source of the less toxic organic arsenic in the form of arsenobetaine. The arsenic reported in 2012 in fruit juice and rice by *Consumer Reports* was primarily inorganic arsenic.

Drinking Water

Chronic arsenic poisoning results from drinking contaminated well water over a long period of time. Many aquifers contain high concentration of arsenic salts. The World

Health Organization (WHO) recommends a limit of 0.01 mg/L (10 parts per billion) of arsenic in drinking water. This recommendation was established based on the limit of detection for most laboratories' testing equipment at the time of publication of the WHO water quality guidelines. More recent findings show that consumption of water with levels as low as 0.00017 mg/L (0.17 parts per billion) over long periods of time can lead to arsenicosis.

From a 1988 study in China, the US protection agency quantified the lifetime exposure of arsenic in drinking water at concentrations of 0.0017 mg/L, 0.00017 mg/L, and 0.000017 mg/L are associated with a lifetime skin cancer risk of 1 in 10,000, 1 in 100,000, and 1 in 1,000,000 respectively. WHO asserts that a level of 0.01 mg/L poses a risk of 6 in 10000 chance of lifetime skin cancer risk and contends that this level of risk is acceptable.

One of the worst incidents of arsenic poisoning via well water occurred in Bangladesh, which the World Health Organization called the largest mass poisoning of a population in history.

Mining techniques such as hydraulic fracturing may mobilize arsenic in groundwater and aquifers due to enhanced methane transport and resulting changes in redox conditions, and inject fluid containing additional arsenic.

Occupational exposures

Because of its high toxicity, arsenic is seldom used in the Western world, although in Asia it is still a popular pesticide. Arsenic is mainly encountered occupationally in the smelting of zinc and copper ores.

Food

It has been found that rice is particularly susceptible to accumulation of arsenic from soil. Rice grown in the U.S. has an average 260 ppb of arsenic, according to a study; but U.S. arsenic intake remains far below World Health Organization-recommended limits. China has set a standard for arsenic limits in food (150 ppb), as levels in rice exceed those in water.

Arsenic is a ubiquitous element present in American drinking water. In the United States, levels of arsenic that are above natural levels, but still well below danger levels set in federal safety standards, have been detected in commercially grown chickens. The source of the arsenic appears to be the feed additives roxarsone and nitarsone, which are used to control the parasitic infection coccidiosis as well as to increase weight and skin coloring of the poultry.

High levels of inorganic arsenic were reportedly found in 83 California wines in 2015.

Pathophysiology

Arsenic interferes with cellular longevity by allosteric inhibition of an essential metabolic enzyme pyruvate dehydrogenase (PDH) complex, which catalyzes the oxidation of pyruvate to acetyl-CoA by NAD^+. With the enzyme inhibited, the energy system of the cell is disrupted resulting in a cellular apoptosis episode. Biochemically, arsenic prevents use of thiamine resulting in a clinical picture resembling thiamine deficiency. Poisoning with arsenic can raise lactate levels and lead to lactic acidosis. Low potassium levels in the cells increases the risk of experiencing a life-threatening heart rhythm problem from arsenic trioxide. Arsenic in cells clearly stimulates the production of hydrogen peroxide (H_2O_2). When the H_2O_2 reacts with certain metals such as iron or manganese it produces a highly reactive hydroxyl radical. Inorganic arsenic trioxide found in ground water particularly affects voltage-gated potassium channels, disrupting cellular electrolytic function resulting in neurological disturbances, cardiovascular episodes such as prolonged QT interval, neutropenia, high blood pressure, central nervous system dysfunction, anemia, and death.

Arsenic exposure plays a key role in the pathogenesis of vascular endothelial dysfunction as it inactivates endothelial nitric oxide synthase, leading to reduction in the generation and bioavailability of nitric oxide. In addition, the chronic arsenic exposure induces high oxidative stress, which may affect the structure and function of cardiovascular system. Further, the arsenic exposure has been noted to induce atherosclerosis by increasing the platelet aggregation and reducing fibrinolysis. Moreover, arsenic exposure may cause arrhythmia by increasing the QT interval and accelerating the cellular calcium overload. The chronic exposure to arsenic upregulates the expression of tumor necrosis factor-α, interleukin-1, vascular cell adhesion molecule and vascular endothelial growth factor to induce cardiovascular pathogenesis.

—Pitchai Balakumarl and Jagdeep Kaur, "Arsenic Exposure and Cardiovascular Disorders: An Overview", Cardiovascular Toxicology, December 2009

Tissue culture studies have shown that arsenic compounds block both IKr and Iks channels and, at the same time, activates IK-ATP channels. Arsenic compounds also disrupt ATP production through several mechanisms. At the level of the citric acid cycle, arsenic inhibits pyruvate dehydrogenase and by competing with phosphate it uncouples oxidative phosphorylation, thus inhibiting energy-linked reduction of NAD+, mitochondrial respiration, and ATP synthesis. Hydrogen peroxide production is also increased, which might form reactive oxygen species and oxidative stress. These metabolic interferences lead to death from multi-system organ failure, probably from necrotic cell death, not apoptosis. A post mortem reveals brick red colored mucosa, due to severe hemorrhage. Although arsenic causes toxicity, it can also play a protective role.

Mechanism

Arsenite inhibits not only the formation of acetyl-CoA but also the enzyme succinic dehydrogenase. Arsenate can replace phosphate in many reactions. It is able to form Glc-6-Arsenate in vitro; therefore it has been argued that hexokinase could be inhibited. (Eventually this may be a mechanism leading to muscle weakness in chronic arsenic poisoning.) In the glyceraldehyde 3-phosphate dehydrogenase reaction arsenate attacks the enzyme-bound thioester. The formed 1-arseno-3-phosphoglycerate is unstable and hydrolyzes spontaneously. Thus, ATP formation in Glycolysis is inhibited while bypassing the phosphoglycerate kinase reaction. (Moreover, the formation of 2,3-bisphosphoglycerate in erythrocytes might be affected, followed by a higher oxygen affinity of hemoglobin and subsequently enhanced cyanosis) As shown by Gresser (1981), submitochondrial particles synthesize Adenosine-5'-diphosphate-arsenate from ADP and arsenate in presence of succinate. Thus, by a variety of mechanisms arsenate leads to an impairment of cell respiration and subsequently diminished ATP formation. This is consistent with observed ATP depletion of exposed cells and histopathological findings of mitochondrial and cell swelling, glycogen depletion in liver cells and fatty change in liver, heart and kidney.

Experiments demonstrated enhanced arterial thrombosis in a rat animal model, elevations of serotonin levels, thromboxane A and adhesion proteins in platelets, while human platelets showed similar responses. The effect on vascular endothelium may eventually be mediated by the arsenic-induced formation of nitric oxide. It was demonstrated that +3 As concentrations substantially lower than concentrations required for inhibition of the lysosomal protease cathepsin L in B cell line TA3 were sufficient to trigger apoptosis in the same B cell line, while the latter could be a mechanism mediating immunosuppressive effects.

Kinetics

The two forms of inorganic arsenic, reduced (trivalent As (III)) and oxidized (pentavalent As(V)), can be absorbed, and accumulated in tissues and body fluids. In the liver, the metabolism of arsenic involves enzymatic and non-enzymatic methylation, the most frequently excreted metabolite ($\geq$ 90%) in the urine of mammals is dimethylarsinic acid or cacodylic acid, DMA(V). Dimethylarsenic acid is also known as Agent Blue and was used as herbicide in the American war in Vietnam.

In humans inorganic arsenic is reduced nonenzymatically from pentoxide to trioxide, using glutathione (GSH) or it is mediated by enzymes. Reduction of arsenic pentoxide to arsenic trioxide increases its toxicity and bio availability, Methylation occurs through methyltransferase enzymes. S-adenosylmethionine (SAM) may serve as methyl donor. Various pathways are used, the principal route being dependent on the current environment of the cell. Resulting metabolites are monomethylarsonous acid, MMA(III), and dimethylarsinous acid, DMA(III).

Methylation had been regarded as a detoxification process but reduction from +5 As to +3 As may be considered as a bioactivation instead. Another suggestion is that methylation might be a detoxification if As[III] intermediates are not permitted to accumulate because the pentavalent organoarsenics have a lower affinity to thiol groups than inorganic pentavalent arsenics. Gebel (2002) stated that methylation is a detoxification through accelerated excretion.With regard to carcinogenicity it has been suggested that methylation should be regarded as a toxification.

Arsenic, especially +3 As, binds to single, but with higher affinity to vicinal sulfhydryl groups, thus reacts with a variety of proteins and inhibits their activity. It was also proposed that binding of arsenite at nonessential sites might contribute to detoxification. Arsenite inhibits members of the disulfide oxidoreductase family like glutathione reductase and thioredoxin reductase.

The remaining unbound arsenic ($\leq$ 10%) accumulates in cells, which over time may lead to skin, bladder, kidney, liver, lung, and prostate cancers. Other forms of arsenic toxicity in humans have been observed in blood, bone marrow, cardiac, central nervous system, gastrointestinal, gonadal, kidney, liver, pancreatic, and skin tissues.

Heat Shock Response

Another aspect is the similarity of arsenic effects to the heat shock response. Short-term arsenic exposure has effects on signal transduction inducing heat shock proteins with masses of 27,60,70,72,90,110 kDa as well as metallotionein, ubiquitin, mitogen-activated [MAP] kinases, extracellular regulated kinase [ERK], c-jun terminal kinases [JNK] and p38. Via JNK and p38 it activates c-fos, c-jun and egr-1 which are usually activated by growth factors and cytokines The effects are largely dependent on the dosing regime and may be as well inversed.

As shown by some experiments reviewed by Del Razo (2001), ROS induced by low levels of inorganic arsenic increase the transcription and the activity of the activator protein 1 (AP-1) and the nuclear factor-κB (NF-κB) (maybe enhanced by elevated MAPK levels), which results in c-fos/c-jun activation, over-secretion of pro-inflammatory and growth promoting cytokines stimulating cell proliferation. Germolec et al. (1996) found an increased cytokine expression and cell proliferation in skin biopsies from individuals chronically exposed to arsenic-contaminated drinking water.

Increased AP-1 and NF-κB obviously also result in an up-regulation of mdm2 protein, which decreases p53 protein levels. Thus, taking into account p53's function, a lack of it could cause a faster accumulation of mutations contributing to carcinogenesis. However, high levels of inorganic arsenic inhibit NF-κB activation and cell proliferation. An experiment of Hu et al. (2002) demonstrated increased binding activity of AP-1 and NF-κB after acute (24 h) exposure to +3 sodium arsenite, whereas long-term exposure (10–12 weeks) yielded the opposite result. The authors conclude that the former may be interpreted as a defense response while the latter could lead to carcinogenesis. As the contradicting findings and connected mechanistic hypotheses indicate, there is a difference in acute and chronic effects of arsenic on signal transduction which is not clearly understood yet.

Oxidative Stress

Studies have demonstrated that the oxidative stress generated by arsenic may disrupt the signal transduction pathways of the nuclear transcriptional factors PPAR's, AP-1, and NF-κB, as well as the pro-inflammatory cytokines IL-8 and TNF-α. The interference of oxidative stress with signal transduction pathways may affect physiological processes associated with cell growth, metabolic syndrome X, glucose homeostasis, lipid metabolism, obesity, insulin resistance, inflammation, and diabetes-2. Recent scientific evidence has elucidated the physiological roles of the PPAR's in the ω- hydroxylation of fatty acids and the inhibition of pro-inflammatory transcription factors (NF-κB and AP-1), pro-inflammatory cytokines (IL-1, -6, -8, -12, and TNF-α), cell4 adhesion molecules (ICAM-1 and VCAM-1), inducible nitric oxide synthase, proinflammatory nitric oxide (NO), and anti-apoptotic factors.

Epidemiological studies have suggested a correlation between chronic consumption of drinking water contaminated with arsenic and the incidence of Type 2-diabetes. The human liver after exposure to therapeutic drugs may exhibit hepatic non-cirrhotic portal hypertension, fibrosis, and cirrhosis.However, the literature provides insufficient scientific evidence to show cause and effect between arsenic and the onset of diabetes mellitus Type 2.

Diagnosis

Arsenic may be measured in blood or urine to monitor excessive environmental or occupational exposure, confirm a diagnosis of poisoning in hospitalized victims or to assist in the forensic investigation in a case of fatal over dosage. Some analytical techniques are capable of distinguishing organic from inorganic forms of the element. Organic arsenic compounds tend to be eliminated in the urine in unchanged form, while inorganic forms are largely converted to organic arsenic compounds in the body prior to urinary excretion. The current biological exposure index for U.S. workers of 35 µg/L total urinary arsenic may easily be exceeded by a healthy person eating a seafood meal.

Tests are available to diagnose poisoning by measuring arsenic in blood, urine, hair, and fingernails. The urine test is the most reliable test for arsenic exposure within the last few days. Urine testing needs to be done within 24–48 hours for an accurate analysis of an acute exposure. Tests on hair and fingernails can measure exposure to high levels of arsenic over the past 6–12 months. These tests can determine if one has been exposed to above-average levels of arsenic. They cannot predict, however, whether the arsenic levels in the body will affect health. Chronic arsenic exposure can remain in the body systems for a longer period of time than a shorter term or more isolated exposure and can be detected in a longer time frame after the introduction of the arsenic, important in trying to determine the source of the exposure.

Hair is a potential bioindicator for arsenic exposure due to its ability to store trace elements from blood. Incorporated elements maintain their position during growth of hair. Thus for a temporal estimation of exposure, an assay of hair composition needs to be carried out with a single hair which is not possible with older techniques requiring homogenization and dissolution of several strands of hair. This type of biomonitoring has been achieved with newer microanalytical techniques like Synchrotron radiation based X ray fluorescence (SXRF) spectroscopy and Microparticle induced X ray emission (PIXE). The highly focused and intense beams study small spots on biological samples allowing analysis to micro level along with the chemical speciation. In a study, this method has been used to follow arsenic level before, during and after treatment with Arsenious oxide in patients with Acute Promyelocytic Leukemia.

Treatment

Chelation

Dimercaprol and dimercaptosuccinic acid are chelating agents that sequester the arsenic away from blood proteins and are used in treating acute arsenic poisoning. The most important side effect is hypertension. Dimercaprol is considerably more toxic than succimer.

DMSA monoesters, e.g. MiADMSA, are promising antidotes for arsenic poisoning. Calcium sodium edetate is also used.

Nutrition

Supplemental potassium decreases the risk of experiencing a life-threatening heart rhythm problem from arsenic trioxide.

In addition to its presence as a poison, for centuries arsenic was used medicinally. It has been used for over 2,400 years as a part of traditional Chinese medicine. In the western world, arsenic compounds, such as salvarsan, were used extensively to treat syphilis before penicillin was introduced. It was eventually replaced as a therapeutic agent by sulfa drugs and then by other antibiotics. Arsenic was also an ingredient in many tonics (or patent medicines).

In addition, during the Elizabethan era, some women used a mixture of vinegar, chalk, and arsenic applied topically to whiten their skin. This use of arsenic was intended to prevent aging and creasing of the skin, but some arsenic was inevitably absorbed into the blood stream.

Some pigments, most notably the popular Emerald Green (known also under several other names), were based on arsenic compounds. Overexposure to these pigments was a frequent cause of accidental poisoning of artists and craftsmen.

Arsenic became a favored method for murder of the Middle Ages and Renaissance, particularly among ruling classes in Italy allegedly. Because the symptoms are similar to those of cholera, which was common at the time, arsenic poisoning often went undetected. By the 19th century, it had acquired the nickname "inheritance powder," perhaps because impatient heirs were known or suspected to use it to ensure or accelerate their inheritances.

In ancient Korea, and particularly in Joseon Dynasty, arsenic-sulfur compounds have been used as a major ingredient of *sayak* (사약; 賜藥), which was a poison cocktail used in capital punishment of high-profile political figures and members of the royal family. Due to social and political prominence of the condemned, many of these events were well-documented, often in the Annals of Joseon Dynasty; they are sometimes portrayed in historical television miniseries because of their dramatic nature.

Notable Cases

Arsenic poisoning, accidental or deliberate, has been implicated in the illness and death of a number of prominent people throughout history.

Francesco I de' Medici, Grand Duke of Tuscany

Recent forensic evidence uncovered by Italian scientists suggests that Francesco (1541-1587) and his wife were poisoned, possibly by his brother and successor Ferdinando.

Eric XIV of Sweden

Towards the end of his life, king Eric XIV (1533-1577) was held prisoner in many different castles in both Sweden and Finland. He died in prison in Örbyhus Castle: according to a tradition starting with Johannes Messenius, his final meal was a poisoned bowl of pea soup. A document signed by his brother, John III of Sweden, and a nobleman, Bengt Bengtsson Gylta (1514–74), gave Eric's guards in his last prison authorization to poison him if anyone tried to release him. His body was exhumed in 1958 and modern forensic analysis revealed evidence of lethal arsenic poisoning.

George III of Great Britain

George III's (1738–1820) personal health was a concern throughout his long reign. He suffered from periodic episodes of physical and mental illness, five of them disabling enough to require the King to withdraw from his duties. In 1969, researchers asserted that the episodes of madness and other physical symptoms were characteristic of the disease porphyria, which was also identified in members of his immediate and extended family. In addition, a 2004 study of samples of the King's hair revealed extremely high levels of arsenic, which is a possible trigger of disease symptoms. A 2005 article in the medical journal *The Lancet* suggested the source of the arsenic could be the antimony used as a consistent element of the King's medical treatment. The two minerals are often found in the same ground, and mineral extraction at the time was not precise enough to eliminate arsenic from compounds containing antimony.

Theodor Ursinus

Theodor Gottlieb Ursinus (1749–1800), a high-ranking Prussian civil servant and justice official, was poisoned by his wife Charlotte Ursinus (1760–1836). At the time, his death was ruled a stroke, but soon after the widow was found to have poisoned, between 1797 and 1801, not only her husband, but also her aunt and her lover, as well as to have attempted to poison her servant in 1803. Her sensational trial led to the first reliable method of identifying arsenic poisoning.

Napoleon Bonaparte

It has been suggested that Napoleon Bonaparte (1769–1821) suffered and died from arsenic poisoning during his imprisonment on the island of Saint Helena. Forensic samples of his hair did show high levels, 13 times the normal amount, of the element. This, however, does not prove deliberate poisoning by Napoleon's enemies: copper arsenite has been used as a pigment in some wallpapers, and microbiological liberation of the arsenic into the immediate environment would be possible. The case is equivocal in the absence of clearly authenticated samples of the wallpaper. Samples of hair taken during Napoleon's lifetime also show levels of arsenic, so that arsenic from the soil could not have polluted the post-mortem sample. Even without contaminated wallpaper or soil, commercial use of arsenic at the time provided many other routes by which Napoleon could have consumed enough arsenic to leave this forensic trace.

Simón Bolívar

South American independence leader Simón Bolívar (1783–1830), according to Paul Auwaerter from the Division of Infectious Diseases in the Department of Medicine at the Johns Hopkins University School of Medicine, may have died due to chronic arsenic poisoning further complicated by bronchiectasis and lung cancer. Auwaerter has considered murder and acute arsenic poisoning unlikely, arguing that gradual environmental contact with arsenic would have been entirely possible as a result of drinking contaminated water in Peru or through the medicinal use of arsenic (which was common at the time) as Bolívar had reportedly resorted to it during the treatment for some of his illnesses.

Charles Francis Hall

American explorer Charles Francis Hall (1821–1871) died unexpectedly during his third Arctic expedition aboard the ship *Polaris*. After returning to the ship from a sledging expedition Hall drank a cup of coffee and fell violently ill. He collapsed in what was described as a fit. He suffered from vomiting and delirium for the next week, then seemed to improve for a few days. He accused several of the ship's company, including ship's physician Emil Bessels with whom he had longstanding disagreements, of having poisoned him. Shortly thereafter, Hall again began suffering the same symptoms, died, and was taken ashore for burial. Following the expedition's return a US Navy investigation ruled that Hall had died from apoplexy.

In 1968, however, Hall's biographer Chauncey C. Loomis, a professor at Dartmouth College, traveled to Greenland to exhume Hall's body. Due to the permafrost, Hall's body, flag shroud, clothing and coffin were remarkably well preserved. Tissue samples of bone, fingernails and hair showed that Hall died of poisoning from large doses of arsenic in the last two weeks of his life, consistent with the symptoms party members reported. It is possible that he was murdered by Bessels or one of the other members of the expedition.

Clare Boothe Luce

Clare Boothe Luce (1903–1987), the American ambassador to Italy from 1953 to 1956, did not die from arsenic poisoning, but suffered an increasing variety of physical and psychological symptoms until arsenic was implicated. Its source was traced to the flaking arsenic-laden paint on the ceiling of her bedroom. She may also have eaten food contaminated by arsenic in flaking ceiling paint in the embassy dining room.

Guangxu Emperor

In 2008, testing in the People's Republic of China confirmed that the Guangxu Emperor (1871–1908) was poisoned with a massive dose of arsenic; suspects include his dying aunt, Empress Dowager Cixi, and her strongman, Yuan Shikai.

Phar Lap

The famous and largely successful New Zealand-bred racehorse Phar Lap died suddenly in 1932. Poisoning was considered as a cause of death and several forensic examinations were completed at the time of death. In a recent examination, 75 years after his death, forensic scientists determined that the horse had ingested a massive dose of arsenic shortly before his death.

King Faisal I of Iraq

According to his British nurse, Lady Badget, King Faisal I of Iraq suffered from symptoms similar to those of arsenic poisoning during his last visit to Switzerland for treatment in 1933, at the age of 48. His Swiss doctors found him in a very healthy situation a day before.

Anderson Mazoka

The popular opposition leader in Zambia, Anderson Mazoka, whose health deteriorated after the 2001 presidential elections, repeatedly accused government agents of poisoning him. His daughter, Mutinta, confirmed after his death on 24 May 2006 that arsenic was found in his body after he died from kidney complications.

Aluminium Phosphide Poisoning

Acute aluminium phosphide poisoning (AAlPP) is a large, though under-reported, problem throughout the world, particularly in the Indian subcontinent. Aluminium phosphide (AlP), which is readily available as a fumigant for stored cereal grains, sold under various brand names such as *QuickPhos* and *Celphos*, is highly toxic, especially when consumed from a freshly opened container. Death results from profound shock, myocarditis and multi-organ failure. Aluminium phosphide has a fatal dose of between 0.15 and 0.5 grams (0.0053 and 0.0176 oz). It has been reported to be the most common cause of suicidal death in North India. Deaths have also been reported in Iran. In January 2017, four children died at a trailer park in Amarillo, Texas, after the pesticide was used under the home to kill rats. Several incidents of death in travelers in Thailand and other parts of Southeast Asia may have been caused by aluminum phosphide or chlorpyrifos, an organophosphate insecticide, used in an attempt to kill bedbugs in hotels. Wired magazine reported on the problem in March 2014. A short film in Arabic on Youtube that focused on the problem in Saudi Arabia had over 3.5 million hits in 2014. The CDC has classified phosphine as immediately dangerous to life at 50 parts per million.

Mortality Rates

The mortality rates from AAlPP vary from 40 to 80 percent. The actual numbers of cases may be much larger, as less than five percent of those with AAlPP eventually reach a tertiary care center.Since 1992, when aluminium phosphide became freely available in the market, it had, reportedly, overtaken all other forms of deliberate poisoning, such as organophosphorus and barbiturate poisoning, in North India. In a 25-year-long study on 5,933 unnatural deaths in northwest India, aluminium phosphide poisoning was found to be the major cause of death among all cases of poisonings.

Mechanism of Toxicity

The toxicity of aluminium phosphide is attributed to the liberation of phosphine gas, a cytotoxic compound that causes free radical mediated injury, inhibits vital cellular enzymes and is directly corrosive to tissues. The following reaction releases phosphine when AlP reacts with water in the body:

$AlP + 3\ H_2O \rightarrow Al(OH)_3 + PH_3$, and

$AlP + 3\ HCl \rightarrow AlCl_3 + PH_3$ (stomach)

Signs, Symptoms, and Diagnosis

After ingestion, toxic features usually develop within a few minutes. The major lethal consequence of aluminium phosphide ingestion is profound circulatory collapse, and is reportedly secondary to these toxins generated, which lead due to direct effects on cardiomyocytes, fluid loss, and adrenal gland damage. The signs and symptoms are non-specific, dose dependent and evolve with time passing. The dominant clinical feature is severe hypotension refractory to dopamine therapy. Other features may include dizziness, fatigue, tightness in the chest, headache, nausea, vomiting, diarrhoea, ataxia, numbness, paraesthesia, tremor, muscle weakness, diplopia and jaundice. If severe inhalation occurs, the patient may develop acute respiratory distress syndrome (ARDS), heart failure, arrhythmias, convulsion and coma. Late manifestation include liver and kidney toxicities.

The diagnosis of AAlP usually depends on the clinical suspicion or history (self-report or by attendants). In some nations, tablets of AlP are also referred to as rice tablets and, if there is a history of rice tablet ingestion, then it should be treated differently from other types of rice tablets that are made up of herbal products. For a silver nitrate test on gastric aspirate, diluted gastric content can be positive.

Management and Outcome

The management of AAlPP remains purely supportive because no specific antidote exists. Mortality rates approach 60%. Correction of metabolic acidosis is a cornerstone of treatment. The role of magnesium sulfate as a potential therapy in AlP poisoning may decrease the likelihood of a fatal outcome, and has been described in many studies. After ingestion, removal of unabsorbed poison from the gut ("gut decontamination"), especially if administered within 1–2 hours, can be effective. Potassium permanganate (1:10,000) gastric lavage can decompose the toxin. All patients of severe AlP poisoning require continuous invasive hemodynamic monitoring and early resuscitation with fluid and vasoactive agents.

REFERENCES

1. Lead poisoning and health. WHO. September 2016. Retrieved 14 October 2016.
2. Lead Information for Workers. CDC. 30 September 2013. Retrieved 14 October 2016.
3. Gracia, RC; Snodgrass, WR (1 January 2007). Lead toxicity and chelation therapy.. American journal of health-system pharmacy : AJHP : official journal of the American Society of Health-System Pharmacists. 64 (1): 45–53. doi:10.2146/ajhp060175. PMID 17189579.
4. Advisory Committee On Childhood Lead Poisoning Prevention (ACCLPP). CDC. May 2012. Retrieved 18 May 2012.
5. The Code of Federal Regulations of the United States of America. U.S. Government Printing Office. 2005. p. 116.
6. Dapul, H; Laraque, D (August 2014). Lead poisoning in children.. Advances in pediatrics. 61 (1): 313–33. doi:10.1016/j.yapd.2014.04.004. PMID 25037135.
7. Needleman, H (2004). Lead poisoning. Annual Review of Medicine. 55: 209–22. doi:10.1146/annurev.med.55.091902.103653. PMID 14746518.
8. Lead Information for Employers. CDC. 30 September 2013. Retrieved 14 October 2016.
9. What Do Parents Need to Know to Protect Their Children?. CDC. 30 October 2012. Retrieved 14 October 2016.
10. Grant (2009) p. 785
11. Guidotti, TL; Ragain, L (2007). Protecting children from toxic exposure: three strategies. Pediatric clinics of North America. 54 (2): 227–35, vii. doi:10.1016/j.pcl.2007.02.002. PMID 17448358.
12. Pearson, Schonfeld (2003) p.369
13. Trevor, Katzung, Masters (2007) p. 479
14. Lowry, Jennifer A. (2010) ORAL CHELATION THERAPY FOR PATIENTS WITH LEAD POISONING. WHO
15. Rossi, E (2008). "Low Level Environmental Lead Exposure – A Continuing Challenge". The Clinical biochemist. Reviews / Australian Association of Clinical Biochemists. 29 (2): 63–70. PMC 2533151. PMID 18787644.
16. Barbosa Jr, F; Tanus-Santos, JE; Gerlach, RF; Parsons, PJ (2005). A Critical Review of Biomarkers Used for Monitoring Human Exposure to Lead: Advantages, Limitations, and Future Needs. Environmental Health Perspectives. 113 (12): 1669–74. doi:10.1289/ehp.7917. PMC 1314903. PMID 16330345.
17. Ragan, P; Turner, T (2009). Working to prevent lead poisoning in children: getting the lead out. JAAPA. 22 (7): 40–5. doi:10.1097/01720610-200907000-00010. PMID 19697571.
18. Grant (2009) p. 761
19. Kosnett (2007) p. 948

20. Karri, SK; Saper, RB; Kales, SN (2008). Lead Encephalopathy Due to Traditional Medicines. Current drug safety. 3 (1): 54–9. doi:10.2174/157488608783333907. PMC 2538609. PMID 18690981.

21. Kosnett (2005) p. 825

22. Mycyk, Hryhorczuk, Amitai (2005) p. 463

23. Dart, Hurlbut, Boyer-Hassen (2004) p. 1426

24. Timbrell, J.A., ed. (2008). Biochemical mechanisms of toxicity: Specific examples. Principles of Biochemical Toxicology (4th ed.). Informa Health Care. ISBN 0-8493-7302-6.

25. Pearce, JM (2007). Burton's line in lead poisoning. European neurology. 57 (2): 118–9. doi:10.1159/000098100. PMID 17179719.

26. Merrill, Morton, Soileau (2007) p. 860

27. Patrick, L (2006). Lead toxicity, a review of the literature. Part 1: Exposure, evaluation, and treatment. Alternative Medicine Review. 11 (1): 2–22. PMID 16597190.

28. Bellinger, DC (2004). Lead. Pediatrics. 113 (4 Suppl): 1016–22. doi:10.1542/peds.113.4.S1.1016. PMID 15060194.

29. Kosnett (2006) p.240

30. Henretig (2006) p. 1314

31. Brunton (2007) p. 1131

32. James, William; Berger, Timothy; Elston, Dirk (2005). Andrews' Diseases of the Skin: Clinical Dermatology. (10th ed.). Saunders. ISBN 0-7216-2921-0. [:859]

33. El Safoury, OmarSoliman; Abd El Fatah, DinaSabry; Ibrahim, Magdy (2009). Treatment of periocular hyperpigmentation due to lead of kohl (surma) by penicillamine: A single group non-randomized clinical trial. Indian Journal of Dermatology. 54 (4): 361. doi:10.4103/0019-5154.57614. ISSN 0019-5154.

34. Rambousek (2008) p.177

35. Review of Ophthalmology® > Wills Eye Resident Case Series. Revophth.com. Retrieved on 2015-04-23.

36. J. Chisolm, H. Harrison. (1956-12-01) The Exposure of Children to Lead, Journal of the American Academy of Pediatrics.Vol. 18. pp. 943 -958

37. Landrigan, PJ; Schechter, CB; Lipton, JM; Fahs, MC; Schwartz, J (2002). Environmental pollutants and disease in American children. Environmental Health Perspectives. 110 (7): 721–8. doi:10.1289/ehp.02110721. PMC 1240919. PMID 12117650.

38. Woolf, AD; Goldman, R; Bellinger, DC (2007). Update on the clinical management of childhood lead poisoning. Pediatric clinics of North America. 54 (2): 271–94, viii. doi:10.1016/j.pcl.2007.01.008. PMID 17448360.

39. Blood Lead Level Testing, Department of Ecology State of Washington. 2011

40. Baran, Robert et al. (2012) Baran and Dawber's Diseases of the Nails and

Their Management. John Wiley & Sons. ISBN 1118286707. p. 417.

41. White, LD; Cory-Slechta, DA; Gilbert, ME; Tiffany-Castiglioni, E; Zawia, NH; Virgolini, M; Rossi-George, A; Lasley, SM; et al. (2007). "New and evolving concepts in the neurotoxicology of lead". Toxicology and applied pharmacology. 225 (1): 1–27. doi:10.1016/j.taap.2007.08.001. PMID 17904601.
42. Lanphear, BP; Hornung, R; Khoury, J; Yolton, K; Baghurst, P; Bellinger, DC; Canfield, RL; Dietrich, KN; et al. (2005). Low-Level Environmental Lead Exposure and Children's Intellectual Function: An International Pooled Analysis. Environmental Health Perspectives. 113 (7): 894–9. doi:10.1289/ehp.7688. PMC 1257652. PMID 16002379.
43. Pokras, MA; Kneeland, MR (2008). Lead poisoning: using transdisciplinary approaches to solve an ancient problem. EcoHealth. 5 (3): 379–85. doi:10.1007/s10393-008-0177-x. PMID 19165554.
44. Brudevold F, Steadman LT (1956). The distribution of lead in human enamel (PDF). J Dent Res. 35 (3): 430–437. doi:10.1177/00220345560350031401. PMID 13332147.
45. Brudevold F, Aasenden R, Srinivasian BN, Bakhos Y (1977). Lead in enamel and saliva, dental caries, and the use of enamel biopsies for mesuring past exposure to lead (PDF). J Dent Res. 56 (10): 1165–1171. doi:10.1177/00220345770560100701. PMID 272374.
46. Goyer RA (1990). Transplacental transport of lead. Environ Health Perspect. Environmental Health Perspectives, Vol. 89. 89: 101–105. doi:10.2307/3430905. JSTOR 3430905. PMC 1567784. PMID 2088735.
47. Moss ME, Lamphear BP, Auinger P (1999). Association of dental caries and blood lead levels. JAMA. 281 (24): 2294–2298. doi:10.1001/jama.281.24.2294. PMID 10386553.
48. Campbell JR, Moss ME, Raubertas RF (2000). The association between caries and childhood lead exposure. Environ Health Perspect. Environmental Health Perspectives, Vol. 108, No. 11. 108 (11): 1099–1102. doi:10.2307/3434965. JSTOR 3434965. PMC 1240169. PMID 11102303.
49. Gemmel A, Tavares M, Alperin S, Soncini J, Daniel D, Dunn J, Crawford S, Braveman N, Clarkson TW, McKinlay S, Bellinger DC (2002). Blood lead level and dental caries in school-age children. Environ Health Perspect. 110 (10): A625–A630. doi:10.1289/ehp.021100625. PMC 1241049. PMID 12361944.
50. Billings RJ, Berkowitz RJ, Watson G (2004). Teeth (PDF). Pediatrics. 113 (4): 1120–1127. PMID 15060208.
51. Agency for Toxic Substances and Disease Registry (August 20, 2007). Lead Toxicity: Who Is at Risk of Lead Exposure?. Environmental Health and Medicine Education. U.S. Department of Health and Human Services. Course: WB 1105.
52. Grant (2009) p. 789
53. Rubin, Strayer (2008) p. 267
54. Ekong, EB; Jaar, BG; Weaver, VM (2006). Lead-related nephrotoxicity: a

review of the epidemiologic evidence. Kidney International. 70 (12): 2074–84. doi:10.1038/sj.ki.5001809. PMID 17063179.

55. Wright, LF; Saylor, RP; Cecere, FA (1984). Occult lead intoxication in patients with gout and kidney disease. The Journal of rheumatology. 11 (4): 517–20. PMID 6434739.

56. Lin JL, Huang PT (1994). Body lead stores and urate excretion in men with chronic renal disease. J. Rheumatol. 21 (4): 705–9. PMID 8035397.

57. Shadick NA, Kim R, Weiss S, Liang MH, Sparrow D, Hu H (2000). Effect of low level lead exposure on hyperuricemia and gout among middle aged and elderly men: the normative aging study. J. Rheumatol. 27 (7): 1708–12. PMID 10914856.

58. Navas-Acien, A; Guallar, E; Silbergeld, EK; Rothenberg, SJ (2007). Lead Exposure and Cardiovascular Disease—A Systematic Review. Environmental Health Perspectives. 115 (3): 472–82. doi:10.1289/ehp.9785. PMC 1849948. PMID 17431501.

59. Park, SK; O'Neill, MS; Vokonas, PS; Sparrow, D; Wright, RO; Coull, B; Nie, H; Hu, H; et al. (2008). Air Pollution and Heart Rate Variability: Effect Modification by Chronic Lead Exposure. Epidemiology (Cambridge, Mass.). 19 (1): 111–20. doi:10.1097/EDE.0b013e31815c408a. PMC 2671065. PMID 18091001.

60. Grant (2009) p. 792

61. Cleveland, LM; Minter, ML; Cobb, KA; Scott, AA; German, VF (2008). Lead hazards for pregnant women and children: part 1: immigrants and the poor shoulder most of the burden of lead exposure in this country. Part 1 of a two-part article details how exposure happens, whom it affects, and the harm it can do. The American journal of nursing. 108 (10): 40–9; quiz 50. doi:10.1097/01.NAJ.0000337736.76730.66. PMID 18827541.

62. Bellinger, DC (2005). Teratogen update: lead and pregnancy. Birth defects research. Part A, Clinical and molecular teratology. 73 (6): 409–20. doi:10.1002/bdra.20127. PMID 15880700.

63. Cecil, KM; Brubaker, CJ; Adler, CM; Dietrich, KN; Altaye, M; Egelhoff, JC; Wessel, S; Elangovan, I; et al. (2008). Balmes, John, ed. Decreased Brain Volume in Adults with Childhood Lead Exposure. PLOS Medicine. 5 (5): e112. doi:10.1371/journal.pmed.0050112. PMC 2689675. PMID 18507499.

64. Meyer, PA; McGeehin, MA; Falk, H (2003). A global approach to childhood lead poisoning prevention. International journal of hygiene and environmental health. 206 (4–5): 363–9. doi:10.1078/1438-4639-00232. PMID 12971691.

65. Bellinger, DC (2008). Very low lead exposures and children's neurodevelopment. Current Opinion in Pediatrics. 20 (2): 172–7. doi:10.1097/MOP.0b013e3282f4f97b. PMID 18332714.

66. Needleman, HL; Schell, A; Bellinger, D; Leviton, A; Allred, EN (1990). The long-term effects of exposure to low doses of lead in childhood. An 11-year follow-up report. The New England Journal of Medicine. 322 (2): 83–8.

doi:10.1056/NEJM199001113220203. PMID 2294437.

67. Merrill, Morton, Soileau (2007) p. 861

68. Casarett, Klaassen, Doull (2007) p. 944

69. Wilson, Ian Harold; Wilson, Simon Barton (2016). Confounding and causation in the epidemiology of lead. International Journal of Environmental Health Research. 26 (5-6): 467–82. doi:10.1080/09603123.2016.1161179. PMID 27009351.

70. Shih, RA; Hu, H; Weisskopf, MG; Schwartz, BS (2007). Cumulative Lead Dose and Cognitive Function in Adults: A Review of Studies That Measured Both Blood Lead and Bone Lead. Environmental Health Perspectives. 115 (3): 483–92. doi:10.1289/ehp.9786. PMC 1849945. PMID 17431502.

71. Kosnett, MJ; Wedeen, RP; Rothenberg, SJ; Hipkins, KL; Materna, BL; Schwartz, BS; Hu, H; Woolf, A (2007). Recommendations for Medical Management of Adult Lead Exposure. Environmental Health Perspectives. 115 (3): 463–71. doi:10.1289/ehp.9784. PMC 1849937. PMID 17431500.

72. Research Links Lead Exposure to Changes in Violent Crime Rates Throughout the 20th century (PDF). ICF International.

73. Nevin, R (2000). How lead exposure relates to temporal changes in IQ, violent crime, and unwed pregnancy. Environmental research. 83 (1): 1–22. Bibcode:2000ER.....83....1N. doi:10.1006/enrs.1999.4045. PMID 10845777.

74. Nevin, R (2007). Understanding international crime trends: the legacy of preschool lead exposure. Environmental research. 104 (3): 315–36. Bibcode:2007ER....104..315N. doi:10.1016/j.envres.2007.02.008. PMID 17451672.

75. Vedantam, Shankar (July 8, 2007). Research links lead exposure, criminal activity. Washington Post. Retrieved September 24, 2009.

76. Mañay, N; Cousillas, AZ; Alvarez, C; Heller, T (2008). Lead contamination in Uruguay: the La Teja neighborhood case. Reviews of environmental contamination and toxicology. Reviews of Environmental Contamination and Toxicology. 195: 93–115. doi:10.1007/978-0-387-77030-7_4. ISBN 978-0-387-77029-1. PMID 18418955.

77. Sanborn, MD; Abelsohn, A; Campbell, M; Weir, E (2002). Identifying and managing adverse environmental health effects: 3. Lead exposure. Canadian Medical Association Journal. 166 (10): 1287–92. PMC 111081. PMID 12041847.

78. Watts, J (2009). Lead poisoning cases spark riots in China. Lancet. 374 (9693): 868. doi:10.1016/S0140-6736(09)61612-3. PMID 19757511.

79. Jack Lewis (May 1985). Lead Poisoning: A Historical Perspective. EPA.

80. Deborah Blum (January 5, 2013). Looney Gas and Lead Poisoning: A Short, Sad History. Wired.

81. Kevin Drum (January 2013). America's Real Criminal Element: Lead. Mother Jones.

82. Dominic Casciani (April 20, 2014). Did removing lead from petrol spark a decline in crime?. BBC.

83. Brodkin, E; Copes, R; Mattman, A; Kennedy, J; Kling, R; Yassi, A (2007). Lead and mercury exposures: interpretation and action. Canadian Medical Association Journal. 176 (1): 59–63. doi:10.1503/cmaj.060790. PMC 1764574. PMID 17200393.

84. Dart, Hurlbut, Boyer-Hassen (2004) p. 1424

85. Castellino, Nicolo; Sannolo, Nicola; Castellino, Pietro (1994). Inorganic Lead Exposure and Intoxications. CRC Press. p. 86. ISBN 9780873719971.

86. Henretig (2006) p. 1310

87. Gilbert, SG; Weiss, B (2006). A rationale for lowering the blood lead action level from 10 to 2 μg/dL. Neurotoxicology. 27 (5): 693–701. doi:10.1016/j.neuro.2006.06.008. PMC 2212280. PMID 16889836.

88. Jacobs, David E.; Clickner, Robert P.; Zhou, Joey Y.; Viet, Susan M.; Marker, David A.; Rogers, John W.; Zeldin, Darryl C.; Broene, Pamela; et al. (2002). The prevalence of lead-based paint hazards in U.S. housing. Environmental Health Perspectives. 110 (10): A599–606. doi:10.1289/ehp.021100599. JSTOR 3455813. PMC 1241046. PMID 12361941.

89. Dart, Hurlbut, Boyer-Hassen (2004) p. 1423

90. Kosnett (2006) p.241

91. Chisolm (2004) pp. 221–22

92. Salvato (2003) p.116

93. Tom Kington. The mystery of Caravaggio's death solved at last – painting killed him. the Guardian.

94. Barltrop D, Strehlow CD, Thornton I, Webb JS (November 1975). Absorption of lead from dust and soil. Postgrad Med J. 51 (601): 801–4. doi:10.1136/pgmj.51.601.801. PMC 2496115. PMID 1208289.

95. Woolf, AD; Goldman, R; Bellinger, DC (2007). Update on the clinical management of childhood lead poisoning. Pediatric clinics of North America. 54 (2): 271–94, viii. doi:10.1016/j.pcl.2007.01.008. PMID 17448360.

96. Murphy, K. (May 13, 2009). For urban gardeners, lead is a concern. New York Times. Retrieved September 18, 2009.

97. Yu (2005) p.188

98. Yu (2005) p.187

99. Menkes (2006) p.703

100. Maas, RP; Patch, SC; Morgan, DM; Pandolfo, TJ (2005). Reducing lead exposure from drinking water: recent history and current status. Public Health Reports. 120 (3): 316–21. PMC 1497727. PMID 16134575.

101. um Wins Investigative Reporting Award with Post Team. University of Maryland. February 25, 2005. Archived from the original on September 12, 2006. Retrieved 2007-11-07.

102. HONORS. The Washington Post. February 23, 2005.

103. Christopher Ingraham (15 January 2016). This is how toxic Flint's water really is. Washington Post.

104. Eliott C. McLaughlin, CNN (18 January 2016). Flint's water crisis: 5 things to know - CNN.com. CNN.

105. Mattel CEO: 'Rigorous standards' after massive toy recall. CNN. November 15, 2007. Retrieved September 26, 2009.

106. Schep, LJ; Fountain, JS; Cox, WM; Pesola, GR (2006). Lead shot in the appendix. The New England Journal of Medicine. 354 (16): 1757; author reply 1757. doi:10.1056/NEJMc060133. PMID 16625019.

107. Madsen, HH; Skjdt, T; Jrgensen, PJ; Grandjean, P (1988). Blood lead levels in patients with lead shot retained in the appendix. Acta radiologica (Stockholm, Sweden : 1987). 29 (6): 745–6. doi:10.1080/02841858809171977. PMID 3190952.

108. Durlach, V; Lisovoski, F; Gross, A; Ostermann, G; Leutenegger, M (1986). Appendicectomy in an unusual case of lead poisoning. Lancet. 1 (8482): 687–8. doi:10.1016/S0140-6736(86)91769-1. PMID 2869380.

109. Centers for Disease Control and Prevention (CDC) (2006). Death of a child after ingestion of a metallic charm—Minnesota, 2006. MMWR. Morbidity and mortality weekly report. 55 (12): 340–1. PMID 16572103.

110. Salvato (2003) p.117

111. The Best Way To Solder Nitinol. Blogs.indium.com (2011-02-28). Retrieved on 2011-12-03.

112. Hunt, WG; Watson, RT; Oaks, JL; Parish, CN; Burnham, KK; Tucker, RL; Belthoff, JR; Hart, G (2009). Zhang, Baohong, ed. Lead Bullet Fragments in Venison from Rifle-Killed Deer: Potential for Human Dietary Exposure. PLoS ONE. 4 (4): e5330. Bibcode:2009PLoSO...4.5330H. doi:10.1371/journal.pone.0005330. PMC 2669501. PMID 19390698.

113. Spitz, M; Lucato, LT; Haddad, MS; Barbosa, ER (2008). Choreoathetosis secondary to lead toxicity. Arquivos de neuro-psiquiatria. 66 (3A): 575–7. doi:10.1590/S0004-282X2008000400031. PMID 18813727.

114. Dimaio, VJ; Dimaio, SM; Garriott, JC; Simpson, P (1983). A fatal case of lead poisoning due to a retained bullet. The American Journal of Forensic Medicine and Pathology. 4 (2): 165–9. doi:10.1097/00000433-198306000-00013. PMID 6859004.

115. Fiorica, V; Brinker, JE (1989). Increased lead absorption and lead poisoning from a retained bullet. The Journal of the Oklahoma State Medical Association. 82 (2): 63–7. PMID 2926538.

116. Doubts over MSG and Lead Content in Maggi Instant Noodles. 19 May 2015.

117. Beware! Eating 2 -Minute Maggi Noodles can ruin your Nervous System. news.biharprabha.com. 18 May 2015. Retrieved 18 May 2015.

118. Maggi Noodles Packets Recalled Across Uttar Pradesh, Say Food Inspectors: Report. NDTV. New Delhi, India. 20 May 2015. Retrieved 20 May 2015.

119. Sushmi Dey (16 May 2015). 'Maggi' under regulatory scanner for lead, MSG

beyond permissible limit. The Times of India. New Delhi, India. Retrieved 20 May 2015.

120. Delhi govt bans sales of Maggi from its stores: Report. Times of India. New Delhi, India. 3 June 2015. Retrieved 3 June 2015.

121. IANS (June 4, 2015). Gujarat bans Maggi noodles for 30 days. The Times of India. (The Times Group). Retrieved June 4, 2015.

122. Future Group bans Maggi too: The two-minute death of a India's favourite noodle brand. FirstPost. 3 June 2015. Retrieved 3 June 2015.

123. Lead Exposure in Wisconsin Birds (PDF). Wisconsin department of natural resources. 3 September 2008. Retrieved 10 December 2012.

124. Iqbal, Shahed; Blumenthal, Wendy; Kennedy, Chinaro; Yip, Fuyuen Y.; Pickard, Stephen; Flanders, W. Dana; Loringer, Kelly; Kruger, Kirby; Caldwell, Kathleen L.; Jean Brown, Mary (2009). Hunting with lead: Association between blood lead levels and wild game consumption. Environmental Research. 109 (8): 952–959. doi:10.1016/j.envres.2009.08.007. ISSN 0013-9351. PMID 19747676.

125. No Danger of Lead Poisoning from Meat Obtained by Hunting. University of Illinois. December 20, 2008. Retrieved March 2, 2011.

126. Iqbal, Shahed. Epi-AID Trip Report: Assessment of human health risk from consumption of wild game meat with possible lead contamination among the residents of the State of North Dakota (PDF). Epi-AID Trip Report. National Center for Environmental Health, Centers for Disease Control and Prevention: Atlanta, Georgia, USA. Retrieved March 2, 2011.

127. Blood lead levels—United States, 1999–2002. MMWR Morb. Mortal. Wkly. Rep. 54 (20): 513–6. May 2005. PMID 15917736.

128. Grant (2009) p. 767

129. Rubin, Strayer (2008) p. 266

130. Hu, H; Shih, R; Rothenberg, S; Schwartz, BS (2007). The Epidemiology of Lead Toxicity in Adults: Measuring Dose and Consideration of Other Methodologic Issues. Environmental Health Perspectives. 115 (3): 455–62. doi:10.1289/ehp.9783. PMC 1849918. PMID 17431499.

131. Kosnett (2006) p.238

132. Flora, SJ; Mittal, M; Mehta, A (2008). Heavy metal induced oxidative stress & its possible reversal by chelation therapy. The Indian journal of medical research. 128 (4): 501–23. PMID 19106443.

133. Yu (2005) p.193

134. Casarett, Klaassen, Doull (2007) p. 946

135. Gourlaouen, Christophe; Parisel, Olivier (15 January 2007). Is an Electronic Shield at the Molecular Origin of Lead Poisoning? A Computational Modeling Experiment. Angewandte Chemie International Edition. 46 (4): 553–556. doi:10.1002/anie.200603037. PMID 17152108.

136. Jaffe, E. K.; Martins, J.; et al. (13 October 2000). The Molecular Mechanism

of Lead Inhibition of Human Porphobilinogen Synthase. Journal of Biological Chemistry. 276 (2): 1531–1537. doi:10.1074/jbc.M007663200. PMID 11032836.

137. Scinicariello, Franco; Murray, H. Edward; et al. (15 September 2006). Lead and δ-Aminolevulinic Acid Dehydratase Polymorphism: Where Does It Lead? A Meta-Analysis. Environmental Health Perspectives. 115 (1): 35–41. doi:10.1289/ehp.9448. PMC 1797830. PMID 17366816.
138. Chhabra, Namrata (November 15, 2015). Effect of Lead poisoning on heme biosynthetic pathway. Clinical Cases: Biochemistry For Medics. Archived from the original on 2016-04-03. Retrieved 30 October 2016.
139. Fujita, H; Nishitani, C; Ogawa, K (February 2002). Lead, chemical porphyria, and heme as a biological mediator.. The Tohoku journal of experimental medicine. 196 (2): 53–64. doi:10.1620/tjem.196.53. PMID 12498316.
140. Mycyk, Hryhorczuk, Amitai (2005) p. 462
141. Kosnett (2005) p. 822
142. Xu, J; Yan, HC; Yang, B; Tong, LS; Zou, YX; Tian, Y (2009). Effects of lead exposure on hippocampal metabotropic glutamate receptor subtype 3 and 7 in developmental rats. Journal of negative results in biomedicine. 8: 5. doi:10.1186/1477-5751-8-5. PMC 2674876. PMID 19374778.
143. Lidsky, Theodore; et al. (2003). Lead neurotoxicity in children: basic mechanisms and clinical correlates. Brain. 126 (Pt 1): 5–19. doi:10.1093/brain/awg014. PMID 12477693.
144. Sanders, T; Liu, Y; Buchner, V; Tchounwou, PB (2009). Neurotoxic Effects and Biomarkers of Lead Exposure: A Review. Reviews on environmental health. 24 (1): 15–45. doi:10.1515/REVEH.2009.24.1.15. PMC 2858639. PMID 19476290.
145. How Lead Changes the Brain to Impair Learning and Memory, How Lead Changes the Brain to Impair Learning and Memory. Johns Hopkins Bloomberg School of Public Health. Retrieved 2007-08-14.
146. Henretig (2006) p. 1316
147. Fred HL, van Dijk HA. Images of Memorable Cases: Case 81. Connexions. Retrieved August 25, 2009.
148. Fischer C (2007). Kaplan Medical USMLE Steps 2 and 3 Notes: Internal Medicine, Hematology. pp. 176–177.
149. Grant (2009) p. 784
150. Vaziri, ND (2008). Mechanisms of lead-induced hypertension and cardiovascular disease. American Journal of Physiology. Heart and Circulatory Physiology. 295 (2): H454–65. doi:10.1152/ajpheart.00158.2008. PMC 2519216. PMID 18567711.
151. Mycyk, Hryhorczuk, Amitai (2005) p. 464
152. Gwiazda, R; Campbell, C; Smith, D (2005). A Noninvasive Isotopic Approach to Estimate the Bone Lead Contribution to Blood in Children: Implications for Assessing the Efficacy of Lead Abatement. Environmental Health Perspectives. 113 (1): 104–10. doi:10.1289/ehp.7241. PMC 1253718. PMID 15626656.

153. Wu, A. (2006) Tietz Clinical Guide to Laboratory Tests, 4th ed., Saunders Elsevier, St. Louis, MO, pp. 658–659.

154. Low Level Lead Exposure Harms Children: A Renewed Call for Primary Prevention (PDF). Centers for Disease Control and Prevention. Retrieved 5 January 2012.

155. NIOSH Adult Blood Lead Epidemiology & Surveillance (ABLES) program description. Cincinnati, OH: US Department of Health and Human Services, CDC, National Institute for Occupational Safety and Health. NIOSH. cdc.gov. 2013.

156. Fourth National Report on Human Exposure to Environmental Chemicals. Updated Tables (PDF). US Department of Health and Human Services. Atlanta, GA: cdc.gov. September 2012.

157. Baselt, Randall Clint (2008). Disposition of Toxic Drugs and Chemicals in Man (8th ed.). Biomedical Publications. pp. 823–6. ISBN 978-0-9626523-7-0.

158. Payne, M (2008). Lead in drinking water. Canadian Medical Association Journal. 179 (3): 253–4. doi:10.1503/cmaj.071483. PMC 2474873. PMID 18663205.

159. National Environmental Public Health Tracking Network, 2010.

160. Yeoh, B; Woolfenden, S; Lanphear, B; Ridley, GF; Livingstone, N (15 December 2014). Household interventions for preventing domestic lead exposure in children.. The Cochrane database of systematic reviews. 12: CD006047. doi:10.1002/14651858.CD006047.pub4. PMID 25506680.

161. Chisamera, D (October 19, 2008). EPA Sets Tightest Lead Air Emission Standard. eFluxMedia.

162. Polluted Kansas Town Seeks Federal Buyout. All things considered. National Public Radio. August 25, 2009. Retrieved August 25, 2009.

163. Treece Journal: Welcome to Our Town. Wish We Weren't Here. Saulny, S. New York Times, September 13, 2009

164. Kosnett (2006) p.242

165. Henretig (2006) p. 1321

166. Mycyk, Hryhorczuk, Amitai (2005) p. 465

167. Olson (2007) p.1658

168. Kosnett (2005) p. 832

169. Kosnett (2007) p. 949

170. Trevor, Katzung, Masters (2007) p. 480

171. Lightfoot, TL; Yeager, JM (2008). Pet bird toxicity and related environmental concerns. The Veterinary Clinics of North America. Exotic Animal Practice. 11 (2): 229–59, vi. doi:10.1016/j.cvex.2008.01.006. PMID 18406386.

172. Menkes (2006) p.706

173. Meyer, PA; Brown, MJ; Falk, H (2008). Global approach to reducing lead exposure and poisoning. Mutation research. 659 (1–2): 166–75. doi:10.1016/j.mrrev.2008.03.003. PMID 18436472.

174. Flora, SJ; Pachauri, V (Jul 2010). Chelation in metal intoxication.. International journal of environmental research and public health. 7 (12): 2745–88. doi:10.3390/ijerph7072745. PMC 2922724. PMID 20717537.

175. Gracia RC, Snodgrass WR (January 2007). Lead toxicity and chelation therapy. Am J Health Syst Pharm. 64 (1): 45–53. doi:10.2146/ajhp060175. PMID 17189579.

176. Bradberry, S; Vale, A (2009). A comparison of sodium calcium edetate (edetate calcium disodium) and succimer (DMSA) in the treatment of inorganic lead poisoning. Clinical toxicology (Philadelphia, Pa.). 47 (9): 841–58. doi:10.3109/15563650903321064. PMID 19852620.

177. Pearson, Schonfeld (2003) p.370

178. Lee, BK; Schwartz, BS; Stewart, W; Ahn, KD (1995). Provocative chelation with DMSA and EDTA: evidence for differential access to lead storage sites. Occupational and Environmental Medicine. 52 (1): 13–9. doi:10.1136/oem.52.1.13. PMC 1128144. PMID 7697134.

179. Herbert L. Needleman (June 28, 1999). The Removal of Lead from Gasoline (PDF). University of North Carolina.

180. Global health risks : mortality and burden of disease attributable to selected major risks. (PDF). Geneva, Switzerland: World Health Organization. 2009. p. 24. ISBN 9789241563871.

181. Konradsen F, van der Hoek W, Cole DC, et al. (November 2003). Reducing acute poisoning in developing countries—options for restricting the availability of pesticides. Toxicology. 192 (2–3): 249–61. doi:10.1016/S0300-483X(03)00339-1. PMID 14580791.

182. Jones, RL; Homa, DM; Meyer, PA; Brody, DJ; Caldwell, KL; Pirkle, JL; Brown, MJ (2009). Trends in blood lead levels and blood lead testing among US children aged 1 to 5 years, 1988–2004. Pediatrics. 123 (3): e376–85. doi:10.1542/peds.2007-3608. PMID 19254973.

183. Murata, K; Iwata, T; Dakeishi, M; Karita, K (2009). Lead toxicity: does the critical level of lead resulting in adverse effects differ between adults and children?. Journal of occupational health. 51 (1): 1–12. doi:10.1539/joh.K8003. PMID 18987427.

184. China to relocate 15,000 from lead-poisoned area. AFP. 2009-10-16. Archived from the original on 2009-10-19. Retrieved 2009-10-20.

185. China to move residents from lead smelter base-report. Reuters. 2009-10-18. Retrieved 2009-10-20.

186. Aid groups say lead poisoning has killed 400 children in Nigeria. Associated Press. 2010-10-05. Retrieved 2010-10-05.

187. Chisolm (2004) p. 223

188. Merrill, Morton, Soileau (2007) p. 862

189. Needleman, H (2009). Low level lead exposure: history and discovery. Annals of Epidemiology. 19 (4): 235–8. doi:10.1016/j.annepidem.2009.01.022. PMID

19344860.

190. Prioreschi, P (1998). A History of Medicine, Volume 3 Of Roman Medicine. Horatius Press. p. 279. ISBN 1-888456-03-5.

191. Couper RTL.; Fernandez, P. L.; Alonso, P. L. (2006). The Severe Gout of Emperor Charles V. N Engl J Med. 355 (18): 1935–36. doi:10.1056/NEJMc062352. PMID 17079773.

192. Hodge 1992, p. 308

193. Delile, H.; Blichert-Toft, J.; Goiran, J. -P.; Keay, S.; Albarede, F. (2014). Lead in ancient Rome's city waters. Proceedings of the National Academy of Sciences. 111 (18): 6594–6599. Bibcode:2014PNAS..111.6594D. doi:10.1073/pnas.1400097111.

194. Ancient Rome's tap water heavily contaminated with lead, researchers say – The Guardian

195. Lead in Ancient Rome's Water Was 100 Times Natural Levels – Discover

196. Director: Chris Warren (2004). Tales of the Living Dead: Poisoned Roman Babies (television). Brighton TV for National Geographic.

197. Nriagu JO (1983). Saturnine gout among Roman aristocrats. Did lead poisoning contribute to the fall of the Empire?. N. Engl. J. Med. 308 (11): 660–3. doi:10.1056/NEJM198303173081123. PMID 6338384.

198. Scarborough, John (1984). The Myth of Lead Poisoning Among the Romans: An Essay Review

199. Hernberg, S (2000). Lead poisoning in a historical perspective. American journal of industrial medicine. 38 (3): 244–54. doi:10.1002/1097-0274(200009)38:3<244::AID-AJIM3>3.0.CO;2-F. PMID 10940962.

200. Eisinger, J (1982). Lead and wine. Eberhard Gockel and the colica Pictonum. Medical History. 26 (3): 279–302. doi:10.1017/s0025727300041508. PMC 1139187. PMID 6750289.

201. Gochfeld, M (2005). Chronologic history of occupational medicine. Journal of occupational and environmental medicine / American College of Occupational and Environmental Medicine. 47 (2): 96–114. doi:10.1097/01.jom.0000152917.03649.0e. PMID 15706170.

202. The mystery of Caravaggio's death solved at last – painting killed him, Tom Kington, The Guardian, Wednesday, 16 June 2010.

203. Varney, Tamara L, Murphy, A. Reginald et al. (October 2012). A Preliminary Investigation of Lead Poisoning in a Napoleonic Era Naval Cemetery in Antigua, W.I. (PDF). Caribbean Connection. 2.

204. Curtin, Philip D. (November 1989). Death by Migration: Europe's Encounter with the Tropical World in the Nineteenth Century. pp. 78–79. ISBN 978-0521389228.

205. Brands, H. W. (2000). The First American: The Life and Times of Benjamin Franklin. New York: Anchor Books. ISBN 9780385495400.

206. The Franklin Institute (2010). Benjamin Franklin's Lead Letter, History's Lead Story

207. Mai, FM (2006). "Beethoven's terminal illness and death". The journal of the Royal College of Physicians of Edinburgh. 36 (3): 258–63. PMID 17214130.

208. Weiss, Rick Study Concludes Beethoven Died From Lead Poisoning, The Washington Post, December 6, 2005

209. Grant (2009) p. 757

210. Mycyk, Hryhorczuk, Amitai (2005) p. 467

211. Chiras, DD (2009). Environmental Science (8th ed.). Jones & Bartlett. p. 394. ISBN 0-7637-5925-2.

212. Grant (2009) p. 758

213. Agency for Toxic Substances and Disease Registry (August 20, 2007). Lead Toxicity Cover Page. Environmental Health and Medicine Education. U.S. Department of Health and Human Services. Course: WB 1105.

214. Denworth, Lydia. Toxic Truth: a scientist, a Doctor, and the battle over Lead. Beacon Press. p. 210. ISBN 9780807000328.

215. Kennedy, Donald (1997). Academic Duty. Harvard University Press. p. 237. ISBN 9780674002227.

216. Rosner, David; Markowitz, Gerald (May–June 2005). Standing Up to the Lead Industry: An Interview with Herber Needleman. Public Health Reports. Association of Schools and Programs of Public Health (ASPPH). 120 (3): 8. Retrieved 31 August 2014.

217. Lead Poisoning Prevention Panel Influenced by Industry. The Center for Science and Democracy. Union of Concerned Scientists. 8 February 2004. Retrieved 8 October 2002.

218. Markey, Edward J. (8 October 2002). Turning Lead Into Gold: How the Bush Administration is Poisoning the Lead Advisory Committee at the CDC (PDF). US House of Representatives. Archived from the original (PDF) on 24 October 2002. Retrieved 28 August 2014.

219. (PDF) https://media2.mofo.com/documents/140113-lead-paint.pdf. Retrieved 21 August 2016. Missing or empty |title= (help)

220. Hall, W (2013). Did the elimination of lead from petrol reduce crime in the USA in the 1990s?. F1000Research. 2: 156. doi:10.12688/f1000research.2-156.v2. PMC 3829390. PMID 24555074.

221. Redig, PT; Arent, LR (2008). Raptor toxicology. The Veterinary Clinics of North America. Exotic Animal Practice. 11 (2): 261–82, vi. doi:10.1016/j.cvex.2007.12.004. PMID 18406387.

222. Grant (2009) pp. 768, 771, 774

223. Neathery, MW; Miller, WJ (1975). Metabolism and toxicity of cadmium, mercury, and lead in animals: a review. Journal of Dairy Science. 58 (12): 1767–81. doi:10.3168/jds.S0022-0302(75)84785-0. PMID 1107364.

224. Ferreyra, H; Romano, M; Uhart, M (2009). Recent and chronic exposure of wild ducks to lead in human-modified wetlands in Santa Fe Province, Argentina. Journal of wildlife diseases. 45 (3): 823–7. doi:10.7589/0090-3558-45.3.823. PMID 19617495.

225. Federal Cartridge Company Waterfowl and Steel Shot Guide. Volume I; 1988.

226. Degernes, LA (2008). Waterfowl toxicology: a review. The Veterinary Clinics of North America. Exotic Animal Practice. 11 (2): 283–300, vi. doi:10.1016/j.cvex.2007.12.001. PMID 18406388.

227. Green, RE; Hunt, WG; Parish, CN; Newton, I; Pizzari, Tom (2008). Pizzari, Tom, ed. Effectiveness of Action to Reduce Exposure of Free-Ranging California Condors in Arizona and Utah to Lead from Spent Ammunition. PLoS ONE. 3 (12): e4022. Bibcode:2008PLoSO...3.4022G. doi:10.1371/journal.pone.0004022. PMC 2603582. PMID 19107211.

228. Get the Lead Out (Protecting the Condor). California Department of Fish and Game. Retrieved 2009-07-28.

CHAPTER 4

Environmental Impact of The Petroleum Industry

Chapter Contents

- **Introduction**
- **Issues**
- **Acid Rain**
- **Mitigation**
- **Environmental Impact of the Energy Industry**

Petroleum sources are usually small pockets of liquid or gas trapped within rock layers deep underground (often under the seafloor). Extracted crude oil is refined and used to manufacture gasoline (used in transportation) and *petrochemicals* (used in the production of plastics, pharmaceuticals, and cleaning products).

INTRODUCTION

The **environmental impact of petroleum** is often negative because it is toxic to almost all forms of life and its extraction fuels climate change. Petroleum, commonly referred to as oil, is closely linked to virtually all aspects of present society, especially for transportation and heating for both homes and for commercial and industrial activities.

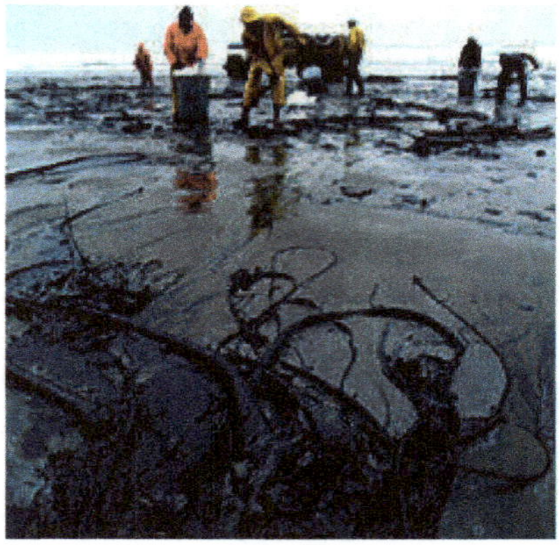

A beach after an oil spill.

ISSUES

Toxicity

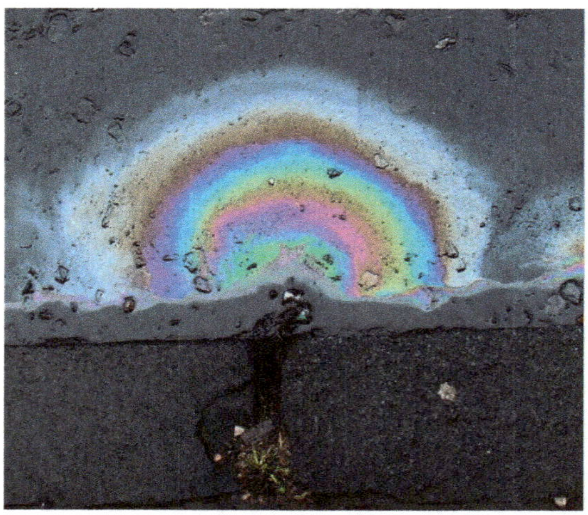

Petroleum distillates can create a sheen on the surface of water as a thin layer creating an optical phenomenon called interphase.

Crude oil is a mixture of many different kinds of organic compounds, many of which are highly toxic and cancer causing (carcinogenic). Oil is acutely lethal to fish - that is, it kills fish quickly, at a concentration of 4000 parts per million (ppm)(0.4%). Crude oil and petroleum distillates cause birth defects.

Benzene is present in both crude oil and gasoline and is known to cause leukaemia in humans. The compound is also known to lower the white blood cell count in humans, which would leave people exposed to it more susceptible to infections. Studies have linked benzene exposure in the mere parts per billion (ppb) range to terminal leukemia, Hodgkin's lymphoma, and other blood and immune system diseases within 5-15 years of exposure."

Exhaust or Air Pollution

Air pollution is the introduction of harmful substances including particulates and biological molecules into Earth's atmosphere. It may cause diseases, allergies or death in humans; it may also cause harm to other living organisms such as animals and food crops, and may damage the natural or built environment. Human activity and natural processes can both generate air pollution.

Indoor air pollution and poor urban air quality are listed as two of the world's worst toxic pollution problems in the 2008 Blacksmith Institute World's Worst Polluted Places report. According to the 2014 WHO report, air pollution in 2012 caused the deaths of around 7 million people worldwide, an estimate roughly matched by the International Energy Agency.

Pollutants

An air pollutant is a substance in the air that can have adverse effects on humans and the ecosystem. The substance can be solid particles, liquid droplets, or gases. A pollutant can be of natural origin or man-made. Pollutants are classified as primary or secondary. Primary pollutants are usually produced from a process, such as ash from a volcanic eruption. Other examples include carbon monoxide gas from motor vehicle exhaust, or the sulfur dioxide released from factories. Secondary pollutants are not emitted directly. Rather, they form in the air when primary pollutants react or interact. Ground level ozone is a prominent example of a secondary pollutant. Some pollutants may be both primary and secondary: they are both emitted directly and formed from other primary pollutants.

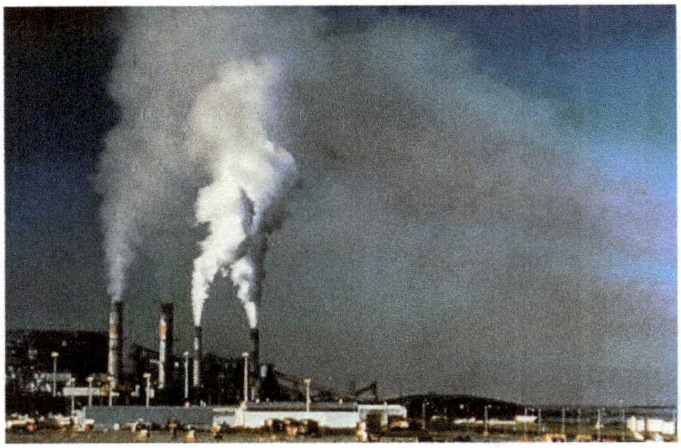

Before flue-gas desulfurization was installed, the emissions from this power plant in New Mexico contained excessive amounts of sulfur dioxide.

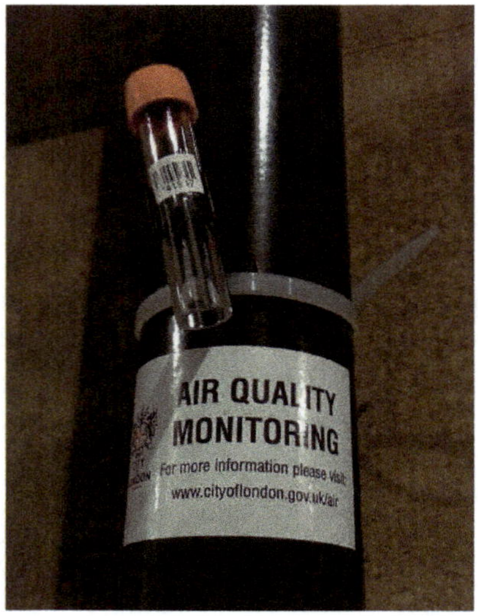

Nitrogen dioxide diffusion tube for air quality monitoring. Positioned in London City.

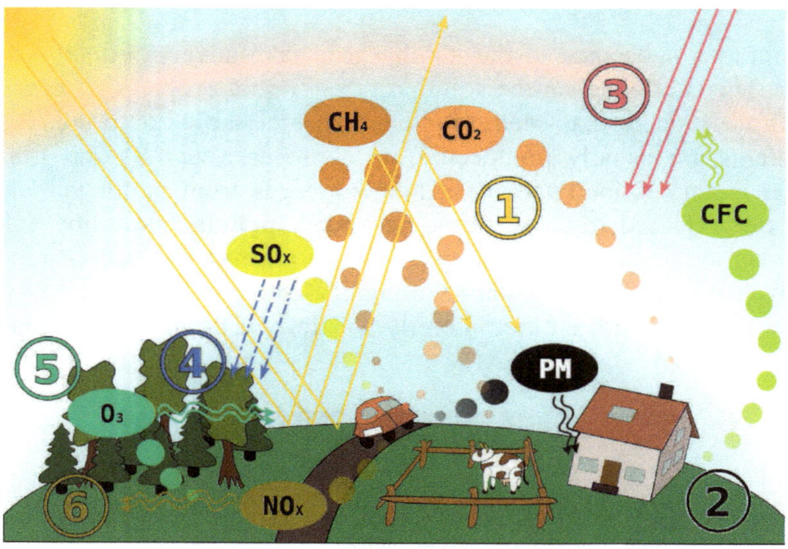

Schematic drawing, causes and effects of air pollution: (1) greenhouse effect, (2) particulate contamination, (3) increased UV radiation, (4) acid rain, (5) increased ground level ozone concentration, (6) increased levels of nitrogen oxides.

Major primary pollutants produced by human activity include:

- Carbon dioxide (CO_2) - This is by far the most emitted form of human caused air pollution. Although CO_2 is currently only about 405 parts per million in earth's atmosphere, billions of metric tons of CO_2 are emitted annually by burning of fossil fuels. CO_2 increase in earth's atmosphere has been accelerating.

- Sulfur oxides (SO_x) - particularly sulfur dioxide, a chemical compound with the formula SO_2. SO_2 is produced by volcanoes and in various industrial processes. Coal and petroleum often contain sulfur compounds, and their combustion generates sulfur dioxide. Further oxidation of SO_2, usually in the presence of a catalyst such as NO_2, forms H_2SO_4, and thus acid rain. This is one of the causes for concern over the environmental impact of the use of these fuels as power sources.
- Nitrogen oxides (NO_x) - Nitrogen oxides, particularly nitrogen dioxide, are expelled from high temperature combustion, and are also produced during thunderstorms by electric discharge. They can be seen as a brown haze dome above or a plume downwind of cities. Nitrogen dioxide is a chemical compound with the formula NO_2. It is one of several nitrogen oxides. One of the most prominent air pollutants, this reddish-brown toxic gas has a characteristic sharp, biting odor.
- Carbon monoxide (CO) - CO is a colorless, odorless, toxic yet non-irritating gas. It is a product of incomplete combustion of fuel such as natural gas, coal or wood. Vehicular exhaust is a major source of carbon monoxide.
- Volatile organic compounds (VOC) - VOCs are a well-known outdoor air pollutant. They are categorized as either methane (CH_4) or non-methane (NMVOCs). Methane is an extremely efficient greenhouse gas which contributes to enhanced global warming. Other hydrocarbon VOCs are also significant greenhouse gases because of their role in creating ozone and prolonging the life of methane in the atmosphere. This effect varies depending on local air quality. The aromatic NMVOCs benzene, toluene and xylene are suspected carcinogens and may lead to leukemia with prolonged exposure. 1,3-butadiene is another dangerous compound often associated with industrial use.
- Particulates, alternatively referred to as particulate matter (PM), atmospheric particulate matter, or fine particles, are tiny particles of solid or liquid suspended in a gas. In contrast, aerosol refers to combined particles and gas. Some particulates occur naturally, originating from volcanoes, dust storms, forest and grassland fires, living vegetation, and sea spray. Human activities, such as the burning of fossil fuels in vehicles, power plants and various industrial processes also generate significant amounts of aerosols. Averaged worldwide, anthropogenic aerosols—those made by human activities—currently account for approximately 10 percent of our atmosphere. Increased levels of fine particles in the air are linked to health hazards such as heart disease, altered lung function and lung cancer.
- Persistent free radicals connected to airborne fine particles are linked to cardiopulmonary disease.
- Toxic metals, such as lead and mercury, especially their compounds.
- Chlorofluorocarbons (CFCs) - harmful to the ozone layer; emitted from products are currently banned from use. These are gases which are released from air conditioners, refrigerators, aerosol sprays, etc. On release into the air, CFCs rise to the stratosphere. Here they come in contact with other gases and damage the

ozone layer. This allows harmful ultraviolet rays to reach the earth's surface. This can lead to skin cancer, eye disease and can even cause damage to plants.

- Ammonia (NH_3) - emitted from agricultural processes. Ammonia is a compound with the formula NH_3. It is normally encountered as a gas with a characteristic pungent odor. Ammonia contributes significantly to the nutritional needs of terrestrial organisms by serving as a precursor to foodstuffs and fertilizers. Ammonia, either directly or indirectly, is also a building block for the synthesis of many pharmaceuticals. Although in wide use, ammonia is both caustic and hazardous. In the atmosphere, ammonia reacts with oxides of nitrogen and sulfur to form secondary particles.
- Odours — such as from garbage, sewage, and industrial processes
- Radioactive pollutants - produced by nuclear explosions, nuclear events, war explosives, and natural processes such as the radioactive decay of radon.

Secondary pollutants include:

- Particulates created from gaseous primary pollutants and compounds in photochemical smog. Smog is a kind of air pollution. Classic smog results from large amounts of coal burning in an area caused by a mixture of smoke and sulfur dioxide. Modern smog does not usually come from coal but from vehicular and industrial emissions that are acted on in the atmosphere by ultraviolet light from the sun to form secondary pollutants that also combine with the primary emissions to form photochemical smog.
- Ground level ozone (O_3) formed from NO_x and VOCs. Ozone (O_3) is a key constituent of the troposphere. It is also an important constituent of certain regions of the stratosphere commonly known as the Ozone layer. Photochemical and chemical reactions involving it drive many of the chemical processes that occur in the atmosphere by day and by night. At abnormally high concentrations brought about by human activities (largely the combustion of fossil fuel), it is a pollutant, and a constituent of smog.
- Peroxyacetyl nitrate (PAN) - similarly formed from NO_x and VOCs.

Minor air pollutants include:

- A large number of minor hazardous air pollutants. Some of these are regulated in USA under the Clean Air Act and in Europe under the Air Framework Directive
- A variety of persistent organic pollutants, which can attach to particulates

Persistent organic pollutants (POPs) are organic compounds that are resistant to environmental degradation through chemical, biological, and photolytic processes. Because of this, they have been observed to persist in the environment, to be capable of long-range transport, bioaccumulate in human and animal tissue, biomagnify in food chains, and to have potentially significant impacts on human health and the environment.

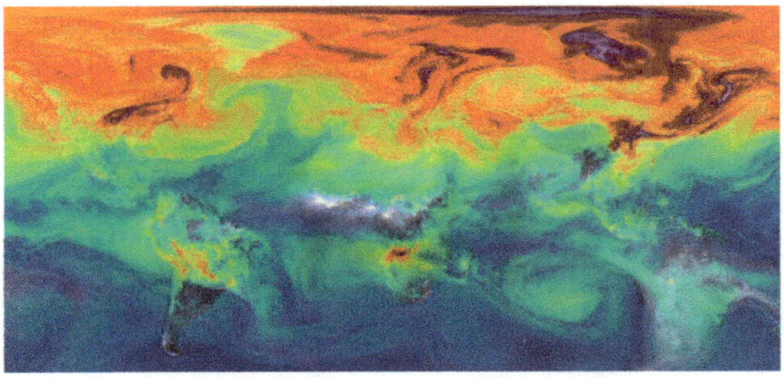

Carbon dioxide in Earth's atmosphere if *half* of global-warming emissions are *not* absorbed. (NASA simulation; 9 November 2015)

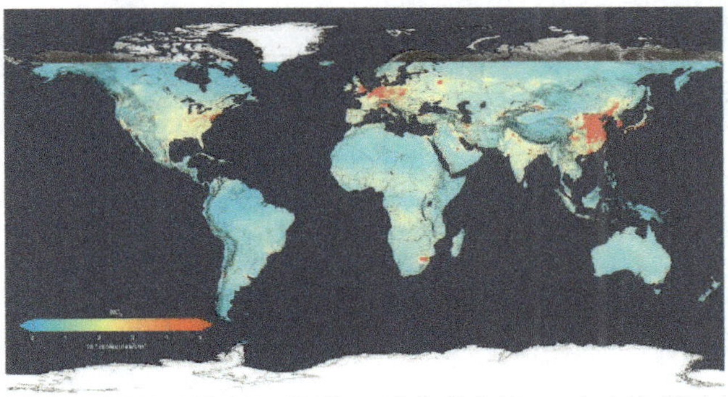

Nitrogen dioxide 2014 - global air quality levels (released 14 December 2015).

Sources

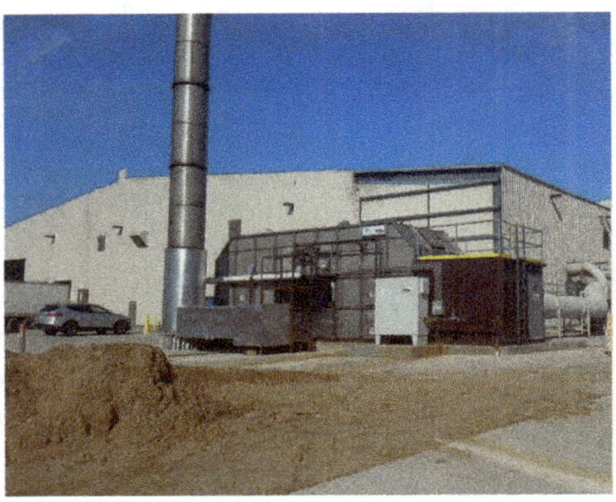

This video provides an overview of a NASA study on the human fingerprint on global air quality.

There are various locations, activities or factors which are responsible for releasing pollutants into the atmosphere. These sources can be classified into two major categories.

Anthropogenic (man-made) Sources:

Controlled burning of a field outside of Statesboro, Georgia in preparation for spring planting.

These are mostly related to the burning of multiple types of fuel.

- **Stationary sources** include smoke stacks of power plants, manufacturing facilities (factories) and waste incinerators, as well as furnaces and other types of fuel-burning heating devices. In developing and poor countries, traditional biomass burning is the major source of air pollutants; traditional biomass includes wood, crop waste and dung.
- **Mobile sources** include motor vehicles, marine vessels, and aircraft.
- **Controlled burn** practices in agriculture and forest management. Controlled or prescribed burning is a technique sometimes used in forest management, farming, prairie restoration or greenhouse gas abatement. Fire is a natural part of both forest and grassland ecology and controlled fire can be a tool for foresters. Controlled burning stimulates the germination of some desirable forest trees, thus renewing the forest.
- **Fumes** from paint, hair spray, varnish, aerosol sprays and other solvents
- **Waste deposition** in landfills, which generate methane. Methane is highly flammable and may form explosive mixtures with air. Methane is also an asphyxiant and may displace oxygen in an enclosed space. Asphyxia or suffocation may result if the oxygen concentration is reduced to below 19.5% by displacement.
- **Military resources,** such as nuclear weapons, toxic gases, germ warfare and rocketry

Natural Sources:

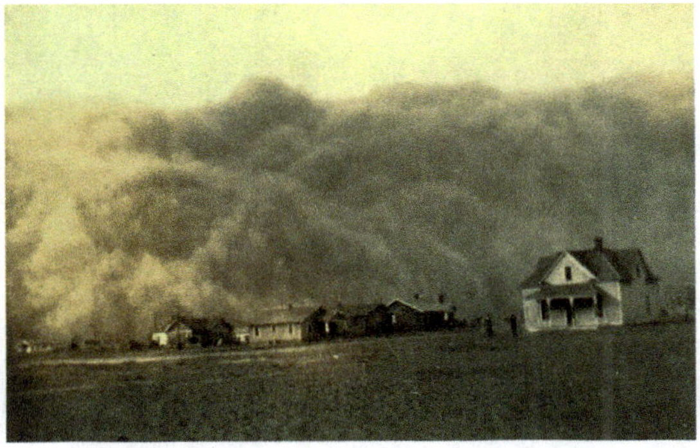

Dust storm approaching Stratford, Texas.

- Dust from natural sources, usually large areas of land with little or no vegetation
- Methane, emitted by the digestion of food by animals, for example cattle
- Radon gas from radioactive decay within the Earth's crust. Radon is a colorless, odorless, naturally occurring, radioactive noble gas that is formed from the decay of radium. It is considered to be a health hazard. Radon gas from natural sources can accumulate in buildings, especially in confined areas such as the basement and it is the second most frequent cause of lung cancer, after cigarette smoking.
- Smoke and carbon monoxide from wildfires
- Vegetation, in some regions, emits environmentally significant amounts of Volatile organic compounds (VOCs) on warmer days. These VOCs react with primary anthropogenic pollutants—specifically, NO_x, SO_2, and anthropogenic organic carbon compounds — to produce a seasonal haze of secondary pollutants. Black gum, poplar, oak and willow are some examples of vegetation that can produce abundant VOCs. The VOC production from these species result in ozone levels up to eight times higher than the low-impact tree species.
- Volcanic activity, which produces sulfur, chlorine, and ash particulates

Emission Factors

Air pollutant emission factors are reported representative values that attempt to relate the quantity of a pollutant released to the ambient air with an activity associated with the release of that pollutant. These factors are usually expressed as the weight of pollutant divided by a unit weight, volume, distance, or duration of the activity emitting the pollutant (e.g., kilograms of particulate emitted per tonne of coal burned). Such factors facilitate estimation of emissions from various sources of air pollution. In most cases, these factors are simply averages of all available data of acceptable quality, and are generally assumed to be representative of long-term averages.

There are 12 compounds in the list of persistent organic pollutants. Dioxins and furans are two of them and intentionally created by combustion of organics, like open burning of plastics. These compounds are also endocrine disruptors and can mutate the human genes.

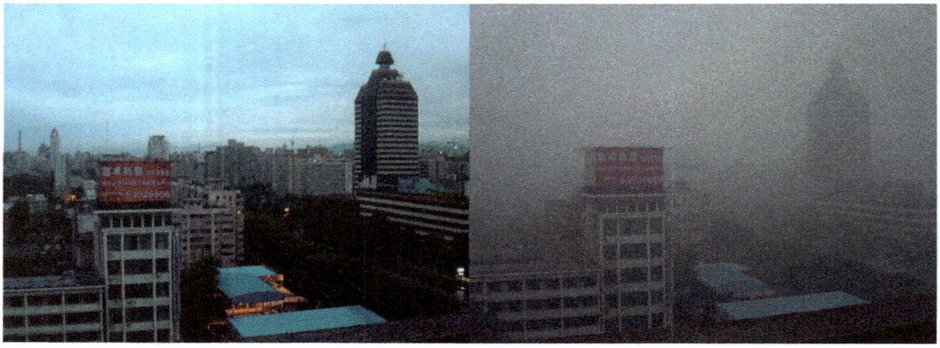

Beijing air on a 2005-day after rain (left) and a smoggy day (right).

The United States Environmental Protection Agency has published a compilation of air pollutant emission factors for a wide range of industrial sources. The United Kingdom, Australia, Canada and many other countries have published similar compilations, as well as the European Environment Agency.

Exposure

Air pollution risk is a function of the hazard of the pollutant and the exposure to that pollutant. Air pollution exposure can be expressed for an individual, for certain groups (e.g. neighborhoods or children living in a country), or for entire populations. For example, one may want to calculate the exposure to a hazardous air pollutant for a geographic area, which includes the various microenvironments and age groups. This can be calculated as an inhalation exposure. This would account for daily exposure in various settings (e.g. different indoor micro-environments and outdoor locations). The exposure needs to include different age and other demographic groups, especially infants, children, pregnant women and other sensitive subpopulations. The exposure to an air pollutant must integrate the concentrations of the air pollutant with respect to the time spent in each setting and the respective inhalation rates for each subgroup for each specific time that the subgroup is in the setting and engaged in particular activities (playing, cooking, reading, working, etc.). For example, a small child's inhalation rate will be less than that of an adult. A child engaged in vigorous exercise will have a higher respiration rate than the same child in a sedentary activity. The daily exposure, then, needs to reflect the time spent in each micro-environmental setting and the type of activities in these settings. The air pollutant concentration in each microactivity/microenvironmental setting is summed to indicate the exposure.

Indoor Air Quality (IAQ)

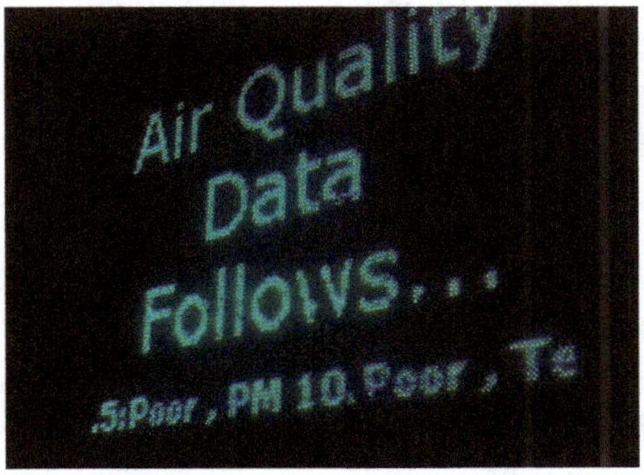

Air quality monitoring, New Delhi, India.

A lack of ventilation indoors concentrates air pollution where people often spend the majority of their time. Radon (Rn) gas, a carcinogen, is exuded from the Earth in certain locations and trapped inside houses. Building materials including carpeting and plywood emit formaldehyde (H_2CO) gas. Paint and solvents give off volatile organic compounds (VOCs) as they dry. Lead paint can degenerate into dust and be inhaled. Intentional air pollution is introduced with the use of air fresheners, incense, and other scented items. Controlled wood fires in stoves and fireplaces can add significant amounts of smoke particulates into the air, inside and out. Indoor pollution fatalities may be caused by using pesticides and other chemical sprays indoors without proper ventilation.

Carbon monoxide poisoning and fatalities are often caused by faulty vents and chimneys, or by the burning of charcoal indoors or in a confined space, such as a tent. Chronic carbon monoxide poisoning can result even from poorly-adjusted pilot lights. Traps are built into all domestic plumbing to keep sewer gas and hydrogen sulfide, out of interiors. Clothing emits tetrachloroethylene, or other dry cleaning fluids, for days after dry cleaning.

Though its use has now been banned in many countries, the extensive use of asbestos in industrial and domestic environments in the past has left a potentially very dangerous material in many localities. Asbestosis is a chronic inflammatory medical condition affecting the tissue of the lungs. It occurs after long-term, heavy exposure to asbestos from asbestos-containing materials in structures. Sufferers have severe dyspnea (shortness of breath) and are at an increased risk regarding several different types of lung cancer. As clear explanations are not always stressed in non-technical literature, care should be taken to distinguish between several forms of relevant diseases. According to the World Health Organisation (WHO), these may defined as; asbestosis, *lung cancer*, and *Peritoneal Mesothelioma* (generally a very rare form of cancer, when more widespread it is almost always associated with prolonged exposure to asbestos).

Biological sources of air pollution are also found indoors, as gases and airborne particulates. Pets produce dander, people produce dust from minute skin flakes and decomposed hair, dust mites in bedding, carpeting and furniture produce enzymes and micrometre-sized fecal droppings, inhabitants emit methane, mold forms on walls and generates mycotoxins and spores, air conditioning systems can incubate Legionnaires' disease and mold, and houseplants, soil and surrounding gardens can produce pollen, dust, and mold. Indoors, the lack of air circulation allows these airborne pollutants to accumulate more than they would otherwise occur in nature.

Health Effects

Air pollution is a significant risk factor for a number of pollution-related diseases and health conditions including respiratory infections, heart disease, COPD, stroke and lung cancer. The health effects caused by air pollution may include difficulty in breathing, wheezing, coughing, asthma and worsening of existing respiratory and cardiac conditions. These effects can result in increased medication use, increased doctor or emergency room visits, more hospital admissions and premature death. The human health effects of poor air quality are far reaching, but principally affect the body's respiratory system and the cardiovascular system. Individual reactions to air pollutants depend on the type of pollutant a person is exposed to, the degree of exposure, and the individual's health status and genetics. The most common sources of air pollution include particulates, ozone, nitrogen dioxide, and sulphur dioxide. Children aged less than five years that live in developing countries are the most vulnerable population in terms of total deaths attributable to indoor and outdoor air pollution.

Mortality

The World Health Organization estimated in 2014 that every year air pollution causes the premature death of some 7 million people worldwide. India has the highest death rate due to air pollution. India also has more deaths from asthma than any other nation according to the World Health Organization. In December 2013 air pollution was estimated to kill 500,000 people in China each year. There is a positive correlation between pneumonia-related deaths and air pollution from motor vehicle emissions.

Annual premature European deaths caused by air pollution are estimated at 430,000. An important cause of these deaths is nitrogen dioxide and other nitrogen oxides (NOx) emitted by road vehicles.Across the European Union, air pollution is estimated to reduce life expectancy by almost nine months. Causes of deaths include strokes, heart disease, COPD, lung cancer, and lung infections.

Urban outdoor air pollution is estimated to cause 1.3 million deaths worldwide per year. Children are particularly at risk due to the immaturity of their respiratory organ systems.

The US EPA estimates that a proposed set of changes in diesel engine technology (*Tier 2*) could result in 12,000 fewer *premature mortalities*, 15,000 fewer heart attacks, 6,000 fewer emergency room visits by children with asthma, and 8,900 fewer respiratory-related hospital admissions each year in the United States.

The US EPA has estimated that limiting ground-level ozone concentration to 65 parts per billion, would avert 1,700 to 5,100 premature deaths nationwide in 2020 compared with the 75-ppb standard. The agency projected the more protective standard would also prevent an additional 26,000 cases of aggravated asthma, and more than a million cases of missed work or school. Following this assessment, the EPA acted to protect public health by lowering the National Ambient Air Quality Standards (NAAQS) for ground-level ozone to 70 parts per billion (ppb).

A new economic study of the health impacts and associated costs of air pollution in the Los Angeles Basin and San Joaquin Valley of Southern California shows that more than 3,800 people die prematurely (approximately 14 years earlier than normal) each year because air pollution levels violate federal standards. The number of annual premature deaths is considerably higher than the fatalities related to auto collisions in the same area, which average fewer than 2,000 per year.

Diesel exhaust (DE) is a major contributor to combustion-derived particulate matter air pollution. In several human experimental studies, using a well-validated exposure chamber setup, DE has been linked to acute vascular dysfunction and increased thrombus formation.

The mechanisms linking air pollution to increased cardiovascular mortality are uncertain, but probably include pulmonary and systemic inflammation.

Cardiovascular Disease

A 2007 review of evidence found ambient air pollution exposure is a risk factor correlating with increased total mortality from cardiovascular events (range: 12% to 14% per 10 microg/m^3 increase).

Air pollution is also emerging as a risk factor for stroke, particularly in developing countries where pollutant levels are highest. A 2007 study found that in women, air pollution is not associated with hemorrhagic but with ischemic stroke. Air pollution was also found to be associated with increased incidence and mortality from coronary stroke in a cohort study in 2011. Associations are believed to be causal and effects may be mediated by vasoconstriction, low-grade inflammation and atherosclerosis Other mechanisms such as autonomic nervous system imbalance have also been suggested.

Lung disease

Chronic obstructive pulmonary disease (COPD) includes diseases such as chronic bronchitis and emphysema.

Research has demonstrated increased risk of developing asthma and COPD from increased exposure to traffic-related air pollution. Additionally, air pollution has been associated with increased hospitalization and mortality from asthma and COPD.

A study conducted in 1960-1961 in the wake of the Great Smog of 1952 compared 293 London residents with 477 residents of Gloucester, Peterborough, and Norwich, three towns with low reported death rates from chronic bronchitis. All subjects were male postal truck drivers aged 40 to 59. Compared to the subjects from the outlying towns, the London subjects exhibited more severe respiratory symptoms (including cough, phlegm, and dyspnea), reduced lung function (FEV_1 and peak flow rate), and increased sputum production and purulence. The differences were more pronounced for subjects aged 50 to 59. The study controlled for age and smoking habits, so concluded that air pollution was the most likely cause of the observed differences.

It is believed that much like cystic fibrosis, by living in a more urban environment serious health hazards become more apparent. Studies have shown that in urban areas patients suffer mucus hypersecretion, lower levels of lung function, and more self-diagnosis of chronic bronchitis and emphysema.

Cancer

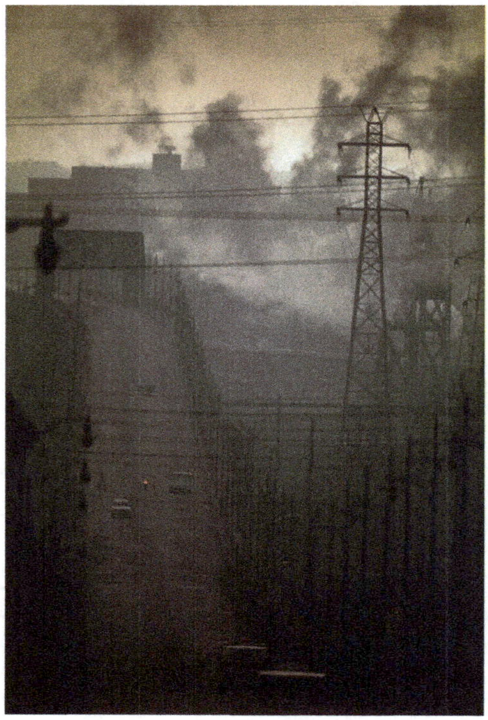

Cancer mainly the result of environmental factors.

A review of evidence regarding whether ambient air pollution exposure is a risk factor for cancer in 2007 found solid data to conclude that long-term exposure to PM2.5 (fine particulates) increases the overall risk of non-accidental mortality by 6% per a 10 microg/m^3 increase. Exposure to PM2.5 was also associated with an increased risk of mortality from lung cancer (range: 15% to 21% per 10 microg/m^3 increase) and total cardiovascular mortality (range: 12% to 14% per a 10 microg/m^3 increase). The review further noted that living close to busy traffic appears to be associated with elevated risks of these three outcomes --- increase in lung cancer deaths, cardiovascular deaths, and overall non-accidental deaths. The reviewers also found suggestive evidence that exposure to PM2.5 is positively associated with mortality from coronary heart diseases and exposure to SO_2 increases mortality from lung cancer, but the data was insufficient to provide solid conclusions. Another investigation showed that higher activity level increases deposition fraction of aerosol particles in human lung and recommended avoiding heavy activities like running in outdoor space at polluted areas.

In 2011, a large Danish epidemiological study found an increased risk of lung cancer for patients who lived in areas with high nitrogen oxide concentrations. In this study, the association was higher for non-smokers than smokers. An additional Danish study, also in 2011, likewise noted evidence of possible associations between air pollution and other forms of cancer, including cervical cancer and brain cancer.

In December 2015, medical scientists reported that cancer is overwhelmingly a result of environmental factors, and not largely down to bad luck. Maintaining a healthy weight, eating a healthy diet, minimizing alcohol and eliminating smoking reduces the risk of developing the disease, according to the researchers.

Children

In the United States, despite the passage of the Clean Air Act in 1970, in 2002 at least 146 million Americans were living in non-attainment areas—regions in which the concentration of certain air pollutants exceeded federal standards. These dangerous pollutants are known as the criteria pollutants, and include ozone, particulate matter, sulfur dioxide, nitrogen dioxide, carbon monoxide, and lead. Protective measures to ensure children's health are being taken in cities such as New Delhi, India where buses now use compressed natural gas to help eliminate the "pea-soup" smog. A recent study in Europe has found that exposure to ultrafine particles can increase blood pressure in children.

Clean areas

Even in the areas with relatively low levels of air pollution, public health effects can be significant and costly, since a large number of people breathe in such pollutants. A 2005 scientific study for the British Columbia Lung Association showed that a small improvement in air quality (1% reduction of ambient PM2.5 and ozone concentrations) would produce $29 million in annual savings in the Metro Vancouver region in 2010. This finding is based on health valuation of lethal (death) and sub-lethal (illness) affects.

Central Nervous System

Data is accumulating that air pollution exposure also affects the central nervous system.

In a June 2014 study conducted by researchers at the University of Rochester Medical Center, published in the journal Environmental Health Perspectives, it was discovered that early exposure to air pollution causes the same damaging changes in the brain as autism and schizophrenia. The study also shows that air pollution also affected short-term memory, learning ability, and impulsivity. Lead researcher Professor Deborah Cory-Slechta said that When we looked closely at the ventricles, we could see that the white matter that normally surrounds them hadn't fully developed. It appears that inflammation had damaged those brain cells and prevented that region of the brain from developing, and the ventricles simply expanded to fill the space. Our findings add to the growing body of evidence that air pollution may play a role in autism, as well as in other neurodevelopmental disorders. Air pollution has a more significant negative effect on males than on females.

In 2015, experimental studies reported the detection of significant episodic (situational) cognitive impairment from impurities in indoor air breathed by test subjects who were not informed about changes in the air quality. Researchers at the Harvard University and SUNY Upstate Medical University and Syracuse University measured the cognitive performance of 24 participants in three different controlled laboratory atmospheres that simulated those found in conventional and green buildings, as well as green buildings with enhanced ventilation. Performance was evaluated objectively using the widely used Strategic Management Simulation software simulation tool, which is a well-validated assessment test for executive decision-making in an unconstrained situation allowing initiative and improvisation. Significant deficits were observed in the performance scores achieved in increasing concentrations of either volatile organic compounds (VOCs) or carbon dioxide, while keeping other factors constant. The highest impurity levels reached are not uncommon in some classroom or office environments.

Agricultural Effects

In India in 2014, it was reported that air pollution by black carbon and ground level ozone had cut crop yields in the most affected areas by almost half in 2010 when compared to 1980 levels.

Economic effects

Air pollution costs the world economy $5 trillion per year as a result of productivity losses and degraded quality of life, according to a joint study by the World Bank and the Institute for Health Metrics and Evaluation (IHME) at the University of Washington These productivity losses are caused by deaths due to diseases caused by air pollution. One out of ten deaths in 2013 was caused by diseases associated with air pollution and the problem is getting worse. The problem is even more acute in the developing world. Children under age 5 in lower-income countries are more than 60 times as likely to die from exposure to air pollution as children in high-income countries. The report states that additional economic losses caused by air pollution, including health costs and the adverse effect on agricultural and other productivity were not calculated in the report, and thus the actual costs to the world economy are far higher than $5 trillion.

Historical Disasters

The world's worst short-term civilian pollution crisis was the 1984 Bhopal Disaster in India. Leaked industrial vapours from the Union Carbide factory, belonging to Union Carbide, Inc., U.S.A. (later bought by Dow Chemical Company), killed at least 3787 people and injured from 150,000 to 600,000. The United Kingdom suffered its worst air pollution event when the December 4 Great Smog of 1952 formed over London. In six days more than 4,000 died and more recent estimates put the figure at nearer 12,000.

An accidental leak of anthrax spores from a biological warfare laboratory in the former USSR in 1979 near Sverdlovsk is believed to have caused at least 64 deaths. The worst single incident of air pollution to occur in the US occurred in Donora, Pennsylvania in late October, 1948, when 20 people died and over 7,000 were injured.

Alternatives to pollution

There are now practical alternatives to the three principal causes of air pollution.

- Combustion of fossil fuels for space heating can be replaced by using ground source heat pumps and seasonal thermal energy storage.
- Electric power generation from burning fossil fuels can be replaced by power generation from nuclear and renewables.
- Motor vehicles driven by fossil fuels, a key factor in urban air pollution, can be replaced by electric vehicles.

Reduction Efforts

There are various air pollution control technologies and strategies available to reduce air pollution.At its most basic level, land-use planning is likely to involve zoning and transport infrastructure planning. In most developed countries, land-use planning is an important part of social policy, ensuring that land is used efficiently for the benefit of the wider economy and population, as well as to protect the environment.

Because a large share of air pollution is caused by combustion of fossil fuels such as coal and oil, the reduction of these fuels can reduce air pollution drastically. Most effective is the switch to clean power sources such as wind power, solar power, hydro power which don't cause air pollution. Efforts to reduce pollution from mobile sources includes primary regulation (many developing countries have permissive regulations), expanding regulation to new sources (such as cruise and transport ships, farm equipment, and small gas-powered equipment such as string trimmers, chainsaws, and snowmobiles), increased fuel efficiency (such as through the use of hybrid vehicles), conversion to cleaner fuels or conversion to electric vehicles.

Titanium dioxide has been researched for its ability to reduce air pollution. Ultraviolet light will release free electrons from material, thereby creating free radicals, which break up VOCs and NOx gases. One form is superhydrophilic.

In 2014, Prof. Tony Ryan and Prof. Simon Armitage of University of Sheffield prepared a 10 meter by 20 meter-sized poster coated with microscopic, pollution-eating nanoparticles of titanium dioxide. Placed on a building, this giant poster can absorb the toxic emission from around 20 cars each day.

A very effective means to reduce air pollution is the transition to renewable energy. According to a study published in Energy and Environmental Science in 2015 the switch to 100% renewable energy in the United States would eliminate about 62,000 premature mortalities per year and about 42,000 in 2050, if no biomass were used. This would save about $600 billion in health costs a year due to reduced air pollution in 2050, or about 3.6% of the 2014 U.S. gross domestic product.

Control Devices

The following items are commonly used as pollution control devices in industry and transportation. They can either destroy contaminants or remove them from an exhaust stream before it is emitted into the atmosphere.

- Particulate control
    - Mechanical collectors (dust cyclones, multicyclones)
    - Electrostatic precipitators An electrostatic precipitator (ESP), or electrostatic air cleaner is a particulate collection device that removes particles from a flowing gas (such as air), using the force of an induced electrostatic charge. Electrostatic precipitators are highly efficient filtration devices that minimally impede the flow of gases through the device, and can easily remove fine particulates such as dust and smoke from the air stream.
    - Baghouses Designed to handle heavy dust loads, a dust collector consists of a blower, dust filter, a filter-cleaning system, and a dust receptacle or dust removal system (distinguished from air cleaners which utilize disposable filters to remove the dust).
    - Particulate scrubbers Wet scrubber is a form of pollution control technology. The term describes a variety of devices that use pollutants from a furnace flue gas or from other gas streams. In a wet scrubber, the polluted gas stream is brought into contact with the scrubbing liquid, by spraying it with the liquid, by forcing it through a pool of liquid, or by some other contact method, so as to remove the pollutants.
- Scrubbers
    - Baffle spray scrubber
    - Cyclonic spray scrubber
    - Ejector venturi scrubber
    - Mechanically aided scrubber
    - Spray tower
    - Wet scrubber
- NOx control
    - Low NOx burners
    - Selective catalytic reduction (SCR)
    - Selective non-catalytic reduction (SNCR)
    - NOx scrubbers
    - Exhaust gas recirculation
    - Catalytic converter (also for VOC control)
- VOC abatement
    - Adsorption systems, using activated carbon, such as Fluidized Bed Concentrator

- Flares
- Thermal oxidizers
- Catalytic converters
- Biofilters
- Absorption (scrubbing)
- Cryogenic condensers
- Vapor recovery systems

■ Acid Gas/SO_2 **control**

- Wet scrubbers
- Dry scrubbers
- Flue-gas desulfurization

■ Mercury **control**

- Sorbent Injection Technology
- Electro-Catalytic Oxidation (ECO)
- K-Fuel

■ Dioxin **and** furan **control**

■ Miscellaneous associated equipment

- Source capturing systems
- Continuous emissions monitoring systems (CEMS)

Regulations

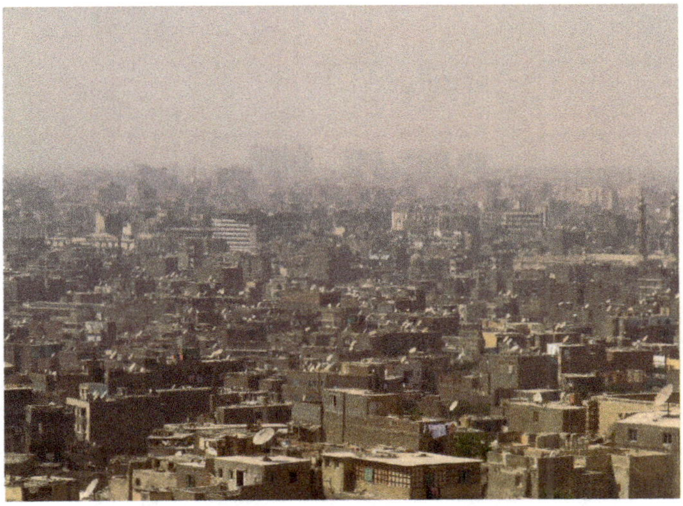

Smog in Cairo.

In general, there are two types of air quality standards. The first class of standards (such as the U.S. National Ambient Air Quality Standards and E.U. Air Quality Directive) set maximum atmospheric concentrations for specific pollutants. Environmental agencies enact regulations which are intended to result in attainment of these target levels. The second class (such as the North American Air Quality Index) take the form of a scale with various thresholds, which is used to communicate to the public the relative risk of outdoor activity. The scale may or may not distinguish between different pollutants.

Canada

In Canada, air pollution and associated health risks are measured with the Air Quality Health Index or (AQHI). It is a health protection tool used to make decisions to reduce short-term exposure to air pollution by adjusting activity levels during increased levels of air pollution.

The Air Quality Health Index or AQHI is a federal program jointly coordinated by Health Canada and Environment Canada. However, the AQHI program would not be possible without the commitment and support of the provinces, municipalities and NGOs. From air quality monitoring to health risk communication and community engagement, local partners are responsible for the vast majority of work related to AQHI implementation. The AQHI provides a number from 1 to 10+ to indicate the level of health risk associated with local air quality. Occasionally, when the amount of air pollution is abnormally high, the number may exceed 10. The AQHI provides a local air quality current value as well as a local air quality maximums forecast for today, tonight and tomorrow and provides associated health advice.

1	2	3	4	5	6	7	8	9	10	+

Risk:	Low **(1-3)**	Moderate **(4-6)**	High **(7-10)**	Very high **(above 10)**

As it is now known that even low levels of air pollution can trigger discomfort for the sensitive population, the index has been developed as a continuum: The higher the number, the greater the health risk and need to take precautions. The index describes the level of health risk associated with this number as 'low', 'moderate', 'high' or 'very high', and suggests steps that can be taken to reduce exposure.

Health Risk	**Air Quality Health Index**	**Health Messages**	
		At Risk population	**General Population**
Low	**1-3**	**Enjoy** your usual outdoor activities.	**Ideal** air quality for outdoor activities

Moderate	**4-6**	**Consider reducing** or rescheduling strenuous activities outdoors if you are experiencing symptoms.	**No need to modify** your usual outdoor activities unless you experience symptoms such as coughing and throat irritation.
High	**7-10**	**Reduce** or reschedule strenuous activities outdoors. Children and the elderly should also take it easy.	**Consider reducing** or rescheduling strenuous activities outdoors if you experience symptoms such as coughing and throat irritation.
Very high	**Above 10**	**Avoid** strenuous activities outdoors. Children and the elderly should also avoid outdoor physical exertion and should stay indoors.	**Reduce** or reschedule strenuous activities outdoors, especially if you experience symptoms such as coughing and throat irritation.

The measurement is based on the observed relationship of Nitrogen Dioxide (NO_2), ground-level Ozone (O_3) and particulates ($PM_{2.5}$) with mortality, from an analysis of several Canadian cities. Significantly, all three of these pollutants can pose health risks, even at low levels of exposure, especially among those with pre-existing health problems.

When developing the AQHI, Health Canada's original analysis of health effects included five major air pollutants: particulates, ozone, and nitrogen dioxide (NO2), as well as sulfur dioxide (SO_2), and carbon monoxide (CO). The latter two pollutants provided little information in predicting health effects and were removed from the AQHI formulation.

The AQHI does not measure the effects of odour, pollen, dust, heat or humidity.

Germany

TA Luft is the German air quality regulation.

Hotspots

Air pollution hotspots are areas where air pollution emissions expose individuals to increased negative health effects. They are particularly common in highly populated, urban areas, where there may be a combination of stationary sources (e.g. industrial facilities) and mobile sources (e.g. cars and trucks) of pollution. Emissions from these sources can cause respiratory disease, childhood asthma, cancer, and other health problems. Fine particulate matter such as diesel soot, which contributes to more than 3.2 million premature deaths around the world each year, is a significant problem. It is very small and can lodge itself within the lungs and enter the bloodstream. Diesel soot is concentrated in densely populated areas, and one in six people in the U.S. live near a diesel pollution hot spot.

While air pollution hotspots affect a variety of populations, some groups are more likely to be located in hotspots. Previous studies have shown disparities in exposure to pollution by race and/or income. Hazardous land uses (toxic storage and disposal facilities, manufacturing facilities, major roadways) tend to be located where property values and income levels are low. Low socioeconomic status can be a proxy for other kinds of social vulnerability, including race, a lack of ability to influence regulation and a lack of ability to move to neighborhoods with less environmental pollution. These communities bear a disproportionate burden of environmental pollution and are more likely to face health risks such as cancer or asthma.

Studies show that patterns in race and income disparities not only indicate a higher exposure to pollution but also higher risk of adverse health outcomes. Communities characterized by low socioeconomic status and racial minorities can be more vulnerable to cumulative adverse health impacts resulting from elevated exposure to pollutants than more privileged communities. Blacks and Latinos generally face more pollution than whites and Asians, and low-income communities bear a higher burden of risk than affluent ones. Racial discrepancies are particularly distinct in suburban areas of the US South and metropolitan areas of the US West. Residents in public housing, who are generally low-income and cannot move to healthier neighborhoods, are highly affected by nearby refineries and chemical plants.

Cities

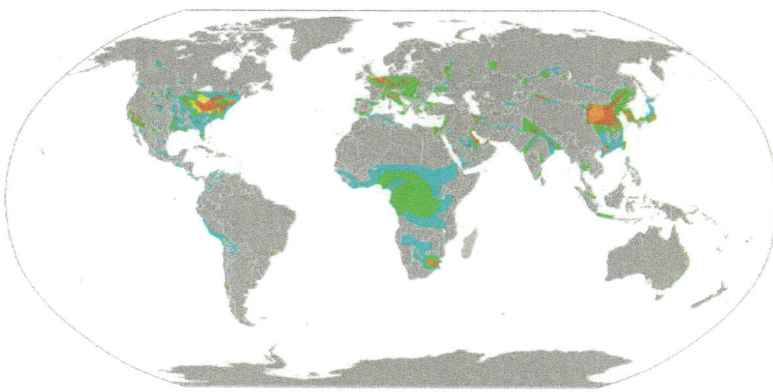

Nitrogen dioxide concentrations as measured from satellite 2002-2004.

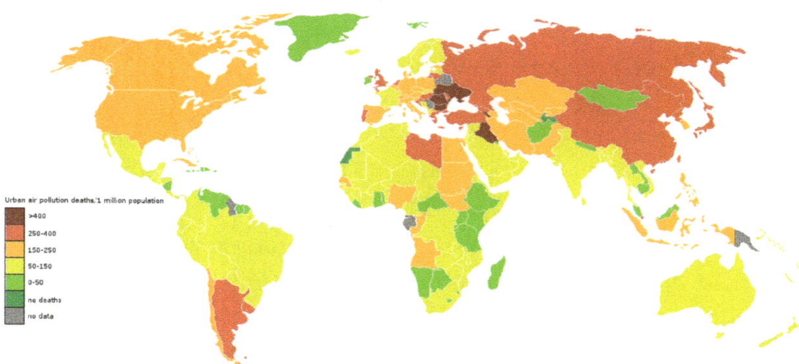

Deaths from air pollution in 2004.

Air pollution is usually concentrated in densely populated metropolitan areas, especially in developing countries where environmental regulations are relatively lax or nonexistent. However, even populated areas in developed countries attain unhealthy levels of pollution, with Los Angeles and Rome being two examples. Between 2002 and 2011 the incidence of lung cancer in Beijing near doubled. While smoking remains the leading cause of lung cancer in China, the number of smokers is falling while lung cancer rates are rising. Another project focusing on the effects on pollution in vegetation has been researched by the local university in Sheffield, UK.

National-scale air toxics assessments 1995-2005

The national-scale air toxics assessment(NATA) is an evaluation of air toxics by the U.S. EPA. EPA has furnished four assessments that characterize nationwide chronic cancer risk estimates and noncancer hazards from inhaling air toxics. The lates was from 2005, and made publicly available in early 2011.

EPA developed the NATA as a state-of-the-science screening tool for State/Local/Tribal Agencies to prioritize pollutants, emission sources and locations of interest for further study, in order to gain a better understanding of the risks. NATA assessments do not incorporate refined information about emission sources, but rather, use general information about sources to develop estimates of risks which are more likely to overestimate impacts than underestimate them. NATA provides estimates of the risk of cancer and other serious health effects from breathing (inhaling) air toxics in order to inform both national and more localized efforts to identify and prioritize air toxics, emission source types and locations which are of greatest potential concern in terms of contributing to population risk. This in turn helps air pollution experts focus limited analytical resources on areas and or populations where the potential for health risks are highest. Assessments include estimates of cancer and non-cancer health effects based on chronic exposure from outdoor sources, including assessments of non-cancer health effects for Diesel Particulate Matter. Assessments provide a snapshot of the outdoor air quality and the risks to human health that would result if air toxic emissions levels remained unchanged.

Most polluted cities by PM	
Particulate matter, µg/m³ (2004)	**City**
168	Cairo, Egypt
150	Delhi, India
128	Kolkata, India (Calcutta)
125	Tianjin, China
123	Chongqing, China
109	Kanpur, India
109	Lucknow, India
104	Jakarta, Indonesia
101	Shenyang, China

Governing Urban Air Pollution

In Europe, Council Directive 96/62/EC on ambient air quality assessment and management provides a common strategy against which member states can "set objectives for ambient air quality in order to avoid, prevent or reduce harmful effects on human health and the environment . . . and improve air quality where it is unsatisfactory".

On 25 July 2008 in the case Dieter Janecek v Freistaat Bayern CURIA, the European Court of Justice ruled that under this directive citizens have the right to require national authorities to implement a short term action plan that aims to maintain or achieve compliance to air quality limit values.

This important case law appears to confirm the role of the EC as centralised regulator to European nation-states as regards air pollution control. It places a supranational legal obligation on the UK to protect its citizens from dangerous levels of air pollution, furthermore superseding national interests with those of the citizen.

In 2010, the European Commission (EC) threatened the UK with legal action against the successive breaching of PM10 limit values. The UK government has identified that if fines are imposed, they could cost the nation upwards of £300 million per year.

In March 2011, the Greater London Built-up Area remains the only UK region in breach of the EC's limit values, and has been given 3 months to implement an emergency action plan aimed at meeting the EU Air Quality Directive. The City of London has dangerous levels of PM10 concentrations, estimated to cause 3000 deaths per year within the city. As well as the threat of EU fines, in 2010 it was threatened with legal action for scrapping the western congestion charge zone, which is claimed to have led to an increase in air pollution levels.

In response to these charges, Boris Johnson, Mayor of London, has criticised the current need for European cities to communicate with Europe through their nation state's central government, arguing that in future A great city like London should be permitted to bypass its government and deal directly with the European Commission regarding its air quality action plan.

This can be interpreted as recognition that cities can transcend the traditional national government organisational hierarchy and develop solutions to air pollution using global governance networks, for example through transnational relations. Transnational relations include but are not exclusive to national governments and intergovernmental organisations, allowing sub-national actors including cities and regions to partake in air pollution control as independent actors.

Particularly promising at present are global city partnerships. These can be built into networks, for example the C40 Cities Climate Leadership Group, of which London is a member. The C40 is a public ‹non-state' network of the world's leading cities that aims to curb their greenhouse emissions. The C40 has been identified as ‹governance from the middle' and is an alternative to intergovernmental policy. It has the potential to improve urban air quality as participating cities exchange information, learn from best practices and consequently mitigate carbon dioxide emissions independently from national government decisions. A criticism of the C40 network is that its exclusive nature limits influence to participating cities and risks drawing resources away from less powerful city and regional actors.

Atmospheric Dispersion

The basic technology for analyzing air pollution is through the use of a variety of mathematical models for predicting the transport of air pollutants in the lower atmosphere. The principal methodologies are:

- Point source dispersion, used for industrial sources
- Line source dispersion, used for airport and roadway air dispersion modeling
- Area source dispersion, used for forest fires or duststorms
- Photochemical models, used to analyze reactive pollutants that form smog

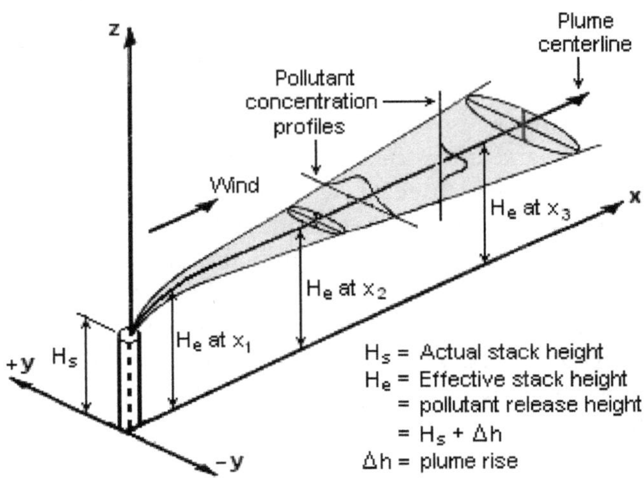

Visualization of a buoyant Gaussian air pollution dispersion plume as used in many atmospheric dispersion models.

The point source problem is the best understood, since it involves simpler mathematics and has been studied for a long period of time, dating back to about the year 1900. It uses a Gaussian dispersion model for continuous buoyant pollution plumes to predict the air pollution isopleths, with consideration given to wind velocity, stack height, emission rate and stability class (a measure of atmospheric turbulence).This model has been extensively validated and calibrated with experimental data for all sorts of atmospheric conditions.

The roadway air dispersion model was developed starting in the late 1950s and early 1960s in response to requirements of the National Environmental Policy Act and the U.S. Department of Transportation (then known as the Federal Highway Administration) to understand impacts of proposed new highways upon air quality, especially in urban areas. Several research groups were active in this model development, among which were: the Environmental Research and Technology (ERT) group in Lexington, Massachusetts, the ESL Inc. group in Sunnyvale, California and the California Air Resources Board group in Sacramento, California. The research of the ESL group received a boost with a contract award from the United States Environmental Protection Agency to validate a line source model using sulfur hexafluoride as a tracer gas. This program was successful in validating the line source model developed by ESL Inc. Some of the earliest uses of the model were in court cases involving highway air pollution; the Arlington, Virginia portion of Interstate 66 and the New Jersey Turnpike widening project through East Brunswick, New Jersey.

Area source models were developed in 1971 through 1974 by the ERT and ESL groups, but addressed a smaller fraction of total air pollution emissions, so that their use and need was not as widespread as the line source model, which enjoyed hundreds of different applications as early as the 1970s. Similarly photochemical models were developed primarily in the 1960s and 70s, but their use was more specialized and for regional needs, such as understanding smog formation in Los Angeles, California.

ACID RAIN

Acid rain is a rain or any other form of precipitation that is unusually acidic, meaning that it possesses elevated levels of hydrogen ions (low pH). It can have harmful effects on plants, aquatic animals and infrastructure. Acid rain is caused by emissions of sulfur dioxide and nitrogen oxide, which react with the water molecules in the atmosphere to produce acids. Some governments have made efforts since the 1970s to reduce the release of sulfur dioxide and nitrogen oxide into the atmosphere with positive results. Nitrogen oxides can also be produced naturally by lightning strikes, and sulfur dioxide is produced by volcanic eruptions. Acid rain has been shown to have adverse impacts on forests, freshwaters and soils, killing insect and aquatic life-forms, causing paint to peel, corrosion of steel structures such as bridges, and weathering of stone buildings and statues as well as having impacts on human health.

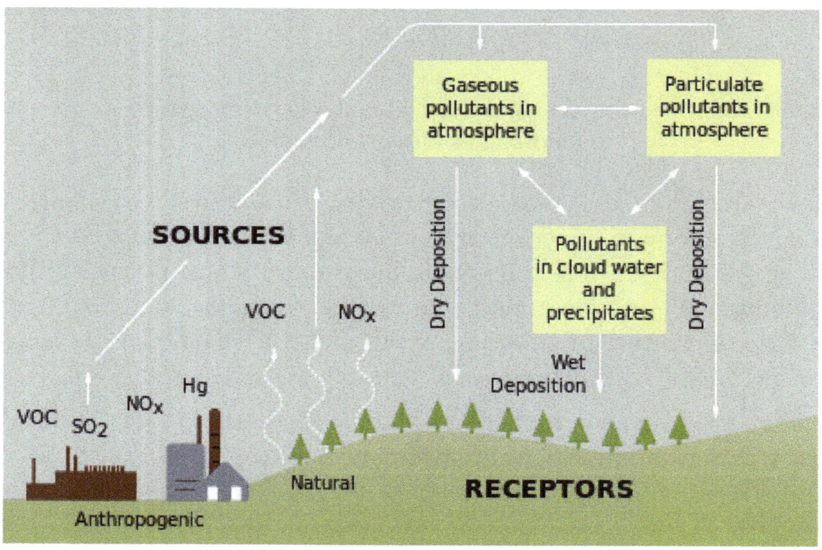

Processes involved in acid deposition (note that only SO_2 and NO_x play a significant role in acid rain).

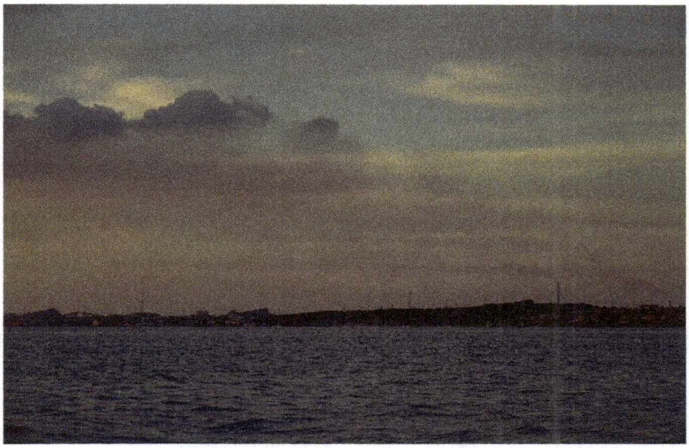

Acid clouds can grow on SO_2 emissions from refineries, as seen here in Curaçao.

Acid rain is a popular term referring to the deposition of a mixture from wet (rain, snow, sleet, fog, cloudwater, and dew) and dry (acidifying particles and gases) acidic components. Distilled water, once carbon dioxide is removed, has a neutral pH of 7. Liquids with a pH less than 7 are acidic, and those with a pH greater than 7 are alkaline. Clean or unpolluted rain has an acidic pH, but usually no lower than 5.7, because carbon dioxide and water in the air react together to form carbonic acid, a weak acid according to the following reaction:

$H_2O\ (l) + CO_2\ (g) \rightleftharpoons H_2CO_3\ (aq)$

Carbonic acid then can ionize in water forming low concentrations of hydronium and carbonate ions:

$H_2O\ (l) + H_2CO_3\ (aq) \rightleftharpoons HCO_3^-\ (aq) + H_3O^+\ (aq)$

However, unpolluted rain can also contain other chemicals which affect its pH (acidity level). A common example is nitric acid produced by electric discharge in the atmosphere such as lightning. Acid deposition as an environmental issue (discussed later in the article) would include additional acids other than H_2CO_3.

The corrosive effect of polluted, acidic city air on limestone and marble was noted in the 17th century by John Evelyn, who remarked upon the poor condition of the Arundel marbles.Since the Industrial Revolution, emissions of sulfur dioxide and nitrogen oxides into the atmosphere have increased. In 1852, Robert Angus Smith was the first to show the relationship between acid rain and atmospheric pollution in Manchester, England.

Though acidic rain was discovered in 1853, it was not until the late 1960s that scientists began widely observing and studying the phenomenon. The term "acid rain" was coined in 1872 by Robert Angus Smith. Canadian Harold Harvey was among the first to research a "dead" lake. Public awareness of acid rain in the U.S increased in the 1970s after The New York Times published reports from the Hubbard Brook Experimental Forest in New Hampshire of the myriad deleterious environmental effects shown to result from it.

Occasional pH readings in rain and fog water of well below 2.4 have been reported in industrialized areas. Industrial acid rain is a substantial problem in China and Russia and areas downwind from them. These areas all burn sulfur-containing coal to generate heat and electricity.

The problem of acid rain has not only increased with population and industrial growth, but has become more widespread. The use of tall smokestacks to reduce local pollution has contributed to the spread of acid rain by releasing gases into regional atmospheric circulation. Often deposition occurs a considerable distance downwind of the emissions, with mountainous regions tending to receive the greatest deposition (simply because of their higher rainfall). An example of this effect is the low pH of rain which falls in Scandinavia.

History of Acid Rain in the United States

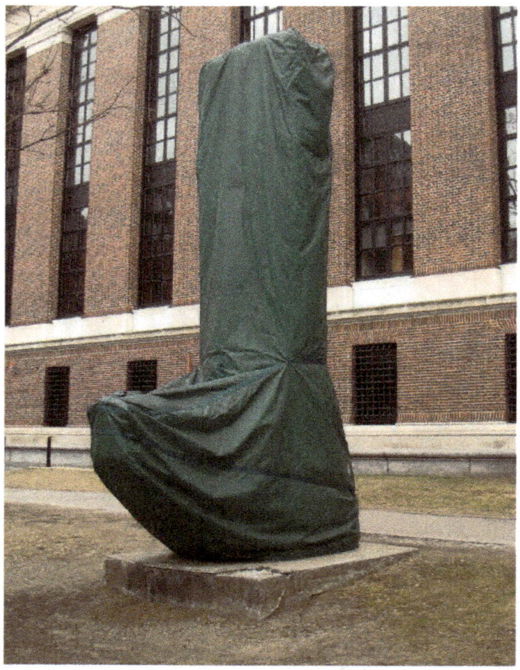

Since 1998, Harvard University wraps some of the bronze and marble statues on its campus, such as this "Chinese stele", with waterproof covers every winter, in order to protect them from erosion caused by acid rain and acid snow

The earliest report about acid rain in the United States was from the chemical evidence from Hubbard Brook Valley. In 1972, a group of scientists including Gene Likens discovered the rain that was deposited at White Mountains of New Hampshire was acidic. The pH of the sample was measured to be 4.03 at Hubbard Brook. The Hubbard Brook Ecosystem Study followed up with a series of research that analyzed the environmental effects of acid rain. Acid rain that mixed with stream water at Hubbard

Brook was neutralized by the alumina from soils. The result of this research indicates the chemical reaction between acid rain and aluminum leads to increasing rate of soil weathering. Experimental research was done to examine the effects of increased acidity in stream on ecological species. In 1980, a group of scientists modified the acidity of Norris Brook, New Hampshire, and observed the change in species' behaviors. There was a decrease in species diversity, an increase in community dominants, and a decrease in the food web complexity.

In 1980, the U.S. Congress passed an Acid Deposition Act. This Act established an 18-year assessment and research program under the direction of the National Acidic Precipitation Assessment Program (NAPAP). NAPAP looked at the entire problem from a scientific perspective. It enlarged a network of monitoring sites to determine how acidic the precipitation actually was, and to determine long-term trends, and established a network for dry deposition. It looked at the effects of acid rain and funded research on the effects of acid precipitation on freshwater and terrestrial ecosystems, historical buildings, monuments, and building materials. It also funded extensive studies on atmospheric processes and potential control programs.

From the start, policy advocates from all sides attempted to influence NAPAP activities to support their particular policy advocacy efforts, or to disparage those of their opponents. For the U.S. Government's scientific enterprise, a significant impact of NAPAP were lessons learned in the assessment process and in environmental research management to a relatively large group of scientists, program managers and the public.

In 1981, the National Academy of Sciences was looking into research about the controversial issues regarding acid rain. President Ronald Reagan did not place a huge attention on the issues of acid rain until his personal visit to Canada and confirmed that Canadian border suffered from the drifting pollution from smokestacks in Midwest of US. Reagan honored the agreement to Canadian Prime Minister Trudeau's enforcement of anti-pollution regulation. In 1982, US President Ronald Reagan commissioned William Nierenberg to sit on National Science Board. Nierenberg selected scientists including Gene Likens to sit on a panel to draft a report on acid rain. In 1983, the panel of scientists came up with a draft report, which concluded that acid rain is a real problem and solutions should be sought. White House Office of Science and Technology Policy reviewed the draft report and sent Fred Singer's suggestions of the report, which cast doubt on the cause of acid rain.The panelists revealed rejections against Singer's positions and submitted the report to Nirenberg in April. In May 1983, the House of Representatives voted against legislations that aimed to control sulfur emissions. There was a debate about whether Nierenberg delayed to release the report. Nierenberg himself denied the saying about his suppression of the report and explained that the withheld of the report after the House's vote was due to the fact that the report was not ready to be published.

In 1991, DENR provided its first assessment of acid rain in the United States. It reported that 5% of New England Lakes were acidic, with sulfates being the most common problem. They noted that 2% of the lakes could no longer support Brook Trout, and 6% of the lakes were unsuitable for the survival of many species of minnow. Subsequent Reports to Congress have documented chemical changes in soil and freshwater ecosystems, nitrogen saturation, decreases in amounts of nutrients in soil, episodic acidification, regional haze, and damage to historical monuments.

Meanwhile, in 1989, the U.S. Congress passed a series of amendments to the Clean Air Act. Title IV of these amendments established the Acid Rain Program, a cap and trade system designed to control emissions of sulfur dioxide and nitrogen oxides. Title IV called for a total reduction of about 10 million tons of SO_2 emissions from power plants. It was implemented in two phases. Phase I began in 1995, and limited sulfur dioxide emissions from 110 of the largest power plants to a combined total of 8.7 million tons of sulfur dioxide. One power plant in New England (Merrimack) was in Phase I. Four other plants (Newington, Mount Tom, Brayton Point, and Salem Harbor) were added under other provisions of the program. Phase II began in 2000, and affects most of the power plants in the country.

During the 1990s, research continued. On March 10, 2005, EPA issued the Clean Air Interstate Rule (CAIR). This rule provides states with a solution to the problem of power plant pollution that drifts from one state to another. CAIR will permanently cap emissions of SO_2 and NO_x in the eastern United States. When fully implemented, CAIR will reduce SO_2emissions in 28 eastern states and the District of Columbia by over 70% and NO_x emissions by over 60% from 2003 levels.

Overall, the program's cap and trade program has been successful in achieving its goals. Since the 1990s, SO_2 emissions have dropped 40%, and according to the Pacific Research Institute, acid rain levels have dropped 65% since 1976. Conventional regulation was used in the European Union, which saw a decrease of over 70% in SO_2 emissions during the same time period.

In 2007, total SO_2 emissions were 8.9 million tons, achieving the program's long-term goal ahead of the 2010 statutory deadline.

In 2007 the EPA estimated that by 2010, the overall costs of complying with the program for businesses and consumers would be $1 billion to $2 billion a year, only one fourth of what was originally predicted. Forbes says: *In 2010, by which time the cap and trade system had been augmented by the George W. Bush administration's Clean Air Interstate Rule, SO2 emissions had fallen to 5.1 million tons.*

The term Citizen science can be traced back as far as January 1989 and a campaign by the Audubon Society to measure Acid rain. Scientist Muki Haklay cites in a policy report for the Wilson Center entitled ‹Citizen Science and Policy: A European Perspective' a first use of the term ‹citizen science' by R. Kerson in the magazine MIT Technology Review from January 1989. Quoting from the Wilson Center report: The new form of engagement in science received the name citizen science. The first recorded example of the use of the term is from 1989, describing how 225 volunteers across the US collected rain samples to assist the Audubon Society in an acid-rain awareness raising campaign. The volunteers collected samples, checked for acidity, and reported back to the organization. The information was then used to demonstrate the full extent of the phenomenon.

Emissions of Chemicals Leading to Acidification

The most important gas which leads to acidification is sulfur dioxide. Emissions of nitrogen oxides which are oxidized to form nitric acid are of increasing importance due to stricter controls on emissions of sulfur containing compounds. 70 Tg(S) per year in the form of SO_2 comes from fossil fuel combustion and industry, 2.8 Tg(S) from wildfires and 7–8 Tg(S) per year from volcanoes.

Natural Phenomena

The principal natural phenomena that contribute acid-producing gases to the atmosphere are emissions from volcanoes. Thus, for example, fumaroles from the Laguna Caliente crater of Poás Volcano create extremely high amounts of acid rain and fog, with acidity as high as a pH of 2, clearing an area of any vegetation and frequently causing irritation to the eyes and lungs of inhabitants in nearby settlements. Acid-producing gasses are also created by biological processes that occur on the land, in wetlands, and in the oceans. The major biological source of sulfur containing compounds is dimethyl sulfide.

Nitric acid in rainwater is an important source of fixed nitrogen for plant life, and is also produced by electrical activity in the atmosphere such as lightning.

Acidic deposits have been detected in glacial ice thousands of years old in remote parts of the globe.

Soils of coniferous forests are naturally very acidic due to the shedding of needles, and the results of this phenomenon should not be confused with acid rain.

Human Activity

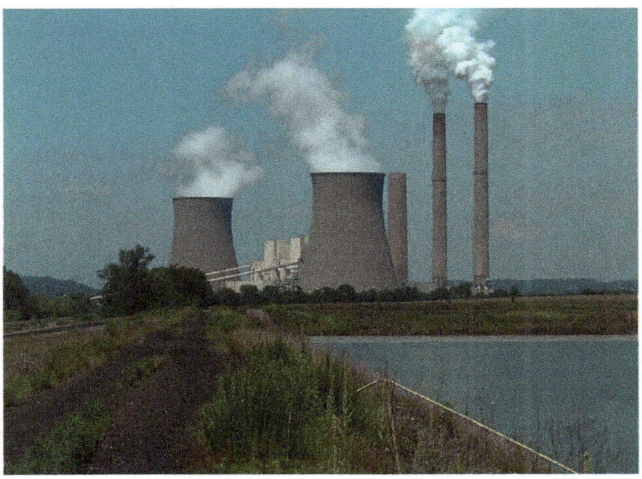

The coal-fired Gavin Power Plant in Cheshire, Ohio.

The principal cause of acid rain is sulfur and nitrogen compounds from human sources, such as electricity generation, factories, and motor vehicles. Electrical power generation using coal is among the greatest contributors to gaseous pollutions that are responsible for acidic rain. The gases can be carried hundreds of kilometers in the atmosphere before they are converted to acids and deposited. In the past, factories had short funnels to let out smoke but this caused many problems locally; thus, factories now have taller smoke funnels. However, dispersal from these taller stacks causes pollutants to be carried farther, causing widespread ecological damage.

Chemical Processes

Combustion of fuels produces sulfur dioxide and nitric oxides. They are converted into sulfuric acid and nitric acid.

Gas Phase Chemistry

In the gas phase sulfur dioxide is oxidized by reaction with the hydroxyl radical via an intermolecular reaction:

$SO_2 + OH\cdot \rightarrow HOSO_2\cdot$

which is followed by:

$HOSO_2\cdot + O_2 \rightarrow HO_2\cdot + SO_3$

In the presence of water, sulfur trioxide (SO_3) is converted rapidly to sulfuric acid:

$SO_3\ (g) + H_2O\ (l) \rightarrow H_2SO_4\ (aq)$

Nitrogen dioxide reacts with OH to form nitric acid:

$NO_2 + OH\cdot \rightarrow HNO_3$

Chemistry in Cloud Droplets

When clouds are present, the loss rate of SO_2 is faster than can be explained by gas phase chemistry alone. This is due to reactions in the liquid water droplets.

Hydrolysis

Sulfur dioxide dissolves in water and then, like carbon dioxide, hydrolyses in a series of equilibrium reactions:

$$SO_2\ (g) + H_2O \rightleftharpoons SO_2{\cdot}H_2O$$

$$SO_2{\cdot}H_2O \rightleftharpoons H^+ + HSO_3^-$$

$$HSO_3^- \rightleftharpoons H^+ + SO_3^{2-}$$

Oxidation

There are a large number of aqueous reactions that oxidize sulfur from S(IV) to S(VI), leading to the formation of sulfuric acid. The most important oxidation reactions are with ozone, hydrogen peroxide and oxygen (reactions with oxygen are catalyzed by iron and manganese in the cloud droplets).

Acid Deposition

Wet Deposition

Wet deposition of acids occurs when any form of precipitation (rain, snow, and so on.) removes acids from the atmosphere and delivers it to the Earth's surface. This can result from the deposition of acids produced in the raindrops (see aqueous phase chemistry above) or by the precipitation removing the acids either in clouds or below clouds. Wet removal of both gases and aerosols are both of importance for wet deposition.

Dry Deposition

Acid deposition also occurs via dry deposition in the absence of precipitation. This can be responsible for as much as 20 to 60% of total acid deposition. This occurs when particles and gases stick to the ground, plants or other surfaces.

Adverse Effects

Acid rain has been shown to have adverse impacts on forests, freshwaters and soils, killing insect and aquatic life-forms as well as causing damage to buildings and having impacts on human health.

Surface Waters and Aquatic Animals

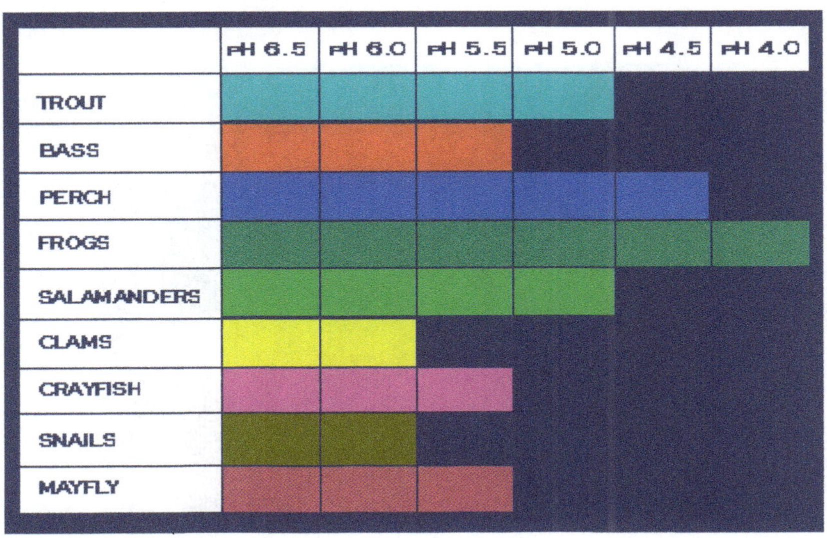

This chart shows that not all fish, shellfish, or the insects that they eat can tolerate the same amount of acid; for example, frogs can tolerate water that is more acidic (i.e., has a lower pH) than trout.

Both the lower pH and higher aluminium concentrations in surface water that occur as a result of acid rain can cause damage to fish and other aquatic animals. At pHs lower than 5 most fish eggs will not hatch and lower pHs can kill adult fish. As lakes and rivers become more acidic biodiversity is reduced. Acid rain has eliminated insect life and some fish species, including the brook trout in some lakes, streams, and creeks in geographically sensitive areas, such as the Adirondack Mountains of the United States. However, the extent to which acid rain contributes directly or indirectly via runoff from the catchment to lake and river acidity (i.e., depending on characteristics of the surrounding watershed) is variable. The United States Environmental Protection Agency's (EPA) website states: "Of the lakes and streams surveyed, acid rain caused acidity in 75% of the acidic lakes and about 50% of the acidic streams".

Soils

Soil biology and chemistry can be seriously damaged by acid rain. Some microbes are unable to tolerate changes to low pH and are killed. The enzymes of these microbes are denatured (changed in shape so they no longer function) by the acid. The hydronium ions of acid rain also mobilize toxins such as aluminium, and leach away essential nutrients and minerals such as magnesium.

$$2\ H^+\ (aq) + Mg^{2+}\ (clay) \rightleftharpoons 2\ H^+\ (clay) + Mg^{2+}\ (aq)$$

Soil chemistry can be dramatically changed when base cations, such as calcium and magnesium, are leached by acid rain thereby affecting sensitive species, such as sugar maple (Acer saccharum).

Forests and Other Vegetation

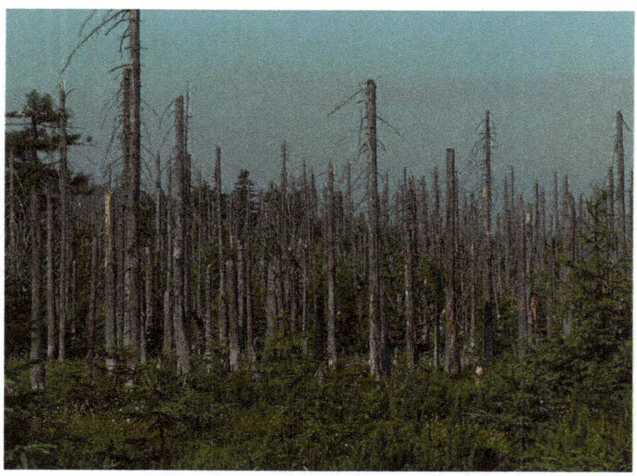

Acid rain can have severe effects on vegetation. A forest in the Black Triangle in Europe.

Adverse effects may be indirectly related to acid rain, like the acid's effects on soil (see above) or high concentration of gaseous precursors to acid rain. High altitude forests are especially vulnerable as they are often surrounded by clouds and fog which are more acidic than rain.

Other plants can also be damaged by acid rain, but the effect on food crops is minimized by the application of lime and fertilizers to replace lost nutrients. In cultivated areas, limestone may also be added to increase the ability of the soil to keep the pH stable, but this tactic is largely unusable in the case of wilderness lands. When calcium is leached from the needles of red spruce, these trees become less cold tolerant and exhibit winter injury and even death.

Ocean Acidification

Coral's limestone skeletal is sensitive to pH drop, because the calcium carbonate, core component of the limestone dissolves in acidic (low pH) solutions.

Human Health Effects

Acid rain does not directly affect human health. The acid in the rainwater is too dilute to have direct adverse effects. However, the particulates responsible for acid rain (sulfur dioxide and nitrogen oxides) do have an adverse effect. Increased amounts of fine particulate matter in the air do contribute to heart and lung problems including asthma and bronchitis.

Other Adverse Effects

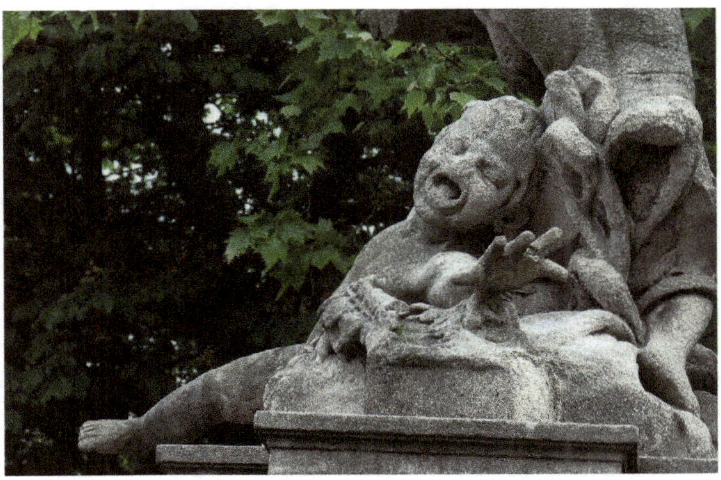

Effect of acid rain on statues.

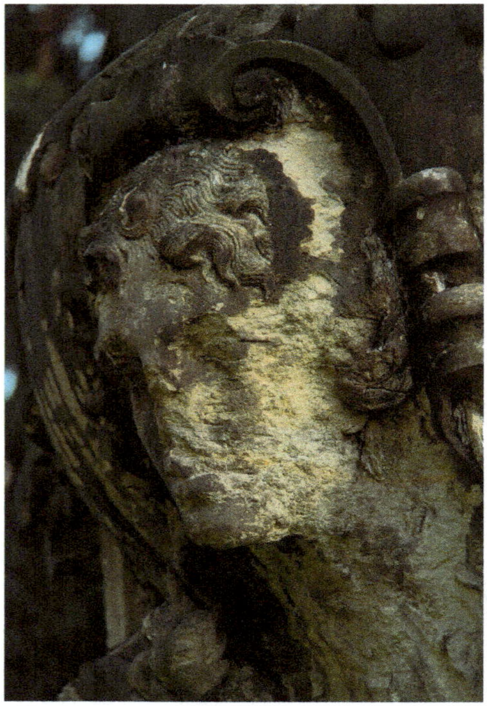

Acid rain and weathering.

Acid rain can damage buildings, historic monuments, and statues, especially those made of rocks, such as limestone and marble, that contain large amounts of calcium carbonate. Acids in the rain react with the calcium compounds in the stones to create gypsum, which then flakes off.

$$CaCO_3\ (s) + H_2SO_4\ (aq) \rightleftharpoons CaSO_4\ (s) + CO_2\ (g) + H_2O\ (l)$$

The effects of this are commonly seen on old gravestones, where acid rain can cause the inscriptions to become completely illegible. Acid rain also increases the corrosion rate of metals, in particular iron, steel, copper and bronze.

Affected Areas

Places significantly impacted by acid rain around the globe include most of eastern Europe from Poland northward into Scandinavia, the eastern third of the United States, and southeastern Canada. Other affected areas include the southeastern coast of China and Taiwan.

Prevention Methods

Technical Solutions

Many coal-firing power stations use flue-gas desulfurization (FGD) to remove sulfur-containing gases from their stack gases. For a typical coal-fired power station, FGD will remove 95% or more of the SO_2 in the flue gases. An example of FGD is the wet scrubber which is commonly used. A wet scrubber is basically a reaction tower equipped with a fan that extracts hot smoke stack gases from a power plant into the tower. Lime or limestone in slurry form is also injected into the tower to mix with the stack gases and combine with the sulfur dioxide present. The calcium carbonate of the limestone produces pH-neutral calcium sulfate that is physically removed from the scrubber. That is, the scrubber turns sulfur pollution into industrial sulfates.

In some areas the sulfates are sold to chemical companies as gypsum when the purity of calcium sulfate is high. In others, they are placed in landfill. However, the effects of acid rain can last for generations, as the effects of pH level change can stimulate the continued leaching of undesirable chemicals into otherwise pristine water sources, killing off vulnerable insect and fish species and blocking efforts to restore native life.

Fluidized bed combustion also reduces the amount of sulfur emitted by power production.

Vehicle emissions control reduces emissions of nitrogen oxides from motor vehicles.

International Treaties

A number of international treaties on the long-range transport of atmospheric pollutants have been agreed for example, the 1985 Helsinki Protocol on the Reduction of Sulphur Emissions under the Convention on Long-Range Transboundary Air Pollution. Canada and the US signed the Air Quality Agreement in 1991. Most European countries and Canada have signed the treaties.

Emissions Trading

In this regulatory scheme, every current polluting facility is given or may purchase on an open market an emissions allowance for each unit of a designated pollutant it emits. Operators can then install pollution control equipment, and sell portions of their emissions allowances they no longer need for their own operations, thereby recovering some of the capital cost of their investment in such equipment. The intention is to give operators economic incentives to install pollution controls.

The first emissions trading market was established in the United States by enactment of the Clean Air Act Amendments of 1990. The overall goal of the Acid Rain Program established by the Act is to achieve significant environmental and public health benefits through reductions in emissions of sulfur dioxide (SO_2) and nitrogen oxides (NO_x), the primary causes of acid rain. To achieve this goal at the lowest cost to society, the program employs both regulatory and market based approaches for controlling air pollution.

Climate Change

Attribution of Recent Climate Change

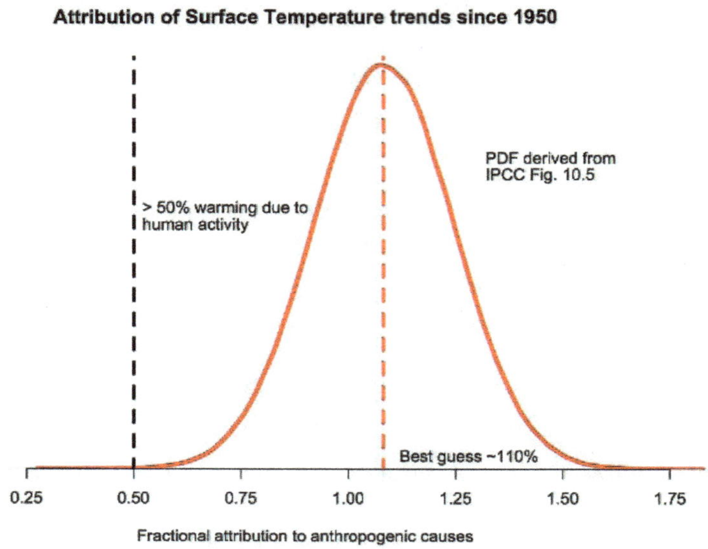

PDF of fraction of surface temperature trends since 1950 attributable to human activity, based on IPCC AR5 10.5.

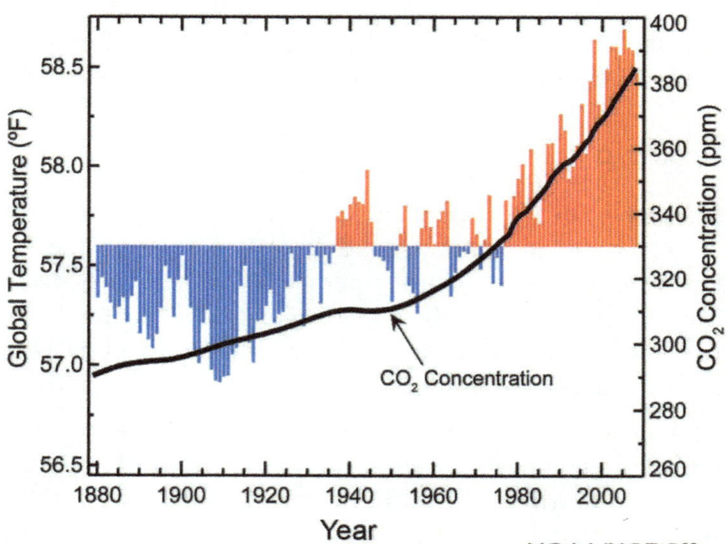

NOAA/NCDC[32]

This graph is known as the Keeling Curve and shows the long-term increase of atmospheric carbon dioxide (CO_2) concentrations from 1958–2015. Monthly CO_2 measurements display seasonal oscillations in an upward trend. Each year's maximum occurs during the Northern Hemisphere's late spring, and declines during its growing season as plants remove some atmospheric CO_2.

Global annual average temperature; year-to-year fluctuations are due to natural processes, such as the effects of El Niños, La Niñas, and the eruption of large volcanoes.

This image shows three examples of internal climate variability measured between 1950 and 2012: the El Niño–Southern oscillation, the Arctic oscillation, and the North Atlantic oscillation.

Attribution of recent climate change is the effort to scientifically ascertain mechanisms responsible for recent climate changes on Earth, commonly known as ‹global warming'. The effort has focused on changes observed during the period of instrumental temperature record, when records are most reliable; particularly in the last 50 years, when human activity has grown fastest and observations of the troposphere have become available. The dominant mechanisms are anthropogenic, i.e., the result of human activity. They are:

- increasing atmospheric concentrations of greenhouse gases
- global changes to land surface, such as deforestation
- increasing atmospheric concentrations of aerosols.

There are also natural mechanisms for variation including climate oscillations, changes in solar activity, and volcanic activity.

According to the Intergovernmental Panel on Climate Change (IPCC), it is "extremely likely" that human influence was the dominant cause of global warming between 1951 and 2010.The IPCC defines "extremely likely" as indicating a probability of 95 to 100%, based on an expert assessment of all the available evidence.

Multiple lines of evidence support attribution of recent climate change to human activities:

- A basic physical understanding of the climate system: greenhouse gas concentrations have increased and their warming properties are well-established.
- Historical estimates of past climate changes suggest that the recent changes in global surface temperature are unusual.
- Computer-based climate models are unable to replicate the observed warming unless human greenhouse gas emissions are included.
- Natural forces alone (such as solar and volcanic activity) cannot explain the observed warming.

The IPCC's attribution of recent global warming to human activities is a view shared by the scientific community, and is also supported by 196 other scientific organizations worldwide (see also: scientific opinion on climate change).

This section introduces some concepts in climate science that are used in the following sections:

Factors affecting Earth's climate can be broken down into feedbacks and forcings.:[7] A forcing is something that is imposed externally on the climate system. External forcings include natural phenomena such as volcanic eruptions and variations in the sun's output. Human activities can also impose forcings, for example, through changing the composition of the atmosphere.

Radiative forcing is a measure of how various factors alter the energy balance of the Earth's atmosphere. A positive radiative forcing will tend to increase the energy of the Earth-atmosphere system, leading to a warming of the system. Between the start of the Industrial Revolution in 1750, and the year 2005, the increase in the atmospheric concentration of carbon dioxide (chemical formula: CO_2) led to a positive radiative forcing, averaged over the Earth's surface area, of about 1.66 watts per square metre (abbreviated $W\ m^{-2}$).

Climate feedbacks can either amplify or dampen the response of the climate to a given forcing.[7] There are many feedback mechanisms in the climate system that can either amplify (a positive feedback) or diminish (a negative feedback) the effects of a change in climate forcing.

Aspects of the climate system will show variation in response to changes in forcings. In the absence of forcings imposed on it, the climate system will still show internal variability (see images opposite). This internal variability is a result of complex interactions between components of the climate system, such as the coupling between the atmosphere and ocean (see also the later section on Internal climate variability and global warming). An example of internal variability is the El Niño-Southern Oscillation.

Detection vs. Attribution

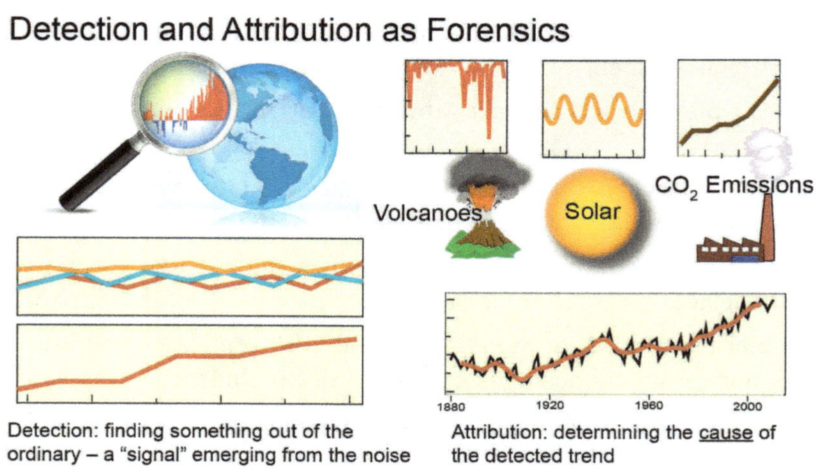

In detection and attribution, the natural factors considered usually include changes in the Sun's output and volcanic eruptions, as well as natural modes of variability such as El Niño and La Niña. Human factors include the emissions of heat-trapping greenhouse gases and particulates as well as clearing of forests and other land-use changes. Figure source: NOAA NCDC.

Detection and attribution of climate signals, as well as its common-sense meaning, has a more precise definition within the climate change literature, as expressed by the IPCC. Detection of a climate signal does not always imply significant attribution. The IPCC's Fourth Assessment Report says "it is *extremely likely* that human activities have exerted a substantial net warming influence on climate since 1750," where "extremely likely" indicates a probability greater than 95%. *Detection* of a signal requires demonstrating that an observed change is statistically significantly different from that which can be explained by natural internal variability.

Attribution requires demonstrating that a signal is:

- unlikely to be due entirely to internal variability;
- consistent with the estimated responses to the given combination of anthropogenic and natural forcing
- not consistent with alternative, physically plausible explanations of recent climate change that exclude important elements of the given combination of forcings.

Key attributions

Greenhouse Gases

Carbon dioxide is the primary greenhouse gas that is contributing to recent climate change. CO 2 is absorbed and emitted naturally as part of the carbon cycle, through animal and plant respiration, volcanic eruptions, and ocean-atmosphere exchange. Human activities, such as the burning of fossil fuels and changes in land use (see below), release large amounts of carbon to the atmosphere, causing CO 2 concentrations in the atmosphere to rise.

The high-accuracy measurements of atmospheric CO_2 concentration, initiated by Charles David Keeling in 1958, constitute the master time series documenting the changing composition of the atmosphere.These data have iconic status in climate change science as evidence of the effect of human activities on the chemical composition of the global atmosphere.

Along with CO_2, methane and nitrous oxide are also major forcing contributors to the greenhouse effect. The Kyoto Protocol lists these together with hydrofluorocarbons (HFCs), perfluorocarbons (PFCs), and sulphur hexafluoride (SF_6), which are entirely artificial (i.e. anthropogenic) gases, which also contribute to radiative forcing in the atmosphere. The chart at right attributes anthropogenic greenhouse gas emissions to eight main economic sectors, of which the largest contributors are power stations (many of which burn coal or other fossil fuels), industrial processes, transportation fuels (generally fossil fuels), and agricultural by-products (mainly methane from enteric fermentation and nitrous oxide from fertilizer use).

Water vapor

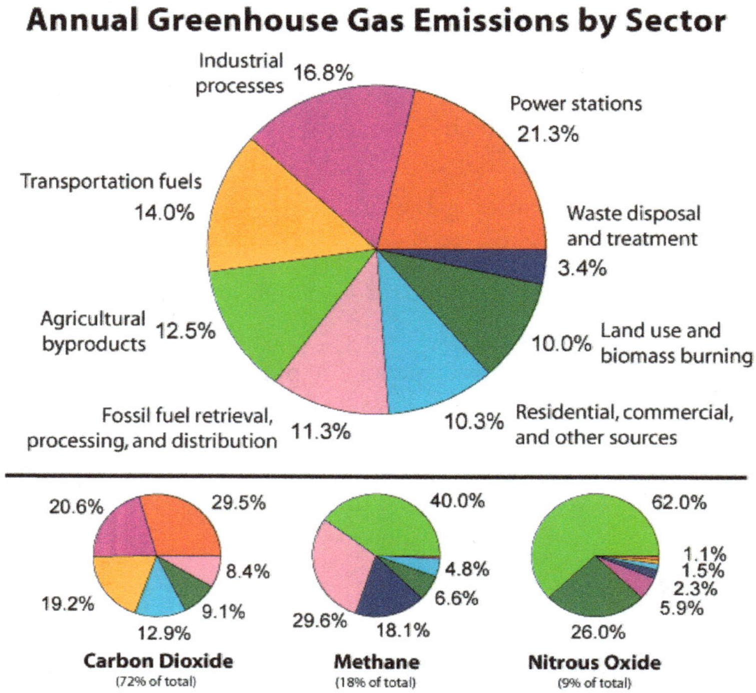

Emission Database for Global Atmospheric Research version 3.2, fast track 2000 project.

Water vapor is the most abundant greenhouse gas and also the most important in terms of its contribution to the natural greenhouse effect, despite having a short atmospheric lifetime (about 10 days). Some human activities can influence local water vapor levels. However, on a global scale, the concentration of water vapor is controlled by temperature, which influences overall rates of evaporation and precipitation.Therefore, the global concentration of water vapor is not substantially affected by direct human emissions.

Land use

Climate change is attributed to land use for two main reasons. Between 1750 and 2007, about two-thirds of anthropogenic CO_2 emissions were produced from burning fossil fuels, and about one-third of emissions from changes in land use, primarily deforestation. Deforestation both reduces the amount of carbon dioxide absorbed by deforested regions and releases greenhouse gases directly, together with aerosols, through biomass burning that frequently accompanies it.

A second reason that climate change has been attributed to land use is that the terrestrial albedo is often altered by use, which leads to radiative forcing. This effect is more significant locally than globally.

Livestock and land use

Worldwide, livestock production occupies 70% of all land used for agriculture, or 30% of the ice-free land surface of the Earth. More than 18% of anthropogenic greenhouse gas emissions are attributed to livestock and livestock-related activities such as deforestation and increasingly fuel-intensive farming practices. Specific attributions to the livestock sector include:

- 9% of global anthropogenic carbon dioxide emissions
- 35–40% of global anthropogenic methane emissions (chiefly due to enteric fermentation and manure)
- 64% of global anthropogenic nitrous oxide emissions, chiefly due to fertilizer use.

Aerosols

With virtual certainty, scientific consensus has attributed various forms of climate change, chiefly cooling effects, to aerosols, which are small particles or droplets suspended in the atmosphere. Key sources to which anthropogenic aerosols are attributed include:

- biomass burning such as slash and burn deforestation. Aerosols produced are primarily black carbon.
- industrial air pollution, which produces soot and airborne sulfates, nitrates, and ammonium
- dust produced by land use effects such as desertification

Attribution of 20th century climate change

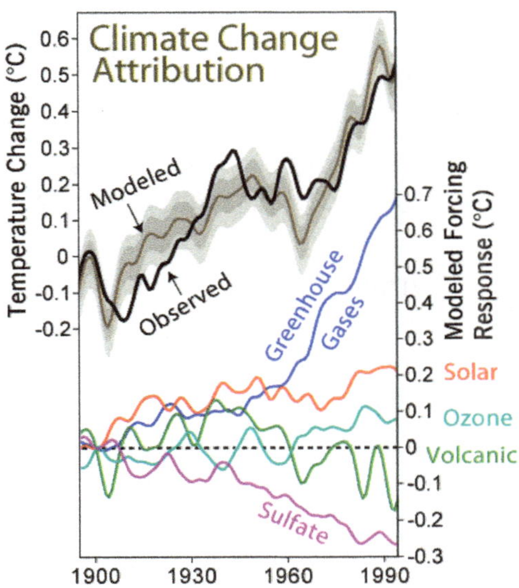

One global climate model's reconstruction of temperature change during the 20th century as the result of five studied forcing factors and the amount of temperature change attributed to each.

Over the past 150 years human activities have released increasing quantities of greenhouse gases into the atmosphere. This has led to increases in mean global temperature, or global warming. Other human effects are relevant—for example, sulphate aerosols are believed to have a cooling effect. Natural factors also contribute. According to the historical temperature record of the last century, the Earth's near-surface air temperature has risen around 0.74 ± 0.18 °Celsius (1.3 ± 0.32 °Fahrenheit).

A historically important question in climate change research has regarded the relative importance of human activity and non-anthropogenic causes during the period of instrumental record. In the 1995 Second Assessment Report (SAR), the IPCC made the widely quoted statement that "The balance of evidence suggests a discernible human influence on global climate". The phrase "balance of evidence" suggested the (English) common-law standard of proof required in civil as opposed to criminal courts: not as high as "beyond reasonable doubt". In 2001 the Third Assessment Report (TAR) refined this, saying "There is new and stronger evidence that most of the warming observed over the last 50 years is attributable to human activities". The 2007 Fourth Assessment Report (AR4) strengthened this finding:

- Anthropogenic warming of the climate system is widespread and can be detected in temperature observations taken at the surface, in the free atmosphere and in the oceans. Evidence of the effect of external influences, both anthropogenic and natural, on the climate system has continued to accumulate since the TAR.

Other findings of the IPCC Fourth Assessment Report include:

- It is *extremely unlikely* (<5%) that the global pattern of warming during the past half century can be explained without external forcing (i.e., it is inconsistent with being the result of internal variability), and *very unlikely* that it is due to known natural external causes alone. The warming occurred in both the ocean and the atmosphere and took place at a time when natural external forcing factors would likely have produced cooling."
- From new estimates of the combined anthropogenic forcing due to greenhouse gases, aerosols, and land surface changes, it is *extremely likely* (>95%) that human activities have exerted a substantial net warming influence on climate since 1750."
- It is *virtually certain* that anthropogenic aerosols produce a net negative radiative forcing (cooling influence) with a greater magnitude in the Northern Hemisphere than in the Southern Hemisphere.

Over the past five decades there has been a global warming of approximately 0.65 °C (1.17 °F) at the Earth's surface (see historical temperature record). Among the possible factors that could produce changes in global mean temperature are internal variability of the climate system, external forcing, an increase in concentration of greenhouse gases, or any combination of these. Current studies indicate that the increase in greenhouse gases, most notably CO_2, is mostly responsible for the observed warming. Evidence for this conclusion includes:

- Estimates of internal variability from climate models, and reconstructions of past temperatures, indicate that the warming is unlikely to be entirely natural.

- Climate models forced by natural factors *and* increased greenhouse gases and aerosols reproduce the observed global temperature changes; those forced by natural factors alone do not.
- Fingerprint methods (see below) indicate that the pattern of change is closer to that expected from greenhouse gas-forced change than from natural change.
- The plateau in warming from the 1940s to 1960s can be attributed largely to sulphate aerosol cooling.

Details on Attribution

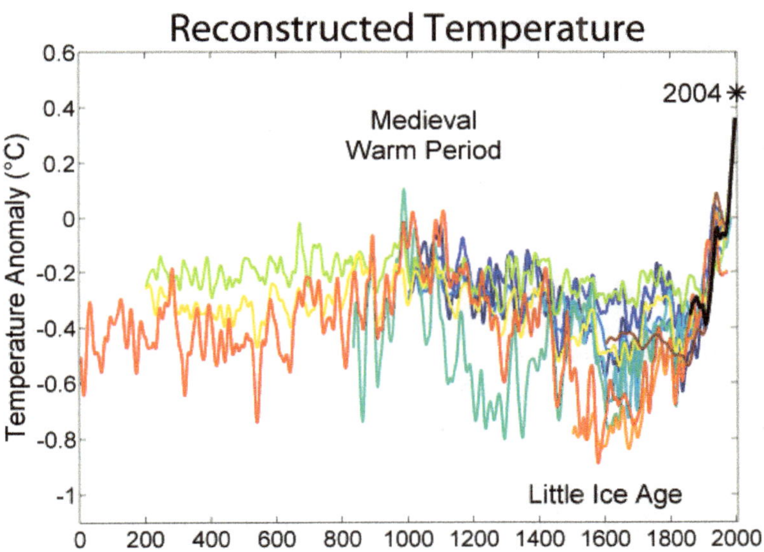

For Northern Hemisphere temperature, recent decades appear to be the warmest since at least about 1000AD, and the warming since the late 19th century is unprecedented over the last 1000 years.Older data are insufficient to provide reliable hemispheric temperature estimates.

Recent scientific assessments find that most of the warming of the Earth's surface over the past 50 years has been caused by human activities (see also the section on scientific literature and opinion). This conclusion rests on multiple lines of evidence. Like the warming "signal" that has gradually emerged from the "noise" of natural climate variability, the scientific evidence for a human influence on global climate has accumulated over the past several decades, from many hundreds of studies. No single study is a "smoking gun." Nor has any single study or combination of studies undermined the large body of evidence supporting the conclusion that human activity is the primary driver of recent warming.

The first line of evidence is based on a physical understanding of how greenhouse gases trap heat, how the climate system responds to increases in greenhouse gases, and how other human and natural factors influence climate. The second line of evidence is from indirect estimates of climate changes over the last 1,000 to 2,000 years. These records are obtained from living things and their remains (like tree rings and corals) and from physical quantities (like the ratio between lighter and heavier isotopes of oxygen in ice cores), which change in measurable ways as climate changes. The lesson from these data is that global surface temperatures over the last several decades are clearly unusual, in that they were higher than at any time during at least the past 400 years. For the Northern Hemisphere, the recent temperature rise is clearly unusual in at least the last 1,000 years (see graph opposite).

The third line of evidence is based on the broad, qualitative consistency between observed changes in climate and the computer model simulations of how climate would be expected to change in response to human activities. For example, when climate models are run with historical increases in greenhouse gases, they show gradual warming of the Earth and ocean surface, increases in ocean heat content and the temperature of the lower atmosphere, a rise in global sea level, retreat of sea ice and snow cover, cooling of the stratosphere, an increase in the amount of atmospheric water vapor, and changes in large-scale precipitation and pressure patterns. These and other aspects of modelled climate change are in agreement with observations.

"Fingerprint" Studies

Reconstructions of global temperature that include greenhouse gas increases and other human influences (red line, based on many models) closely match measured temperatures (dashed line). Those that only include natural influences (blue line, based on many models) show a slight cooling, which has not occurred. The ability of models to generate reasonable histories of global temperature is verified by their response to four 20th-century volcanic eruptions: each eruption caused brief cooling that appeared in observed as well as modeled records.

Finally, there is extensive statistical evidence from so-called "fingerprint" studies. Each factor that affects climate produces a unique pattern of climate response, much as each person has a unique fingerprint. Fingerprint studies exploit these unique signatures, and allow detailed comparisons of modelled and observed climate change patterns. Scientists rely on such studies to attribute observed changes in climate to a particular cause or set of causes. In the real world, the climate changes that have occurred since the start of the Industrial Revolution are due to a complex mixture of human and natural causes. The importance of each individual influence in this mixture changes over time. Of course, there are not multiple Earths, which would allow an experimenter to change one factor at a time on each Earth, thus helping to isolate different fingerprints. Therefore, climate models are used to study how individual factors affect climate. For example, a single factor (like greenhouse gases) or a set of factors can be varied, and the response of the modelled climate system to these individual or combined changes can thus be studied.

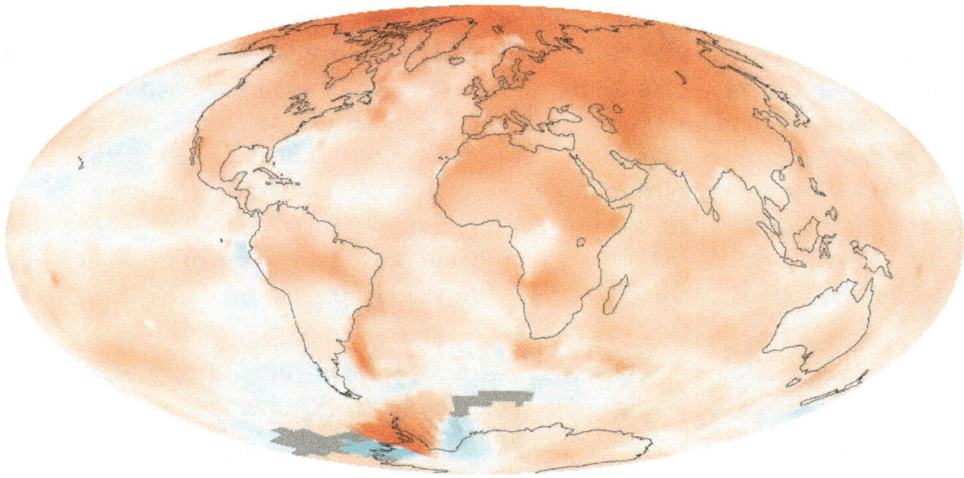

Two fingerprints of human activities on the climate are that land areas will warm more than the oceans, and that high latitudes will warm more than low latitudes. These projections have been confirmed by observations (shown above).

For example, when climate model simulations of the last century include all of the major influences on climate, both human-induced and natural, they can reproduce many important features of observed climate change patterns. When human influences are removed from the model experiments, results suggest that the surface of the Earth would actually have cooled slightly over the last 50 years (see graph, opposite). The clear message from fingerprint studies is that the observed warming over the last half-century cannot be explained by natural factors, and is instead caused primarily by human factors.

Another fingerprint of human effects on climate has been identified by looking at a slice through the layers of the atmosphere, and studying the pattern of temperature changes from the surface up through the stratosphere (see the section on solar activity). The earliest fingerprint work focused on changes in surface and atmospheric temperature. Scientists then applied fingerprint methods to a whole range of climate variables, identifying human-caused climate signals in the heat content of the oceans, the height of the tropopause (the boundary between the troposphere and stratosphere, which has shifted upward by hundreds of feet in recent decades), the geographical patterns of precipitation, drought, surface pressure, and the runoff from major river basins.

Studies published after the appearance of the IPCC Fourth Assessment Report in 2007 have also found human fingerprints in the increased levels of atmospheric moisture (both close to the surface and over the full extent of the atmosphere), in the decline of Arctic sea ice extent, and in the patterns of changes in Arctic and Antarctic surface temperatures.

The message from this entire body of work is that the climate system is telling a consistent story of increasingly dominant human influence – the changes in temperature, ice extent, moisture, and circulation patterns fit together in a physically consistent way, like pieces in a complex puzzle.

Increasingly, this type of fingerprint work is shifting its emphasis. As noted, clear and compelling scientific evidence supports the case for a pronounced human influence on global climate. Much of the recent attention is now on climate changes at continental and regional scales, and on variables that can have large impacts on societies. For example, scientists have established causal links between human activities and the changes in snowpack, maximum and minimum (diurnal) temperature, and the seasonal timing of runoff over mountainous regions of the western United States. Human activity is likely to have made a substantial contribution to ocean surface temperature changes in hurricane formation regions. Researchers are also looking beyond the physical climate system, and are beginning to tie changes in the distribution and seasonal behaviour of plant and animal species to human-caused changes in temperature and precipitation.

For over a decade, one aspect of the climate change story seemed to show a significant difference between models and observations. In the tropics, all models predicted that with a rise in greenhouse gases, the troposphere would be expected to warm more rapidly than the surface. Observations from weather balloons, satellites, and surface thermometers seemed to show the opposite behaviour (more rapid warming of the surface than the troposphere). This issue was a stumbling block in understanding the causes of climate change. It is now largely resolved. Research showed that there were large uncertainties in the satellite and weather balloon data. When uncertainties in models and observations are properly accounted for, newer observational data sets (with better treatment of known problems) are in agreement with climate model results.

This set of graphs shows the estimated contribution of various natural and human factors to changes in global mean temperature between 1889–2006. Estimated contributions are based on multivariate analysis rather than model simulations. The graphs show that human influence on climate has eclipsed the magnitude of natural temperature changes over the past 120 years. Natural influences on temperature—El Niño, solar variability, and volcanic aerosols—have varied approximately plus and minus 0.2 °C (0.4 °F), (averaging to about zero), while human influences have contributed roughly 0.8 °C (1 °F) of warming since 1889.

This does not mean, however, that all remaining differences between models and observations have been resolved. The observed changes in some climate variables, such as Arctic sea ice, some aspects of precipitation, and patterns of surface pressure, appear to be proceeding much more rapidly than models have projected. The reasons for these differences are not well understood. Nevertheless, the bottom-line conclusion from climate fingerprinting is that most of the observed changes studied to date are consistent with each other, and are also consistent with our scientific understanding of how the climate system would be expected to respond to the increase in heat-trapping gases resulting from human activities.

Extreme Weather Events

One of the subjects discussed in the literature is whether or not extreme weather events can be attributed to human activities. Seneviratne *et al.* (2012) stated that attributing individual extreme weather events to human activities was challenging. They were, however, more confident over attributing changes in long-term trends of extreme weather. For example, Seneviratne *et al.* (2012) concluded that human activities had likely led to a warming of extreme daily minimum and maximum temperatures at the global scale.

Another way of viewing the problem is to consider the effects of human-induced climate change on the probability of future extreme weather events. Stott *et al.* (2003), for example, considered whether or not human activities had increased the risk of severe heat waves in Europe, like the one experienced in 2003. Their conclusion was that human activities had very likely more than doubled the risk of heat waves of this magnitude.

An analogy can be made between an athlete on steroids and human-induced climate change. In the same way that an athlete's performance may increase from using steroids, human-induced climate change increases the risk of some extreme weather events.

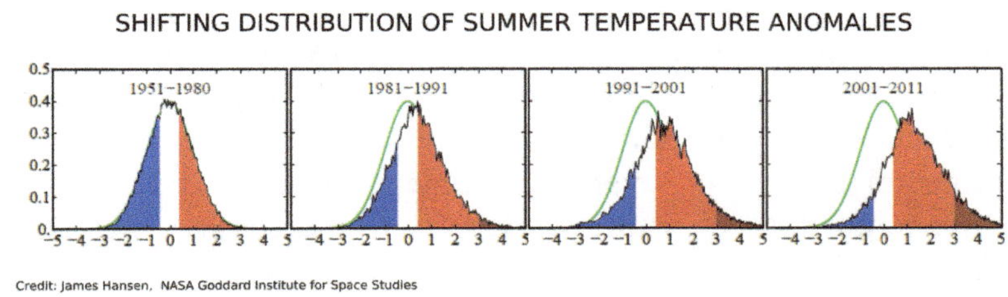

Frequency of occurrence (vertical axis) of local June–July–August temperature anomalies (relative to 1951–1980 mean) for Northern Hemisphere land in units of local standard deviation (horizontal axis).According to Hansen *et al.* (2012),the distribution of anomalies has shifted to the right as a consequence of global warming, meaning that unusually hot summers have become more common. This is analogous to the rolling of a dice: cool summers now cover only half of one side of a six-sided die, white covers one side, red covers four sides, and an extremely hot (red-brown) anomaly covers half of one side.

Hansen *et al.* (2012) suggested that human activities have greatly increased the risk of summertime heat waves. According to their analysis, the land area of the Earth affected by very hot summer temperature anomalies has greatly increased over time (refer to graphs on the left). In the base period 1951-1980, these anomalies covered a few tenths of 1% of the global land area. In recent years, this has increased to around 10% of the global land area. With high confidence, Hansen *et al.* (2012) attributed the 2010 Moscow and 2011 Texas heat waves to human-induced global warming.

An earlier study by Dole *et al.* (2011) concluded that the 2010 Moscow heatwave was mostly due to natural weather variability. While not directly citing Dole *et al.* (2011), Hansen *et al.* (2012) rejected this type of explanation. Hansen *et al.* (2012) stated that a combination of natural weather variability and human-induced global warming was responsible for the Moscow and Texas heat waves.

Scientific literature and opinion

There are a number of examples of published and informal support for the consensus view. As mentioned earlier, the IPCC has concluded that most of the observed increase in globally averaged temperatures since the mid-20th century is "very likely" due to human activities. The IPCC's conclusions are consistent with those of several reports produced by the US National Research Council. A report published in 2009 by the U.S. Global Change Research Program concluded that "[global] warming is unequivocal and primarily human-induced." A number of scientific organizations have issued statements that support the consensus view. Two examples include:

- a joint statement made in 2005 by the national science academies of the G8, and Brazil, China and India;
- a joint statement made in 2008 by the Network of African Science Academies.

Detection and Attribution Studies

The IPCC Fourth Assessment Report (2007), concluded that attribution was possible for a number of observed changes in the climate (see effects of global warming). However, attribution was found to be more difficult when assessing changes over smaller regions (less than continental scale) and over short time periods (less than 50 years). Over larger regions, averaging reduces natural variability of the climate, making detection and attribution easier.

- In 1996, in a paper in *Nature* titled "A search for human influences on the thermal structure of the atmosphere", Benjamin D. Santer et al. wrote: "The observed spatial patterns of temperature change in the free atmosphere from 1963 to 1987 are similar to those predicted by state-of-the-art climate models incorporating various combinations of changes in carbon dioxide, anthropogenic sulphate aerosol and stratospheric ozone concentrations. The degree of pattern similarity between models and observations increases through this period. It is likely that this trend is partially due to human activities, although many uncertainties remain, particularly relating to estimates of natural variability.
- A 2002 paper in the *Journal of Geophysical Research* says "Our analysis suggests that the early twentieth century warming can best be explained by a combination of warming due to increases in greenhouse gases and natural forcing, some cooling due to other anthropogenic forcings, and a substantial, but not implausible, contribution from internal variability. In the second half of the century we find that the warming is largely caused by changes in greenhouse gases, with changes in sulphates and, perhaps, volcanic aerosol offsetting approximately one third of the warming.
- A 2005 review of detection and attribution studies by the International Ad Hoc Detection and Attribution Group found that "natural drivers such as solar variability and volcanic activity are at most partially responsible for the large-scale temperature changes observed over the past century, and that a large fraction of the warming over the last 50 yr can be attributed to greenhouse gas increases. Thus, the recent research supports and strengthens the IPCC Third Assessment Report conclusion that ‹most of the global warming over the past 50 years is likely due to the increase in greenhouse gases.'
- Barnett and colleagues (2005) say that the observed warming of the oceans cannot be explained by natural internal climate variability or solar and volcanic forcing, but is well simulated by two anthropogenically forced climate models,"

concluding that "it is of human origin, a conclusion robust to observational sampling and model differences".

- Two papers in the journal *Science* in August 2005 resolve the problem, evident at the time of the TAR, of tropospheric temperature trends (see also the section on fingerprint studies) . The UAH version of the record contained errors, and there is evidence of spurious cooling trends in the radiosonde record, particularly in the tropics. See satellite temperature measurements for details; and the 2006 US CCSP report.
- Multiple independent reconstructions of the temperature record of the past 1000 years confirm that the late 20th century is probably the warmest period in that time (see the preceding section -details on attribution).

Reviews of Scientific Opinion

- An essay in *Science* surveyed 928 abstracts related to climate change, and concluded that most journal reports accepted the consensus. This is discussed further in scientific opinion on climate change.
- A 2010 paper in the Proceedings of the National Academy of Sciences found that among a pool of roughly 1,000 researchers who work directly on climate issues and publish the most frequently on the subject, 97% agree that anthropogenic climate change is happening.
- A 2011 paper from George Mason University published in the *International Journal of Public Opinion Research*, "The Structure of Scientific Opinion on Climate Change," collected the opinions of scientists in the earth, space, atmospheric, oceanic or hydrological sciences. The 489 survey respondents—representing nearly half of all those eligible according to the survey's specific standards – work in academia, government, and industry, and are members of prominent professional organizations. The study found that 97% of the 489 scientists surveyed agreed that global temperatures have risen over the past century. Moreover, 84% agreed that "human-induced greenhouse warming" is now occurring." Only 5% disagreed with the idea that human activity is a significant cause of global warming.

As described above, a small minority of scientists do disagree with the consensus: see list of scientists opposing global warming consensus. For example, Willie Soon and Richard Lindzen say that there is insufficient proof for anthropogenic attribution. Generally this position requires new physical mechanisms to explain the observed warming.

Solar Activity

Solar radiation at the top of our atmosphere, and global temperature

Modelled simulation of the effect of various factors (including GHGs, Solar irradiance) singly and in combination, showing in particular that solar activity produces a small and nearly uniform warming, unlike what is observed.

Solar sunspot maximum occurs when the magnetic field of the sun collapses and reverse as part of its average 11 year solar cycle (22 years for complete North to North restoration).

The role of the sun in recent climate change has been looked at by climate scientists. Since 1978, output from the Sun has been measured by satellites[6] significantly more accurately than was previously possible from the surface. These measurements indicate that the Sun's total solar irradiance has not increased since 1978, so the warming during the past 30 years cannot be directly attributed to an increase in total solar energy reaching the Earth (see graph above, left). In the three decades since 1978, the combination of solar and volcanic activity probably had a slight cooling influence on the climate.

Climate models have been used to examine the role of the sun in recent climate change. Models are unable to reproduce the rapid warming observed in recent decades when they only take into account variations in total solar irradiance and volcanic activity. Models are, however, able to simulate the observed 20th century changes in temperature when they include all of the most important external forcings, including human influences and natural forcings. As has already been stated, Hegerl *et al.* (2007) concluded that greenhouse gas forcing had "very likely" caused most of the observed global warming since the mid-20th century. In making this conclusion, Hegerl *et al.* (2007) allowed for the possibility that climate models had been underestimated the effect of solar forcing.

The role of solar activity in climate change has also been calculated over longer time periods using "proxy" datasets, such as tree rings. Models indicate that solar and volcanic forcings can explain periods of relative warmth and cold between A.D. 1000 and 1900, but human-induced forcings are needed to reproduce the late-20th century warming.

Another line of evidence against the sun having caused recent climate change comes from looking at how temperatures at different levels in the Earth's atmosphere have changed. Models and observations (see figure above, middle) show that greenhouse gas results in warming of the lower atmosphere at the surface (called the troposphere) but cooling of the upper atmosphere (called the stratosphere). Depletion of the ozone layer by chemical refrigerants has also resulted in a cooling effect in the stratosphere. If the sun was responsible for observed warming, warming of the troposphere at the surface and warming at the top of the stratosphere would be expected as increase solar activity would replenish ozone and oxides of nitrogen. The stratosphere has a reverse temperature gradient than the troposphere so as the temperature of the troposphere cools with altitude, the stratosphere rises with altitude. Hadley cells are the mechanism by which equatorial generated ozone in the tropics (highest area of UV irradiance in the stratosphere) is moved poleward. Global climate models suggest that climate change may widen the Hadley cells and push the jetstream northward thereby expanding the tropics region and resulting in warmer, dryer conditions in those areas overall.

Non-Consensus Views

Habibullo Abdussamatov (2004), head of space research at St. Petersburg's Pulkovo Astronomical Observatory in Russia, has argued that the sun is responsible for recently observed climate change. Journalists for news sources canada.com (Solomon, 2007b), National Geographic News (Ravillious, 2007), and LiveScience (Than, 2007) reported on the story of warming on Mars. In these articles, Abdussamatov was quoted. He stated that warming on Mars was evidence that global warming on Earth was being caused by changes in the sun.

Ravillious (2007) quoted two scientists who disagreed with Abdussamatov: Amato Evan, a climate scientist at the University of Wisconsin-Madison, in the US, and Colin Wilson, a planetary physicist at Oxford University in the UK. According to Wilson, Wobbles in the orbit of Mars are the main cause of its climate change in the current era (see also orbital forcing). Than (2007) quoted Charles Long, a climate physicist at Pacific Northwest National Laboratories in the US, who disagreed with Abdussamatov.

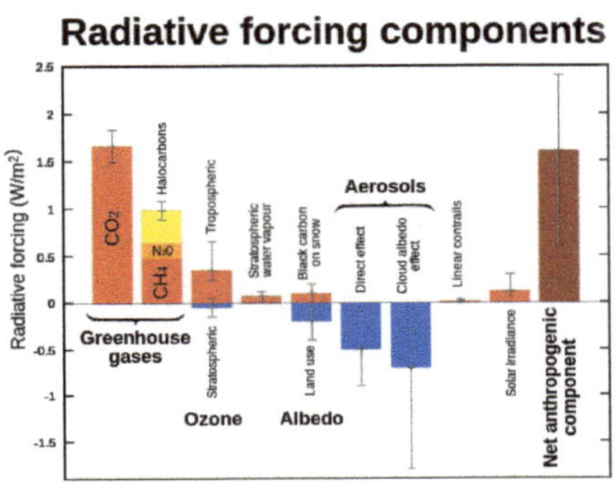

Contribution of natural factors and human activities to radiative forcing of climate change. Radiative forcing values are for the year 2005, relative to the pre-industrial era (1750). The contribution of solar irradiance to radiative forcing is 5% the value of the combined radiative forcing due to increases in the atmospheric concentrations of carbon dioxide, methane and nitrous oxide.

Than (2007) pointed to the view of Benny Peiser, a social anthropologist at Liverpool John Moores University in the UK. In his newsletter, Peiser had cited a blog that had commented on warming observed on several planetary bodies in the Solar system. These included Neptune's moon Triton,Jupiter, Pluto and Mars. In an e-mail interview with Than (2007), Peiser stated that:

I think it is an intriguing coincidence that warming trends have been observed on a number of very diverse planetary bodies in our solar system, (...) Perhaps this is just a fluke.

Than (2007) provided alternative explanations of why warming had occurred on Triton, Pluto, Jupiter and Mars.

The US Environmental Protection Agency (US EPA, 2009) responded to public comments on climate change attribution. A number of commenters had argued that recent climate change could be attributed to changes in solar irradiance. According to the US EPA (2009), this attribution was not supported by the bulk of the scientific literature. Citing the work of the IPCC (2007), the US EPA pointed to the low contribution of solar irradiance to radiative forcing since the start of the Industrial Revolution in 1750. Over this time period (1750 to 2005), the estimated contribution of solar irradiance to radiative forcing was 5% the value of the combined radiative forcing due to increases in the atmospheric concentrations of carbon dioxide, methane and nitrous oxide (see graph opposite).

Effect of Cosmic Rays

Henrik Svensmark has suggested that the magnetic activity of the sun deflects cosmic rays, and that this may influence the generation of cloud condensation nuclei, and thereby have an effect on the climate.The website ScienceDaily reported on a 2009 study that looked at how past changes in climate have been affected by the Earth's magnetic field. Geophysicist Mads Faurschou Knudsen, who co-authored the study, stated that the study's results supported Svensmark's theory. The authors of the study also acknowledged that CO_2 plays an important role in climate change.

Consensus View on Cosmic Rays

The view that cosmic rays could provide the mechanism by which changes in solar activity affect climate is not supported by the literature. Solomon *et al.* (2007) state:

> [..] the cosmic ray time series does not appear to correspond to global total cloud cover after 1991 or to global low-level cloud cover after 1994. Together with the lack of a proven physical mechanism and the plausibility of other causal factors affecting changes in cloud cover, this makes the association between galactic cosmic ray-induced changes in aerosol and cloud formation controversial

Studies by Lockwood and Fröhlich (2007) and Sloan and Wolfendale (2008) found no relation between warming in recent decades and cosmic rays. Pierce and Adams (2009) used a model to simulate the effect of cosmic rays on cloud properties. They concluded that the hypothesized effect of cosmic rays was too small to explain recent climate change. Pierce and Adams (2009) noted that their findings did not rule out a possible connection between cosmic rays and climate change, and recommended further research.

Erlykin *et al.* (2009) found that the evidence showed that connections between solar variation and climate were more likely to be mediated by direct variation of insolation rather than cosmic rays, and concluded: "Hence within our assumptions, the effect of varying solar activity, either by direct solar irradiance or by varying cosmic ray rates, must be less than 0.07 °C since 1956, i.e. less than 14% of the observed global warming." Carslaw (2009) and Pittock (2009) review the recent and historical literature in this field and continue to find that the link between cosmic rays and climate is tenuous, though they encourage continued research. US EPA (2009) commented on research by Duplissy *et al.* (2009):

The CLOUD experiments at CERN are interesting research but do not provide conclusive evidence that cosmic rays can serve as a major source of cloud seeding. Preliminary results from the experiment (Duplissy et al., 2009) suggest that though there was some evidence of ion mediated nucleation, for most of the nucleation events observed the contribution of ion processes appeared to be minor. These experiments also showed the difficulty in maintaining sufficiently clean conditions and stable temperatures to prevent spurious aerosol bursts. There is no indication that the earlier Svensmark experiments

could even have matched the controlled conditions of the CERN experiment. We find that the Svensmark results on cloud seeding have not yet been shown to be robust or sufficient to materially alter the conclusions of the assessment literature, especially given the abundance of recent literature that is skeptical of the cosmic ray-climate linkage

Oil Spills

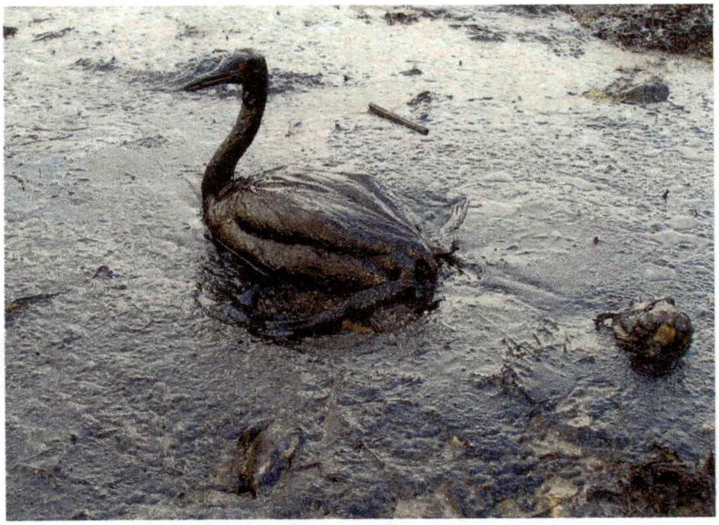

A bird covered in oil from the Black Sea oil spill.

An oil spill is the release of a liquid petroleum hydrocarbon into the environment, especially marine areas, due to human activity, and is a form of pollution. The term is usually applied to marine oil spills, where oil is released into the ocean or coastal waters, but spills may also occur on land. Oil spills may be due to releases of crude oil from tankers, pipelines, railcars, offshore platforms, drilling rigs and wells, as well as spills of refined petroleum products (such as gasoline, diesel) and their by-products, heavier fuels used by large ships such as bunker fuel, or the spill of any oily refuse or waste oil.

Major oil spills include the Kuwaiti oil fires, Kuwaiti oil lakes, Lakeview Gusher, Gulf War oil spill, and the Deepwater Horizon oil spill. Spilt oil penetrates into the structure of the plumage of birds and the fur of mammals, reducing its insulating ability, and making them more vulnerable to temperature fluctuations and much less buoyant in the water. Cleanup and recovery from an oil spill is difficult and depends upon many factors, including the type of oil spilled, the temperature of the water (affecting evaporation and biodegradation), and the types of shorelines and beaches involved. Spills may take weeks, months or even years to clean up.

Volatile Organic Compounds

Volatile organic compounds (VOCs) are gases or vapours emitted by various solids and liquids, many of which have short- and long-term adverse effects on human health and the environment. VOCs from petroleum are toxic and foul the air, and some like benzene are extremely toxic, carcinogenic and cause DNA damage. Benzene often makes up about 1% of crude oil and gasoline. Benzene is present in automobile exhaust. More important for vapors from spills of diesel and crude oil are aliphatic, volatile compounds. Although less toxic than compounds like benzene, their overwhelming abundance can still cause health concerns even when benzene levels in the air are relatively low. The compounds are sometimes collectively measured as total petroleum hydrocarbons or TPH. Petroleum hydrocarbons such as gasoline, diesel, or jet fuel intruding into indoor spaces from underground storage tanks or brownfields threaten safety (e.g., explosive potential) and causes adverse health effects from inhalation.

Waste Oil

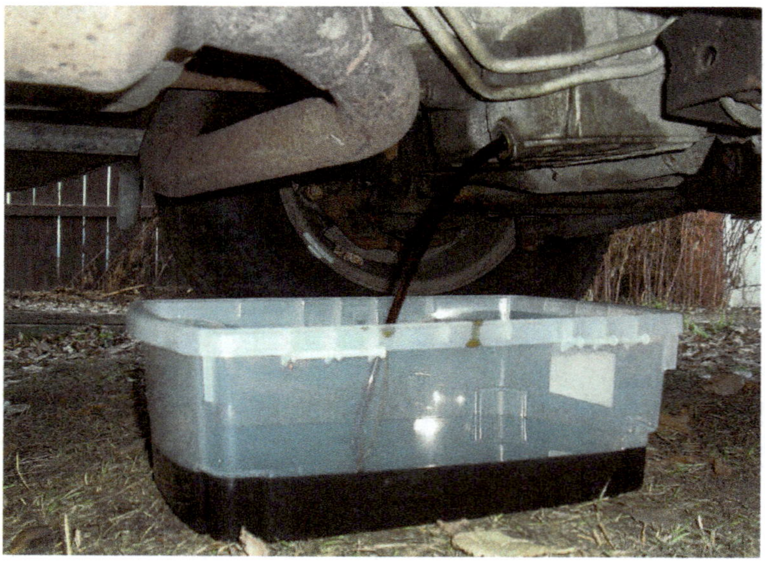

Waste oil in the form of motor oil.

Waste oil is used oil containing not only breakdown products but also impurities from use. Some examples of waste oil are used oils such as hydraulic oil, transmission oil, brake fluids, motor oil, crankcase oil, gear box oil and synthetic oil. Many of the same problems associated with natural petroleum exist with waste oil. When waste oil from vehicles drips out engines over streets and roads, the oil travels into the water table bringing with it such toxins as benzene. This poisons both soil and drinking water. Runoff from storms carries waste oil into rivers and oceans, poisoning them as well.

MITIGATION

Conservation and Phasing Out

- Creating laws to completely phase out the use of petroleum (Sweden's 15-year plan)
- Making use of petroleum more efficiently via better technology

Substitution of other Energy Sources

- Using "cleaner" energy sources such as natural gas and biodiesel, especially in critical areas like cities where there are people.

Use of Biomass Instead of Petroleum

- It is suggested that cellulose from fibrous plant material, such as hemp, can be used to produce alternatives to many oil-based products.
- Plastics can be created from cellulose instead of from oil.
- Lubricants like motor oil and grease can be made from plants and animal fat.

Safety Measures

- Decreasing the risk of spills
- False floors at gasoline stations to catch gasoline and oil drips from making it into the water table
- Double-hulled tanker ships

ENVIRONMENTAL IMPACT OF THE ENERGY INDUSTRY

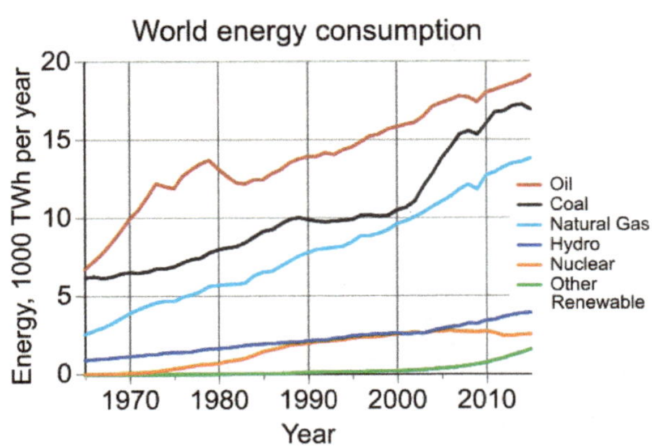

World consumption of primary energy by energy type.

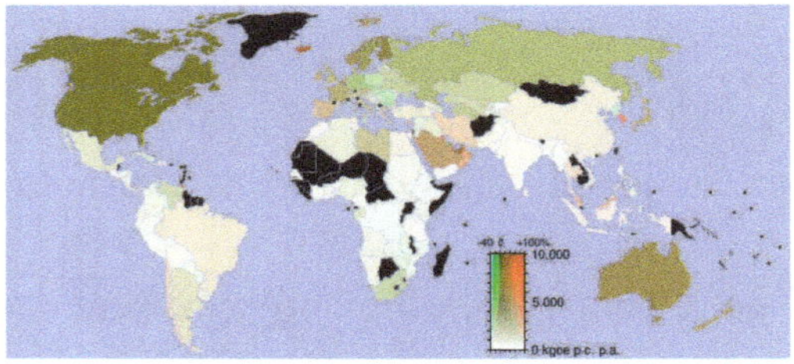

Energy consumption per capita per country (2001). Red hues indicate increase, green hues decrease of consumption during the 1990s.

The **environmental impact of the energy industry** is diverse. Energy has been harnessed by human beings for millennia. Initially it was with the use of fire for light, heat, cooking and for safety, and its use can be traced back at least 1.9 million years. In recent years there has been a trend towards the increased commercialization of various renewable energy sources.

Consumption of fossil fuel resources leads to global warming and climate change. In most parts of the world little change is being made to slow these changes. If the peak oil theory proves true, and more explorations of viable alternative energy sources are made, our impact could be less hostile to our environment.

Rapidly advancing technologies can achieve a transition of energy generation, water and waste management, and food production towards better environmental and energy usage practices using methods of systems ecology and industrial ecology.

Issues

Climate Change

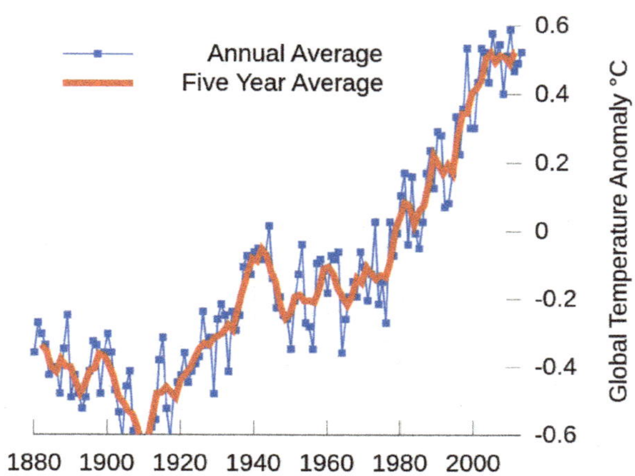

Global mean surface temperature anomaly relative to 1961–1990.

The scientific consensus on global warming and climate change is that it is caused by anthropogenic greenhouse gas emissions, the majority of which comes from burning fossil fuels with deforestation and some agricultural practices being also major contributors. A 2013 study showed that two thirds of the industrial greenhouse gas emissions are due to the fossil-fuel (and cement) production of just ninety companies around the world (between 1751 and 2010, with half emitted since 1986).

Although there is a highly publicized denial of climate change, the vast majority of scientists working in climatology accept that it is due to human activity. The IPCC report *Climate Change 2007: Climate Change Impacts, Adaptation and Vulnerability* predicts that climate change will cause shortages of food and water and increased risk of flooding that will affect billions of people, particularly those living in poverty.

One measurement of greenhouse gas related and other Externality comparisons between energy sources can be found in the ExternE project by the Paul Scherrer Institut and the University of Stuttgart which was funded by the European Commission. According to that study, hydroelectric electricity produces the lowest CO2 emissions, wind produces the second-lowest, nuclear energy produces the third-lowest and solar photovoltaic produces the fourth-lowest.

Similarly, the same research study (ExternE, Externalities of Energy), undertaken from 1995 to 2005 found that the cost of producing electricity from coal or oil would double over its present value, and the cost of electricity production from gas would increase by 30% if external costs such as damage to the environment and to human health, from the airborne particulate matter, nitrogen oxides, chromium VI and arsenic emissions produced by these sources, were taken into account. It was estimated in the study that these external, downstream, fossil fuel costs amount up to 1%-2% of the EU's entire Gross Domestic Product (GDP), and this was before the external cost of global warming from these sources was even included. The study also found that the environmental and health costs of nuclear power, per unit of energy delivered, was €0.0019/kWh, which was found to be lower than that of many renewable sources including that caused by biomass and photovoltaic solar panels, and was thirty times lower than coal at €0.06/kWh, or 6 cents/kWh, with the energy sources of the lowest external environmental and health costs associated with it being wind power at €0.0009/kWh.

Biofuel use

Biofuel is defined as solid, liquid or gaseous fuel obtained from relatively recently lifeless or living biological material and is different from fossil fuels, which are derived from long-dead biological material. Various plants and plant-derived materials are used for biofuel manufacturing.

Bio-diesel

High use of bio-diesel leads to land use changes including deforestation.

Firewood

Unsustainable firewood harvesting can lead to loss of biodiversity and erosion due to loss of forest cover. An example of this is a 40-year study done by the University of Leeds of African forests, which account for a third of the world's total tropical forest which demonstrates that Africa is a significant carbon sink. A climate change expert, Lee White states that "To get an idea of the value of the sink, the removal of nearly 5 billion tonnes of carbon dioxide from the atmosphere by intact tropical forests is at issue.

According to the U.N. the African continent is losing forest twice as fast as the rest of the world. "Once upon a time, Africa boasted seven million square kilometers of forest but a third of that has been lost, most of it to charcoal.

Fossil Fuel Use

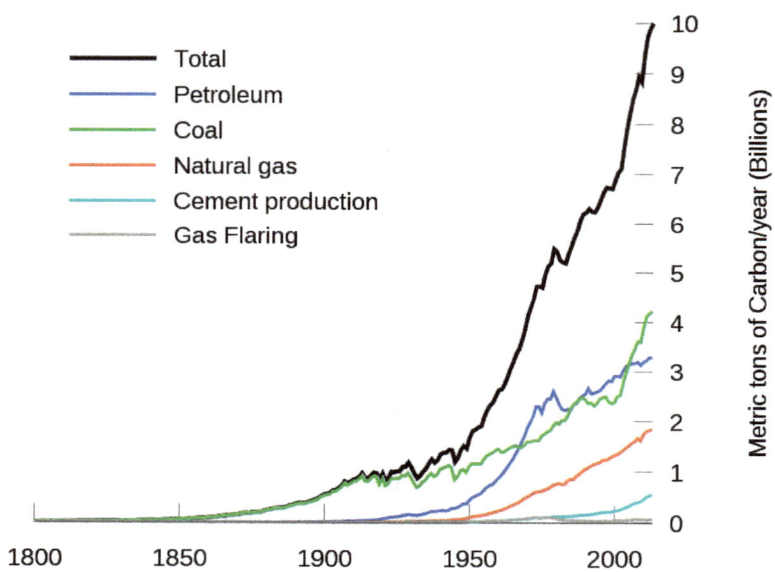

Global fossil carbon emission by fuel type, 1800-2007 AD.

The three fossil fuel types are coal, petroleum and natural gas. It was estimated by the Energy Information Administration that in 2006 primary sources of energy consisted of petroleum 36.8%, coal 26.6%, natural gas 22.9%, amounting to an 86% share for fossil fuels in primary energy production in the world.

In 2013 the burning of fossil fuels produced around 32 billion tonnes (32 gigatonnes) of carbon dioxide and additional air pollution. This caused negative externalities of $4.9 trillion due to global warming and health problems (> 150 $/ton carbon dioxide). Carbon dioxide is one of the greenhouse gases that enhances radiative forcing and contributes to global warming, causing the average surface temperature of the Earth to rise in response, which climate scientists agree will cause major adverse effects.

Coal

The environmental impact of coal mining and burning is diverse. Legislation passed by the U.S. Congress in 1990 required the United States Environmental Protection Agency (EPA) to issue a plan to alleviate toxic pollution from coal-fired power plants. After delay and litigation, the EPA now has a court-imposed deadline of March 16, 2011, to issue its report.

Petroleum

Environmental impact of the petroleum industry

The environmental impact of petroleum is often negative because it is toxic to almost all forms of life. The possibility of climate change exists. Petroleum, commonly referred to as oil, is closely linked to virtually all aspects of present society, especially for transportation and heating for both homes and for commercial activities.

Gas

Natural gas is often described as the cleanest fossil fuel, producing less carbon dioxide per joule delivered than either coal or oil., and far fewer pollutants than other fossil fuels. However, in absolute terms it does contribute substantially to global carbon emissions, and this contribution is projected to grow. According to the IPCC Fourth Assessment Report, in 2004 natural gas produced about 5,300 Mt/yr of CO_2 emissions, while coal and oil produced 10,600 and 10,200 respectively (Figure 4.4); but by 2030, according to an updated version of the SRES B2 emissions scenario, natural gas would be the source of 11,000 Mt/yr, with coal and oil now 8,400 and 17,200 respectively. (Total global emissions for 2004 were estimated at over 27,200 Mt.)

In addition, natural gas itself is a greenhouse gas far more potent than carbon dioxide when released into the atmosphere but is released in smaller amounts.

Electricity Generation

The environmental impact of electricity generation is significant because modern society uses large amounts of electrical power. This power is normally generated at power plants that convert some other kind of energy into electrical power. Each such system has advantages and disadvantages, but many of them pose environmental concerns.

Reservoirs

The environmental impact of reservoirs is coming under ever increasing scrutiny as the world demand for water and energy increases and the number and size of reservoirs increases. Dams and the reservoirs can be used to supply drinking water, generate hydroelectric power, increasing the water supply for irrigation, provide recreational opportunities and for flood control. However, adverse environmental and sociological impacts have also been identified during and after many reservoir constructions. Whether reservoir projects are ultimately beneficial or detrimental—to both the environment and surrounding human populations— has been debated since the 1960s and probably long before that. In 1960 the construction of Llyn Celyn and the flooding of Capel Celyn provoked political uproar which continues to this day. More recently, the construction of Three Gorges Dam and other similar projects throughout Asia, Africa and Latin America have generated considerable environmental and political debate.

Nuclear Power

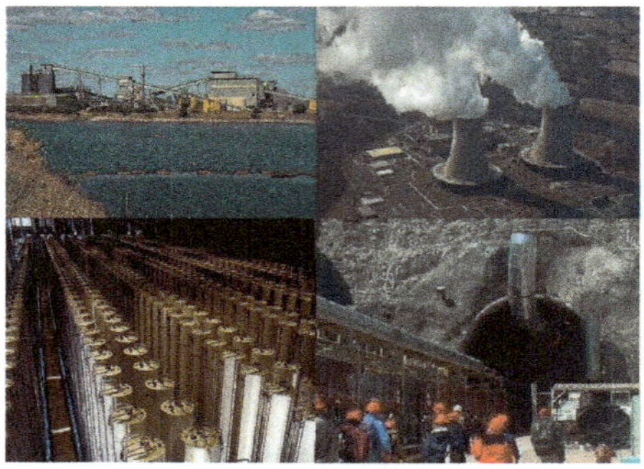

Nuclear power activities involving the environment; mining, enrichment, generation and geological disposal.

The environmental impact of nuclear power results from the nuclear fuel cycle, operation, and the effects of nuclear accidents.

The routine health risks and greenhouse gas emissions from nuclear fission power are smaller than those associated with coal, oil and gas. However, there is a "catastrophic risk" potential if containment fails, which in nuclear reactors can be brought about by over-heated fuels melting and releasing large quantities of fission products into the environment. The most long-lived radioactive wastes, including spent nuclear fuel, must be contained and isolated from humans and the environment for hundreds of thousands of years. The public is sensitive to these risks and there has been considerable public opposition to nuclear power. Despite this potential for disaster, normal fossil fuel related pollution is still considerably more harmful than any previous nuclear disaster.

The 1979 Three Mile Island accident and 1986 Chernobyl disaster, along with high construction costs, ended the rapid growth of global nuclear power capacity. A further disastrous release of radioactive materials followed the 2011 Japanese tsunami which damaged the Fukushima I Nuclear Power Plant, resulting in hydrogen gas explosions and partial meltdowns classified as a Level 7 event. The large-scale release of radioactivity resulted in people being evacuated from a 20 km exclusion zone set up around the power plant, similar to the 30 km radius Chernobyl Exclusion Zone still in effect.

Wind Power

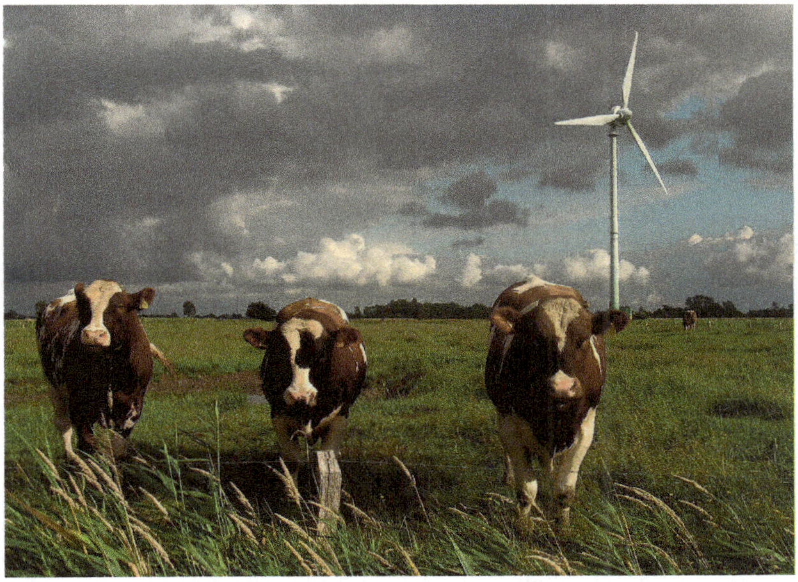

Livestock grazing near a wind turbine.

The **environmental impact of wind power** when compared to the environmental impacts of fossil fuels, is relatively minor. According to the IPCC, in assessments of the life-cycle global warming potential of energy sources, wind turbines have a median value of between 12 and 11 (gCO_2eq/kWh) depending, respectively, on if offshore or onshore turbines are being assessed. Compared with other low carbon power sources, wind turbines have some of the lowest global warming potential per unit of electrical energy generated.

While a wind farm may cover a large area of land, many land uses such as agriculture are compatible with it, as only small areas of turbine foundations and infrastructure are made unavailable for use.

There are reports of bird and bat mortality at wind turbines as there are around other artificial structures. The scale of the ecological impact may or may not be significant, depending on specific circumstances. Prevention and mitigation of wildlife fatalities, and protection of peat bogs, affect the siting and operation of wind turbines.

There are anecdotal reports of negative health effects from noise on people who live very close to wind turbines. Peer-reviewed research has generally not supported these claims.

Aesthetic aspects of wind turbines and resulting changes of the visual landscape are significant.Conflicts arise especially in scenic and heritage protected landscapes.

Mitigation

Energy Conservation

Energy conservation refers to efforts made to reduce energy consumption. Energy conservation can be achieved through increased efficient energy use, in conjunction with decreased energy consumption and/or reduced consumption from conventional energy sources.

Energy conservation can result in increased financial capital, environmental quality, national security, personal security, and human comfort. Individuals and organizations that are direct consumers of energy choose to conserve energy to reduce energy costs and promote economic security. Industrial and commercial users can increase energy use efficiency to maximize profit.

Energy Policy

Energy policy is the manner in which a given entity (often governmental) has decided to address issues of energy development including energy production, distribution and consumption. The attributes of energy policy may include legislation, international treaties, incentives to investment, guidelines for energy conservation, taxation and other public policy techniques.

REFERENCES

1. Likens, Gene E.; Keene, William C.; Miller, John M.; Galloway, James N. (1987). "Chemistry of precipitation from a remote, terrestrial site in Australia". Journal of Geophysical Research. 92: 13299. doi:10.1029/JD092iD11p13299.
2. E. S. de Beer, ed. The Diary of John Evelyn, III, 1955 (19 September 1667) p. 495.
3. Glossary, United States: NASA Earth Observatory, acid rain, archived from the original on 2011-12-13, retrieved 2013-02-15
4. Weathers, K. C. and Likens, G. E. (2006). "Acid rain", pp. 1549–1561 in: W. N. Rom and S. Markowitz (eds.). Environmental and Occupational Medicine. Lippincott-Raven Publ., Philadelphia. Fourth Edition, ISBN 0-7817-6299-5.
5. Seinfeld, John H.; Pandis, Spyros N (1998). Atmospheric Chemistry and Physics — From Air Pollution to Climate Change. John Wiley and Sons, Inc. ISBN 978-0-471-17816-3
6. Likens, G. E.; Bormann, F. H.; Johnson, N. M. (1972). "Acid rain". Environment. 14 (2): 33–40. doi:10.1080/00139157.1972.9933001.
7. Acid Rain in New England, A Brief History ArchivedSeptember 25, 2010, at the Wayback Machine.. Epa.gov. Retrieved on 2013-02-09.
8. Likens, G. E.; Bormann, F. H. (1974). "Acid Rain: A Serious Regional Environmental Problem". Science. 184 (4142): 1176–9. doi:10.1126/

science.184.4142.1176. PMID 17756304.

9. Keller, C. K.; White, T. M.; O'Brien, R.; Smith, J. L. (2006). "Soil CO2 dynamics and fluxes as affected by tree harvest in an experimental sand ecosystem". Journal of Geophysical Research. 111. doi:10.1029/2005JG000157.
10. Galloway, JN; Dianwu, Z; Jiling, X; Likens, GE (1987). "Acid rain: China, United States, and a remote area". Science. 236 (4808): 1559–62. doi:10.1126/science.236.4808.1559. PMID 17835740.
11. Chandru (2006-09-09). "CHINA: Industrialization pollutes its country side with Acid Rain". Southasiaanalysis.org. Archived from the original on June 20, 2010. Retrieved 2010-11-18.
12. Lefohn, A.S.; Husar, J.D.; Husar, R.B. (1999), Global Sulfur Emissions Database, United States: A.S.L. & Associates
13. Likens, G. E.; Wright, R. F.; Galloway, J. N.; Butler, T. J. (1979). "Acid rain". Scientific American. 241 (4): 43–51. doi:10.1038/scientificamerican1079-43.
14. Likens, G. E. (1984). "Acid rain: the smokestack is the "smoking gun"". Garden. 8 (4): 12–18.
15. "Art Under Wraps", Harvard Magazine, March–April 2000
16. Likens, Gene E.; Bormann, F. Herbert; Johnson, Noye M. "Acid Rain". Environment: Science and Policy for Sustainable Development. 14 (2): 33–40. doi:10.1080/00139157.1972.9933001.
17. Johnson, Noye M.; Driscoll, Charles T.; Eaton, John S.; Likens, Gene E.; McDowell, William H. (1981-09-01). "'Acid rain', dissolved aluminum and chemical weathering at the Hubbard Brook Experimental Forest, New Hampshire". Geochimica et Cosmochimica Acta. 45 (9): 1421–1437. doi:10.1016/0016-7037(81)90276-3.
18. Hall, Ronald J.; Likens, Gene E.; Fiance, Sandy B.; Hendrey, George R. (1980-08-01). "Experimental Acidification of a Stream in the Hubbard Brook Experimental Forest, New Hampshire". Ecology. 61 (4): 976–989. doi:10.2307/1936765. ISSN 1939-9170.
19. Lackey, R.T. (1997). "Science, policy, and acid rain: lessons learned" (PDF). Renewable Resources Journal. 15 (1): 9–13.
20. Winstanley, Derek; Lackey, Robert T.; Warnick, Walter L.; Malanchuk, John (1998). "Acid rain: Science and policy making". Environmental Science & Policy. 1: 51. doi:10.1016/S1462-9011(98)00006-9.
21. Times, Robert Reinhold, Special To The New York (1982-06-08). "ACID RAIN ISSUE CREATES STRESS BETWEEN ADMINISTRATION AND SCIENCE ACADEMY". The New York Times. ISSN 0362-4331. Retrieved 2016-11-16.
22. "Ronald Reagan on Environment". www.ontheissues.org. Retrieved 2016-11-16.
23. "HYSTERIA ABOUT ACID RAIN Even Ronald Reagan now casts it as the villain. He is overriding a lot of scientific evidence. - April 14, 1986". archive.fortune.com. Retrieved 2016-11-16.

24. "Ronald Reagan: Nomination of William A. Nierenberg To Be a Member of the National Science Board". www.presidency.ucsb.edu. Retrieved 2016-11-16.
25. "Report of the Acid Rain Peer Review Panel". Document Display | NEPIS | US EPA. July 1984. Retrieved 2016-11-16.
26. "From tobacco to climate change, 'merchants of doubt' undermined the science". Grist. 2010-04-17. Retrieved 2016-11-16.
27. Franklin, Ben A. (1984-08-18). "LEGISLATORS SAT WHITE HOUSE SUPPRESSED ACID RAIN REPORT". The New York Times. ISSN 0362-4331. Retrieved 2016-11-16.
28. "US EPA: A Brief History of Acid Rain". Epa.gov. Archived from the original on 2010-09-25. Retrieved 2010-11-18.
29. 'Cap-and-trade' model eyed for cutting greenhouse gases, San Francisco Chronicle, December 3, 2007.
30. "Facts On File News Services Databases". 2facts.com. Retrieved 2010-11-18.
31. Gilberston, T. and Reyes, O. 2009. Carbon Trading: how it works and why it fails. Dag Hammerskjold Foundation: 22
32. Acid Rain Program 2007 Progress Report, United States Environmental Protection Agency, January 2009.
33. Gerdes, Justin. "Cap and Trade Curbed Acid Rain: 7 Reasons Why It Can Do The Same For Climate Change". Forbes. Forbes. Retrieved 27 Oct 2014.
34. Muki Haklay (2015). "Citizen Science and Policy: A European Perspective" (PDF). Woodrow Wilson International Center for Scholars. p. 11. Retrieved 3 June 2016.
35. R. Kerson (1989). "Lab for the Environnment". MIT Technology Review. Vol. 92 no. 1. pp. 11–12.
36. Berresheim, H.; Wine, P.H. and Davies D.D. (1995). "Sulfur in the Atmosphere". In Composition, Chemistry and Climate of the Atmosphere, ed. H.B. Singh. Van Nostrand Rheingold ISBN 0-442-01264-0
37. Clean Air Act Reduces Acid Rain In Eastern United States, ScienceDaily, September 28, 1998
38. "UK National Air Quality Archive: Air Pollution Glossary". Airquality.co.uk. 2002-04-01. Retrieved 2010-11-18.
39. US EPA: Effects of Acid Rain – Surface Waters and Aquatic Animals
40. Rodhe, H., et al. The global distribution of acidifying wet deposition. Environmental Science and TEchnology. vlo. 36, no. 20 (October) p. 4382–8
41. US EPA: Effects of Acid Rain – Forests Archived July 26, 2008, at the Wayback Machine.
42. Likens, G.E.; Driscoll, C.T.; Buso, D.C.; Mitchell, M.J.; Lovett, G.M.; Bailey, S.W.; Siccama, T.G.; Reiners, W.A.; Alewell, C. (2002). "The biogeochemistry of sulfur at Hubbard Brook" (PDF). Biogeochemistry. 60 (3): 235. doi:10.1023/A:1020972100496.

43. Likens, G. E.; Driscoll, C. T.; Buso, D. C. (1996). "Long-Term Effects of Acid Rain: Response and Recovery of a Forest Ecosystem" (PDF). Science. 272 (5259): 244. doi:10.1126/science.272.5259.244.
44. DeHayes, D.H., Schaberg, P.G. and G.R. Strimbeck. (2001). Red Spruce Hardiness and Freezing Injury Susceptibility. In: F. Bigras, ed. Conifer Cold Hardiness. Kluwer Academic Publishers, the Netherlands ISBN 0-7923-6636-0.
45. Lazarus, Brynne E.; Schaberg, Paul G.; Hawley, Gary J.; DeHayes, Donald H. (2006). "Landscape-scale spatial patterns of winter injury to red spruce foliage in a year of heavy region-wide injury" (PDF). Can. J. For. Res. 36: 142–152. doi:10.1139/x05-236. highbeam copy
46. Effects of Acid Rain – Human Health. Epa.gov (2006-06-02). Retrieved on 2013-02-09.
47. "ICP on effects on materials". Springerlink.com. Retrieved 2010-11-18.
48. "Approaches in modeling the impact of air pollution-induced material degradation" (PDF). Retrieved 2010-11-18.
49. Ed. Hatier (1993). "Acid Rain in Europe". United Nations Environment Programme GRID Arendal. Retrieved 2010-01-31.
50. US Environmental Protection Agency (2008). "Clean Air Markets 2008 Highlights". Retrieved 2010-01-31.
51. Clean Air Act Amendments of 1990, 42 U.S. Code 7651
52. Halldór Björnsson. "Global circulation". Retrieved September 2, 2016. Veðurstofa Íslands. Retrieved on 2008-06-15.
53. Polar vortex. Glossary of Meteorology. American Meteorological Society. June 2000. Retrieved 15 June 2008.
54. Stratospheric Polar Vortex Influences Winter Cold, Researchers Say (Press release). American Association for the Advancement of Science. December 3, 2001. Retrieved May 23, 2015.
55. Air Maps, Littell's Living Age No. 495, 12 November 1853, p. 430.
56. GEOS-5 Analyses and Forecasts of the Major Stratospheric Sudden Warming of January 2013 (Press release). Goddard Space Flight Center. Retrieved January 8, 2014.
57. http://blog.quarkexpeditions.com/polar-vortex-the-science-myth-media-hype-behind-north-american-weather-phenomen.
58. Hartmann, D; Schoeberl, M (1991). Mixing of polar vortex air into middle latitudes as revealed by tracer-tracer scatterplots. Journal of Geophysical Research. 102: 13119. Bibcode:1997JGR...10213119W. doi:10.1029/96JD03715.
59. Cavallo, Steven M.; Hakim, Gregory J. (April 2009). Potential Vorticity Diagnosis of a Tropopause Polar Cyclone. Monthly Weather Review. 137 (4): 1358–1371. Bibcode:2009MWRv..137.1358C. doi:10.1175/2008MWR2670.1.
60. Kolstad, Erik W.; Breiteig, Tarjei; Scaife, Adam A. (April 2010). The association between stratospheric weak polar vortex events and cold air outbreaks in the

Northern Hemisphere. Quarterly Journal of the Royal Meteorological Society. Royal Meteorological Society. 136: 887. Bibcode:2010EGUGA..12.5739K. doi:10.1002/qj.620.

61. Abdolreza Kashki & Javad Khoshhal (2013-11-22). Investigation of the Role of Polar Vortex in Iranian First and Last Snowfalls. Journal of Geology and Geography. Canadian Center of Science and Education. 5 (4). ISSN 1916-9779.
62. Erik A. Rasmussen and John Turner (2003). Polar lows: mesoscale weather systems in the polar regions. Cambridge University Press. p. 174. ISBN 978-0-521-62430-5.
63. Robock, Alan (2000). Volcanic eruptions and climate. Reviews of Geophysics. 38 (2): 191–219. Bibcode:2000RvGeo..38..191R. doi:10.1029/1998RG000054.
64. Todd Mitchell (2004). Arctic Oscillation (AO) time series, 1899 – June 2002. University of Washington. Retrieved on 2009-03-02.
65. Kevin Myatt (2005-01-17). Cold enough for snow, and more's on the way. Roanoke Times. Retrieved on 2012-02-24.
66. Nash, E; Newman, P; Rosenfield, J; Schoeberl, M (2012). An objective determination of the polar vortex using Ertel's potential vorticity. Journal of Geophysical Research. 101 (D5): 9471–9478. Bibcode:1996JGR...101.9471N. doi:10.1029/96JD00066.
67. Li, L; Li, C; Pan, Y (2012). On the differences and climate impacts of early and late stratospheric polar vortex breakup. Advances in Atmospheric Sciences. 29 (5): 1119–1128. Bibcode:2012AdAtS..29.1119L. doi:10.1007/s00376-012-1012-4.
68. Wei, K; Chen, W; Huang, R (2007). Dynamical diagnosis of the breakup of the stratospheric polar vortex in the northern hemisphere. Science in China Series D (Earth Sciences). 50 (9): 1369–1379. doi:10.1007/s11430-007-0100-2.
69. Reichler, Tom; Kim, J; Manzini, E; Kroger, J (2012). A stratospheric connection to Atlantic climate variability. Nature Geoscience. 5: 783–787. Bibcode:2012NatGe...5..783R. doi:10.1038/ngeo1586.
70. Ripesi, Patrizio; et al. (2012). The February 2010 Artcic Oscillation Index and its stratospheric connection (PDF). Quarterly Journal of the Royal Meteorological Society. 138: 1961–1969. Bibcode:2012QJRMS.138.1961R. doi:10.1002/qj.1935.
71. Reichler, Tom; Kim, J; Manzini, E; Kroger, J (2012). A stratospheric connection to Atlantic climate variability. Nature Geoscience. 5: 783–787. Bibcode:2012NatGe...5..783R. doi:10.1038/ngeo1586.
72. Limpasuvan, Varavut; Hartmann, Dennis L.; Thompson, David W. J.; Jeev, Kumar; Yung, Yuk L. (2005). Stratosphere-troposphere evolution during polar vortex intensification(PDF). Journal of Geophysical Research. 110 (D24): 27. Bibcode:2005JGRD..11024101L. doi:10.1029/2005JD006302.
73. Cavallo, S; Hakim, G.J. (2013). Physical mechanisms of tropopause polar vortex intensity change. Journal of the Atmospheric Sciences. 70 (11): 3359–3373. doi:10.1175/JAS-D-13-088.1.
74. Hartmann, D; Schoeberl, M (1991). The dynamics of the stratospheric polar

vortex and its relation to springtime ozone depletions. Science. 251 (4989): 46–52. Bibcode:1991Sci...251...46S. doi:10.1126/science.251.4989.46. PMID 17778602.

75. Widnall, S; Sullivan, J (1973). On the stability of vortex rings. Proceedings of the Royal Society of London. Series A, Mathematical and Physical Sciences. 332 (1590): 335–353. Bibcode:1973RSPSA.332..335W. doi:10.1098/rspa.1973.0029.
76. Manney, G; Zurek, R; O'Neill, A; Swinbank, R (1994). On the motion of air through the stratospheric polar vortex. Journal of the Atmospheric Sciences. 51 (20): 2973–2994. Bibcode:1994JAtS...51.2973M. doi:10.1175/1520-0469(1994)051<2973:otmoat>2.0.co;2.
77. Waugh, D; Plumb, R; Elkins, J; Fahey, D; Boering, K; Dutton, G; Lait, L (2012). Mixing of polar vortex air into middle latitudes as revealed by tracer-tracer scatterplots. Journal of Geophysical Research: Atmospheres. 102 (D11): 13199–1314. Bibcode:1997JGR...10213119W. doi:10.1029/96JD03715.
78. Archived copy. Archived from the original on 2015-12-07. Retrieved 2015-11-26.
79. Erdman, Jon (2014). What's a Polar Vortex?: The Science Behind Arctic Outbreaks. wunderground. Retrieved 25 February 2014.
80. Baldwin, M. P.; Dunkerton, TJ (2001). Stratospheric Harbingers of Anomalous Weather Regimes. Science. 294 (5542): 581–4. Bibcode:2001Sci...294..581B. doi:10.1126/science.1063315. PMID 11641495.
81. NASA (December 21, 2001). Stratospheric Polar Vortex Influences Winter Cold. Earth Observatory. Retrieved January 7, 2014.
82. Song, Yucheng; Robinson, Walter A. (2004). Dynamical Mechanisms for Stratospheric Influences on the Troposphere. Journal of the Atmospheric Sciences. 61 (14): 1711–25. Bibcode:2004JAtS...61.1711S. doi:10.1175/1520-0469(2004)061<1711:DMFSIO>2.0.CO;2.
83. Overland, James E. (2013). Atmospheric science: Long-range linkage. Nature Climate Change. 4: 11–2. Bibcode:2014NatCC...4...11O. doi:10.1038/nclimate2079.
84. Tang, Qiuhong; Zhang, Xuejun; Francis, Jennifer A. (2013). Extreme summer weather in northern mid-latitudes linked to a vanishing cryosphere. Nature Climate Change. 4: 45–50. Bibcode:2014NatCC...4...45T. doi:10.1038/nclimate2065.
85. Screen, J A (2013). Influence of Arctic sea ice on European summer precipitation. Environmental Research Letters. 8 (4): 044015. Bibcode:2013ERL.....8d4015S. doi:10.1088/1748-9326/8/4/044015.
86. Francis, Jennifer A.; Vavrus, Stephen J. (2012). Evidence linking Arctic amplification to extreme weather in mid-latitudes. Geophysical Research Letters. 39 (6): n/a. Bibcode:2012GeoRL..39.6801F. doi:10.1029/2012GL051000.
87. Petoukhov, Vladimir; Semenov, Vladimir A. (2010). A link between reduced Barents-Kara sea ice and cold winter extremes over northern continents. Journal of Geophysical Research. 115. Bibcode:2010JGRD..11521111P. doi:10.1029/2009JD013568.
88. Masato, Giacomo; Hoskins, Brian J.; Woollings, Tim (2013). Winter and Summer

Northern Hemisphere Blocking in CMIP5 Models. Journal of Climate. 26 (18): 7044–59. doi:10.1175/JCLI-D-12-00466.1.

89. Friedlander, Blaine (March 4, 2013). Arctic ice loss amplified Superstorm Sandy violence. Cornell Chronicle.
90. J. A. Pyle (1997-04-08). The Arctic and environmental change. CRC Press. pp. 42–44. ISBN 978-90-5699-020-6.
91. Rolf Müller (2010). Tracer-tracer Relations as a Tool for Research on Polar Ozone Loss. Forschungszentrum Jülich. p. 47. ISBN 978-3-89336-614-9.
92. K. Mohanakuma (2008). Stratosphere troposphere interactions: an introduction. Springer. p. 34. ISBN 978-1-4020-8216-0.
93. Double vortex at Venus South Pole unveiled. European Space Agency. Retrieved June 2006. Check date values in: |access-date= (help)
94. Saturn's Bull's-Eye Marks Its Hot Spot. NASA. 2005. Retrieved January 8, 2014.
95. J. B, ed. (1905). The Two Widecombe Tracts, 1638 giving a Contemporary Account of the great Storm, reprinted with an Introduction. Exeter: James G Commin. Retrieved 29 June 2013.
96. Day, Jeremiah (January 1813). A view of the theories which have been proposed to explain the origin of meteoric stones. The General Repository and Review. Cambridge, Massachusetts: William Hilliard. 3 (1): 156–157. Retrieved 29 June 2013.
97. How Stuff Works entry. Retrieved 21 January 2014.
98. Anna Salleh (2008-03-20). Ball lightning bamboozles physicist. 35.2772;149.1292: Abc.net.au. Retrieved 21 January 2014.
99. Cen, Jianyong; Yuan, Ping; Xue, Simin (17 January 2014). Observation of the Optical and Spectral Characteristics of Ball Lightning. Physical Review Letters. American Physical Society. 112 (3): 035001. Bibcode:2014PhRvL.112c5001C. doi:10.1103/PhysRevLett.112.035001. Retrieved 19 January 2014.
100. Slezak, Michael (16 January 2014). Natural ball lightning probed for the first time. New Scientist. Retrieved 22 January 2014.
101. Anon. Ask the experts. Scientific American. Retrieved 4 April 2007.
102. McNally, J. R. (1960). Preliminary Report on Ball Lightning. Proceedings of the Second Annual Meeting of the Division of Plasma Physics of the American Physical Society (Paper J-15 ed.). Gatlinburg. pp. 1–25.
103. Grigoriev, A. I. (1988). Y. H. Ohtsuki, ed. Statistical Analysis of the Ball Lightning Properties. Science of Ball Lightning. Singapore: World Scientific Publishing Co.: 88–134.
104. Anon. Foreign Affairs: Bristol 17 December. Weekly Journal or British Gazetteer. 24 December 1726.
105. Anon (24 December 1726). Foreign Affairs: London 24 December. London Journal.
106. Clarke, Ronald W. (1983). Benjamin Franklin, A Biography. Random House. p.

87. ISBN 978-1-84212-272-3. Archived from the original on 12 January 2012.

107. Simons, Paul (17 February 2009). Weather Eye Charles Darwin the meteorologist. The Times. London. Retrieved 16 April 2010.

108. http://www.thenational.ae/article/20090223/FRONTIERS/646186738/1036

109. Brewer, Ebenezer Cobham (1864). A Guide to the Scientific Knowledge of Things Familiar. pp. 13–14. Retrieved 22 January 2014.

110. de Fonvielle, Wilfrid (1875). Chapter X Globular lightning. Thunder and lightning (full text). translated by T L Phipson. pp. 32–39. ISBN 978-1-142-61255-9. Retrieved 22 January 2014.

111. Anon (24 December 1867). Globular lightning. The Leeds mercury. Leeds, UK.

112. Tsar-Martyr Nicholas II And His Family. Orthodox.net. Archived from the original on 17 June 2009. Retrieved 13 July 2009.

113. There is no present-day Lake Pasquaney in New Hampshire, United States. New Hampshire's Newfound Lake has a Camp Pasquaney. However, part of the lake is known as Pasquaney Bay.

114. Crowley, Aleister (5 December 1989). Chp. 83. The Confessions of Aleister Crowley: An Autobiography. Penguin. ISBN 0-14-019189-5.

115. Jennison, R. C. (1969). Ball Lightning. Nature. 224 (5222): 895. Bibcode:1969Natur.224..895J. doi:10.1038/224895a0.

116. Miracle saved panth. Sikhnet.com. 2009-12-21. Retrieved 21 January 2014.

117. Golden Globe, 24 November 1894.

118. Mark Stenhoff, Ball Lightning: An Unsolved Problem in Atmospheric Physics (Springer Science & Business Media, 2006) p70

119. The Cape Naturaliste Lighthouse. Lighthouses of Western Australia. Lighthouses of Australia Inc. Retrieved 13 July 2009.

120. Wilder, Laura Ingalls (1937). On the Banks of Plum Creek. Harper Trophy. ISBN 0-06-440005-0.

121. Getline, Meryl (17 October 2005). Playing with (St. Elmo's) fire. USA Today.

122. Ball lightning – and the charge sheath vortex. Peter-thomson.co.uk. Retrieved 13 July 2009.

123. This may be an incorrect translation of the word blixtlokaliseringssystem from the university article cited in the sources

124. Larsson, Anders (23 April 2002). Ett fenomen som gäckar vetenskapen (in Swedish). Uppsala University. Retrieved 19 November 2007.

125. Fizikai Szemle 2004/10. Kfki.hu. Retrieved 21 January 2014.

126. Domokos Tar (2009). Observation of Lightning Ball (Ball Lightning): A new phenomenological description of the phenomenon. Proceedings of the 9th International Symposium on Ball Lightning, Aug. Eindhoven. 0910: 783. arXiv:0910.0783 . Bibcode:2009arXiv0910.0783T.

127. Domokos Tar (2010). Lightning Ball (Ball Lightning) Created by Thunder,

Shock-Wave. arXiv:1007.3348 .

128. Domokos Tar (2009). New Revelation of Lightning Ball Observation and Proposal for a Nuclear Reactor Fusion Experiment. Proceedings 10th International Symposium on Ball Lightning (ISBL-08), July 7–12 Kaliningrad, Russia, pp. 135–141, Eds. Vladimir L. Bychkov & Anatoly I. Nikitin. 0910: 2089. arXiv:0910.2089 . Bibcode:2009arXiv0910.2089T.
129. Source (in Czech). Zpravy.idnes.cz. Retrieved 21 January 2014.
130. The Aviation Herald. avherald.com.
131. BL_Info_10. Ernmphotography.com. Retrieved 13 July 2009.
132. Unusual Phenomea Reports: Ball Lightning. Amasci.com. Retrieved 13 July 2009.
133. Barry, James Dale: Ball lightning and bead lightning: extreme forms of atmospheric electricity, ISBN 0-306-40272-6, 1980, Plenum Press (p. 35)
134. Barry, J.D. (1980a) Ball Lightning and Bead Lightning: Extreme Forms of Atmospheric Electricity. 8–9. New York and London: Plenum Press. ISBN 0-306-40272-6
135. Charman, Neil (14 December 1972). The enigma of ball Lightning. New Scientist. Reed Business information. 56 (824): 632–635. Retrieved 10 May 2010.
136. Ball, Philip (17 January 2014). Focus: First Spectrum of Ball Lightning. Focus. American Physical Society. doi:10.1103/Physics.7.5. Retrieved 19 January 2014.
137. The New Wizard of the West. Homepage.ntlworld.com. Retrieved 13 July 2009.
138. Tesla, Nikola (1978). Nikola Tesla – Colorado Springs Notes 1899–1900. Nolit (Beograd, Yugoslavia), 368–370. ISBN 978-0-913022-26-9
139. Anon (2008). Tenth international syposium on ball lightning/ International symposium III on unconventional plasmas. ICBL. Retrieved 10 May 2010.
140. https://web.archive.org/web/20120604074802/http://www.cose.txstate.edu/isbl_12.html. Archived from the original on 4 June 2012. Retrieved 4 June 2012. Missing or empty |title=(help)
141. Ohtsuki, Y. H.; H. Ofuruton (1991). Plasma fireballs formed by microwave interference in air. Nature. 350 (6314): 139–141. Bibcode:1991Natur.350..139O. doi:10.1038/350139a0.
142. Ohtsuki, Y. H.; H. Ofuruton (1991). Plasma fireballs formed by microwave interference in air (Corrections). Nature. 353 (6347): 868. Bibcode:1991Natur.353..868O. doi:10.1038/353868a0.
143. 'Ball lightning' created in German laboratory | COSMOS magazine. COSMOS magazine. 7 June 2006. Retrieved 13 July 2009.
144. Youichi Sakawa; Kazuyoshi Sugiyama; Tetsuo Tanabe; Richard More (12 July 2006). Fireball Generation in a Water Discharge. Plasma and Fusion Research: Rapid Communications. Retrieved 13 July 2009.
145. How to make a Stable Plasmoid (Ball Lightning) with the GMR (Graphite Microwave Resonator) by Jean-Louis Naudin. Jlnlabs.online.fr. 22 December 2005. Archivedfrom the original on 26 June 2009. Retrieved 13 July 2009.

146. Creating the 4th state of matter with microwaves by Halina Stanley. scienceinschool.org. 13 August 2009. Archivedfrom the original on 31 October 2009. Retrieved 6 October 2009.
147. Universidade Federal de Pernambuco. Ufpe.br. Archived from the original on 21 June 2009. Retrieved 13 July 2009.
148. Pesquisadores da UFPE geram, em laboratório, fenômeno atmosférico conhecido como bolas luminosas. Ufpe.br. 16 January 2007. Archived from the original on 20 December 2008. Retrieved 13 July 2009.
149. Ball Lightning Mystery Solved? Electrical Phenomenon Created in Lab. News. nationalgeographic.com. 21 November 2005. Retrieved 13 July 2009.
150. Snow Harris, William (2008). Section I. On the nature of thunderstorms (originally published in 1843) (Reprint ed.). Bastian Books. pp. 34–43. ISBN 0-554-87861-5. Retrieved 11 May 2010.
151. François Arago, Meteorological Essays by , Longman, 1855
152. Paiva, Gerson Silva; Antonio Carlos Pavão; Elder Alpes de Vasconcelos; Odim Mendes, Jr.; Eronides Felisberto da Silva, Jr. (2007). Production of Ball-Lightning-Like Luminous Balls by Electrical Discharges in Silicon. Phys. Rev. Lett. 98 (4): 048501. Bibcode:2007PhRvL..98d8501P. doi:10.1103/PhysRevLett.98.048501. PMID 17358820.
153. Lightning balls created in the lab. New Scientist. 10 January 2007.
154. Ball Lightning Mystery Solved? Electrical Phenomenon Created in Lab. National Geographic News. 22 January 2007.
155. ftp://ftp.aip.org/epaps/phys_rev_lett/E-PRLTAO-98-047705/
156. Slezak, Michael. Natural ball lightning probed for the first time. New Scientist. Retrieved 17 January 2014.
157. Abrahamson, John; Dinniss, James (2000). Ball lightning caused by oxidation of nanoparticle networks from normal lightning strikes on soil. Nature. 403 (6769): 519–21. Bibcode:2000Natur.403..519A. doi:10.1038/35000525. PMID 10676954.
158. Muldrew, D. B. (1990). The Physical Nature of Ball Lightning. Geophysical Research Letters. 17 (12): 2277–2280. Bibcode:1990GeoRL..17.2277M. doi:10.1029/GL017i012p02277.
159. Muldrew, D. B. (2010). Solid charged-core model of ball lightning. Annales Geophysicae. 28: 223–2010. Bibcode:2010AnGeo..28..223M. doi:10.5194/angeo-28-223-2010.
160. Капица, П. Л. (1955). О природе шаровой молнии. Докл. Акад. наук СССР (in Russian). 101: 245.
161. Kapitsa, Peter L. (1955). The Nature of Ball Lightning. In Donald J. Ritchie. Ball Lightning: A Collection of Soviet Research in English Translation (1961 ed.). Consultants Bureau, New York. pp. 11–16. Retrieved 22 January 2014.
162. Handel, Peter H.; Jean-François Leitner (1994). Development of the maser-caviton ball lightning theory. J. Geophys. Res. 99: 10689. Bibcode:1994JGR....9910689H. doi:10.1029/93JD01021.

163. Dvornikov, Maxim; Dvornikov, Sergey (2006). Gerard, F., ed. Electron gas oscillations in plasma. Theory and applications. Advances in Plasma Physics Research. New York, USA: Nova Science Publishers, Inc.: 197–212. arXiv:physics/0306157 . Bibcode:2003physics...6157D. ISBN 1-59033-928-2.

164. Dvornikov, Maxim (2010). Formation of bound states of electrons in spherically symmetric oscillations of plasma. Physica Scripta. 81 (5): 055502. arXiv:1002.0764 . Bibcode:2010PhyS...81e5502D. doi:10.1088/0031-8949/81/05/055502.

165. Dvornikov, Maxim (2011-12-01). Axially and spherically symmetric solitons in warm plasma. Journal of Plasma Physics. 77 (6): 749–764. arXiv:1010.0701 . Bibcode:2011JPlPh..77..749D. doi:10.1017/S002237781100016X. ISSN 1469-7807.

166. Dvornikov, Maxim (2012-02-08). Effective attraction between oscillating electrons in a plasmoid via acoustic wave exchange. Proc. R. Soc. A. 468 (2138): 415–428. arXiv:1102.0944 . doi:10.1098/rspa.2011.0276. ISSN 1364-5021.

167. Dvornikov, Maxim (2012-11-01). Quantum exchange interaction of spherically symmetric plasmoids. Journal of Atmospheric and Solar-Terrestrial Physics. 89: 62–66. arXiv:1112.0239 . Bibcode:2012JASTP..89...62D. doi:10.1016/j.jastp.2012.08.005.

168. Dvornikov, Maxim (2013). Pairing of charged particles in a quantum plasmoid. Journal of Physics A: Mathematical and Theoretical. 46 (4): 045501. arXiv:1208.2208 . Bibcode:2013JPhA...46d5501D. doi:10.1088/1751-8113/46/4/045501.

169. Dvornikov, M. (2013). Stable Langmuir solitons in plasma with diatomic ions. Nonlinear Processes in Geophysics. 20 (4): 581–588. arXiv:1203.0258 . Bibcode:2013NPGeo..20..581D. doi:10.5194/npg-20-581-2013.

170. Davydova, T. A.; Yakimenko, A. I.; Zaliznyak, Yu. A. (2005-02-28). Stable spatial Langmuir solitons. Physics Letters A. 336 (1): 46–52. Bibcode:2005PhLA..336...46D. doi:10.1016/j.physleta.2004.11.063.

171. Dijkhuis, G. C. (1980-03-13). A model for ball lightning. Nature. 284 (5752): 150–151. Bibcode:1980Natur.284..150D. doi:10.1038/284150a0.

172. Zelikin, M. I. (2008). Superconductivity of plasma and fireballs. Journal of Mathematical Sciences. 151 (6): 3473–3496. doi:10.1007/s10958-008-9047-x.

173. Tar, Domokos (2009-10-05). Observation of Lightning Ball (Ball Lightning): A new phenomenological description of the phenomenon. Proceedings of the -th International Symposium on Ball Lightning, Aug. Eindhoven. 9 (2006). arXiv:0910.0783 .

174. Tar, Domokos (2010-07-20). Lightning Ball (Ball Lightning) Created by Thunder, Shock-Wave. arXiv:1007.3348.

175. Coleman, PF (1993). An explanation for ball lightning?. Weather. 48: 30. Bibcode:1993Wthr...48...27.. doi:10.1002/j.1477-8696.1993.tb07221.x.

176. Meshcheryakov, Oleg (2007). Ball Lightning–Aerosol Electrochemical Power Source or A Cloud of Batteries(PDF). Nanoscale Res. Lett. 2 (3): 319–330.

Bibcode:2007NRL.....2..319M. doi:10.1007/s11671-007-9068-2. Retrieved 27 June 2007.

177. Ball lightning's frightening . . . but finally explained. EE Times. 29 August 2007.

178. Meshcheryakov, Oleg (1 August 2010). How and why electrostatic charge of combustible nanoparticles can radically change the mechanism and rate of their oxidation in humid atmosphere. arXiv:1008.0162 .

179. Meshcheryakov, Oleg (17 Jul 2013). Why not only electric discharge but even a minimum charge on the surface of highly sensitive explosives can catalyze their gradual exothermic decomposition and how a cloud of unipolar charged explosive particles turns into ball lightning. arXiv:1402.3214 .

180. Mario Rabinowitz (11 December 2002). Little Black Holes:Dark Matter And Ball Lightning. Astrophys. Space Sci. 262 (4): 391–410. arXiv:astro-ph/0212251 . Bibcode:1998Ap&SS.262..391R. doi:10.1023/A:1001865715833.

181. Muir, Hazel (23 December 2006). Blackholes in your backyard. New Scientist. 192 (2583/2584): 48–51. doi:10.1016/S0262-4079(06)61459-0.

182. http://www.disclosureproject.org/docs/pdf/uap_exec_summary_dec00.pdf | UAP in the UK Air Defence Region, Executive Summary, Page 7, Defence Intelligence Staff, 2000

183. Could some ball lightning observations be optical hallucinations caused by epileptic seizures, Cooray, G. and V. Cooray, The open access atmospheric science journal, vol. 2, pp. 101–105 (2008)

184. Peer, J.; Kendl, A. (2010). Transcranial stimulability of phosphenes by long lightning electromagnetic pulses. Physics Letters A. 374 (29): 2932–2935. arXiv:1005.1153 . Bibcode:2010PhLA..374.2932P. doi:10.1016/j.physleta.2010.05.023.

185. Ball lightning is all in the mind, say Austrian physicists, The Register, 19 May 2010.

186. Emerging Technology (2010-05-11). Magnetically Induced Hallucinations Explain Ball Lightning, Say Physicists – Technology Review. Technologyreview.com. Retrieved 21 January 2014.

187. Seward, C., Chen, C., Ware, K. Ball Lightning Explained as a Stable Plasma Toroid. PPPS- 2001 Pulsed Power Plasma Science Conference. June 2001.

188. Chen, C., Pakter, R., Seward, D. C. Equilibrium and Stability Properties of Self-Organized Electron Spiral Toroids. Physics of Plasmas. Vol. 8, No. 10, pp. 4441–4449. October 2001.

189. Seward, Clint. Ball Lightning Explanation Leading to Clean Energy. Amazon. com. 2011.

190. Manykin, E. A.; Ojovan, M. I.; Poluektov, P. P. (2006). Samartsev, Vitaly V, ed. Rydberg matter: Properties and decay. Proceedings of the SPIE. SPIE Proceedings. 6181: 618105. Bibcode:2006SPIE.6181E..05M. doi:10.1117/12.675004.

191. Norman, G. É. (2001). Rydberg matter as a metastable state of strongly nonideal plasma. Journal of Experimental and Theoretical Physics Letters. 73: 10–12. Bibcode:2001JETPL..73...10N. doi:10.1134/1.1355396.

192. Manykin, E. A.; Zelener, B. B.; Zelener, B. V. (2011). Thermodynamic and kinetic properties of nonideal Rydberg matter. JETP Letters. 92 (9): 630. Bibcode:2011JETPL..92..630M. doi:10.1134/S0021364010210125.

193. Holmlid, L. (2007). Direct observation of circular Rydberg electrons in a Rydberg matter surface layer by electronic circular dichroism. Journal of Physics: Condensed Matter. 19 (27): 276206–276202. Bibcode:2007JPCM...19A6206H. doi:10.1088/0953-8984/19/27/276206.

194. Endean, V. G. (1976). Ball lightning as electromagnetic energy. Nature. 263 (5580): 753–755. Bibcode:1976Natur.263..753E. doi:10.1038/263753a0.

195. Singer, Stanley (1971). The Nature of Ball Lightning. New York: Plenum Press.

196. The IEEE, Plasma Cosmology and Extreme Ball Lightning. Thunderbolts.info. Retrieved 13 July 2009.

197. Smirnov 1987, Physics Reports, (Review Section of Physical Letters), 152, No. 4, pp. 177–226.

198. Torchigin, V.P. (2009). Ball Lightning as an Optical Incoherent Space Spherical Soliton in Handbook of Solitons: Research, Technology and Applications editors S.P. Lang and S.H. Bedore. New York: Novapublishers: 3–54.

199. Wu, H.-C. (2016). Relativistic-microwave theory of ball lightning. Scientific Reports. Retrieved 22 June 2016.

CHAPTER 5

Pesticide Poisoning

Chapter Contents

Pesticides are selective poisons chosen for use because of their relative safety for humans and animals. It islikely that they will poison these species if they are used in sufficient quantity or in special circumstances, forexample when the water intake of the subject animals is limited.

INTRODUCTION

A **pesticide poisoning** occurs when chemicals intended to control a pest affect non-target organisms such as humans, wildlife, or bees. There are three types of pesticide poisoning. The first of the three is a single and short-term very high level of exposure which can be experienced by individuals who commit suicide, as well as pesticide formulators. The second type of poisoning is long-term high-level exposure, which can occur in pesticide formulators and manufacturers. The third type of poisoning is a long-term low-level exposure, which individuals are exposed to from sources such as pesticide residues in food as well as contact with pesticide residues in the air, water, soil, sediment, food materials, plants and animals.

In developing countries, such as Sri Lanka, pesticide poisonings from short-term very high level of exposure (acute poisoning) is the most worrisome type of poisoning. However, in developed countries, such as Canada, it is the complete opposite: acute pesticide poisoning is controlled, thus making the main issue long-term low-level exposure of pesticides.

CAUSE

The most common exposure scenarios for pesticide-poisoning cases are accidental or suicidal poisonings, occupational exposure, by-stander exposure to off-target drift, and the general public who are exposed through environmental contamination.

Accidental or Suicidal?

Self-poisoning with agricultural pesticides represents a major hidden public health problem accounting for approximately one-third of all suicides worldwide. It is one of the most common forms of self-injury in the Global South. The World Health Organization estimates that 300,000 people die from self-harm each year in the Asia-Pacific region alone. Most cases of intentional pesticide poisoning appear to be impulsive acts undertaken during stressful events, and the availability of pesticides strongly influences the incidence of self poisoning. Pesticides are the agents most frequently used by farmers and students in India to commit suicide.

Occupational

Pesticide poisoning is an important occupational health issue because pesticides are used in a large number of industries, which puts many different categories of workers at risk. Extensive use puts agricultural workers in particular at increased risk for pesticide illnesses. Workers in other industries are at risk for exposure as well. For example, commercial availability of pesticides in stores puts retail workers at risk for exposure and illness when they handle pesticide products. The ubiquity of pesticides puts emergency responders such as fire-fighters and police officers at risk, because they are often the first responders to emergency events and may be unaware of the presence of a poisoning hazard. The process of aircraft disinsection, in which pesticides are used on inbound international flights for insect and disease control, can also make flight attendants sick.

Different job functions can lead to different levels of exposure. Most occupational exposures are caused by absorption through exposed skin such as the face, hands, forearms, neck, and chest. This exposure is sometimes enhanced by inhalation in settings including spraying operations in greenhouses and other closed environments, tractor cabs, and the operation of rotary fan mist sprayers.

Residential

When thinking of pesticide poisoning, one does not take into consideration the contribution that is made of their own household. The majority of households in Canada use pesticides while taking part in activities such as gardening. In Canada 96 percent of households report having a lawn or a garden.56 percent of the households who have a lawn or a garden utilize fertilizer or pesticide. This form of pesticide use may contribute to the third type of poisoning, which is caused by long-term low-level exposure. As mentioned before, long-term low-level exposure affects individuals from sources such as pesticide residues in food as well as contact with pesticide residues in the air, water, soil, sediment, food materials, plants and animals.

Pathophysiology

Organochlorines

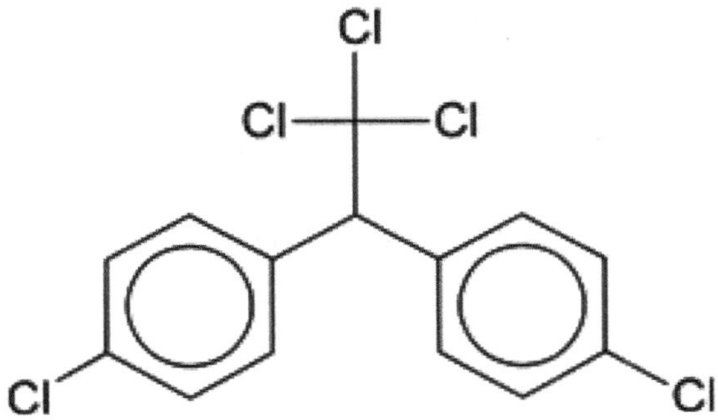

DDT, an organochlorine.

The organochlorine pesticides, like DDT, aldrin, and dieldrin are extremely persistent and accumulate in fatty tissue. Through the process of bioaccumulation (lower amounts in the environment get magnified sequentially up the food chain), large amounts of organochlorines can accumulate in top species like humans. There is substantial evidence to suggest that DDT, and its metabolite DDE, act as endocrine disruptors, interfering with hormonal function of estrogen, testosterone, and other steroid hormones.

Anticholinesterase Compounds

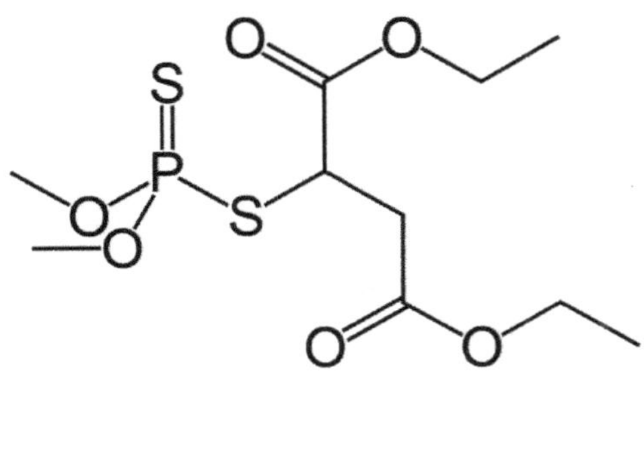

Malathion, an organophosphate anticholinesterase.

Certain organophosphates have long been known to cause a delayed-onset toxicity to nerve cells, which is often irreversible. Several studies have shown persistent deficits in cognitive function in workers chronically exposed to pesticides. Newer evidence suggests that these pesticides may cause developmental neurotoxicity at much lower doses and without depression of plasma cholinesterase levels.

DIAGNOSIS

Most pesticide-related illnesses have signs and symptoms that are similar to common medical conditions, so a complete and detailed environmental and occupational history is essential for correctly diagnosing a pesticide poisoning. A few additional screening questions about the patient's work and home environment, in addition to a typical health questionnaire, can indicate whether there was a potential pesticide poisoning.

If one is regularly using carbamate and organophosphate pesticides, it is important to obtain a baseline cholinesterase test. Cholinesterase is an important enzyme of the nervous system, and these chemical groups kill pests and potentially injure or kill humans by inhibiting cholinesterase. If one has had a baseline test and later suspects a poisoning, one can identify the extent of the problem by comparison of the current cholinesterase level with the baseline level.

PREVENTION

Accidental poisonings can be avoided by proper labeling and storage of containers. When handling or applying pesticides, exposure can be significantly reduced by protecting certain parts of the body where the skin shows increased absorption, such as the scrotal region, underarms, face, scalp, and hands.Using chemical-resistant gloves has been shown to reduce contamination by 33–86%.

Further methods in order to aid prevention of acute pesticide poisoning, concerning both accidental death and suicides, there could be a method for national governments to control accessibility. The pesticides most toxic to humans if restricted has the possibility to reduce deaths. There could also be designated locations in rural living areas and cities used to safely store toxic pesticides in order to gain control over usage.

TREATMENT

Specific treatments for acute pesticide poisoning are often dependent on the pesticide or class of pesticide responsible for the poisoning. However, there are basic management techniques that are applicable to most acute poisonings, including skin decontamination, airway protection, gastrointestinal decontamination, and seizure treatment.

Decontamination of the skin is performed while other life-saving measures are taking place. Clothing is removed, the patient is showered with soap and water, and the hair is shampooed to remove chemicals from the skin and hair. The eyes are flushed with water for 10–15 minutes. The patient is intubated and oxygen administered, if necessary. In more severe cases, pulmonary ventilation must sometimes be supported mechanically. Seizures are typically managed with lorazepam, phenytoin and phenobarbitol, or diazepam (particularly for organochlorine poisonings).

Gastric lavage is not recommended to be used routinely in pesticide poisoning management, as clinical benefit has not been confirmed in controlled studies; it is indicated only when the patient has ingested a potentially life-threatening amount of poison and presents within 60 minutes of ingestion. An orogastric tube is inserted and the stomach is flushed with saline to try to remove the poison. If the patient is neurologically impaired, a cuffed endotracheal tube inserted beforehand for airway protection. Studies of poison recovery at 60 minutes have shown recovery of 8%–32%. However, there is also evidence that lavage may flush the material into the small intestine, increasing absorption. Lavage is contra-indicated in cases of hydrocarbon ingestion.

Activated charcoal is sometimes administered as it has been shown to be successful with some pesticides. Studies have shown that it can reduce the amount absorbed if given within 60 minutes,though there is not enough data to determine if it is effective if time from ingestion is prolonged. Syrup of ipecac is no longer recommended for most pesticide poisonings.

Urinary alkalinisation has been used in acute poisonings from chlorophenoxy herbicides (such as 2,4-D, MCPA, 2,4,5-T and mecoprop); however, evidence to support its use is poor.

EPIDEMIOLOGY

Acute pesticide poisoning is a large-scale problem, especially in developing countries.

"Most estimates concerning the extent of acute pesticide poisoning have been based on data from hospital admissions which would include only the more serious cases. The latest estimate by a WHO task group indicates that there may be 1 million serious unintentional poisonings each year and in addition 2 million people hospitalized for suicide attempts with pesticides. This necessarily reflects only a fraction of the real problem. On the basis of a survey of self-reported minor poisoning carried out in the Asian region, it is estimated that there could be as many as 25 million agricultural workers in the developing world suffering an episode of poisoning each year." In Canada in 2007 more than 6000 cases of acute pesticide poisoning occurred.

Estimating the numbers of chronic poisonings worldwide is more difficult.

SOCIETY AND CULTURE

Rachel Carson's *Silent Spring* brought about the first major wave of public concern over the chronic effects of pesticides.

IN OTHER ANIMALS

An obvious side effect of using a chemical meant to kill is that one is likely to kill more than just the desired organism. Contact with a sprayed plant or "weed" can have an effect upon local wildlife, most notably insects. A cause for concern is how pests, the reason for pesticide use, are building up a resistance. Phytophagous insects are able to build up this resistance because they are easily capable of evolutionary diversification and adaptation. The problem this presents is that in order to obtain the same desired effect of the pesticides they have to be made increasingly stronger as time goes on. Repercussions of the use of stronger pesticides on vegetation has a negative result on the surrounding environment, but also would contribute to consumers' long-term low-level exposure.

Environmental Impact of Pesticides

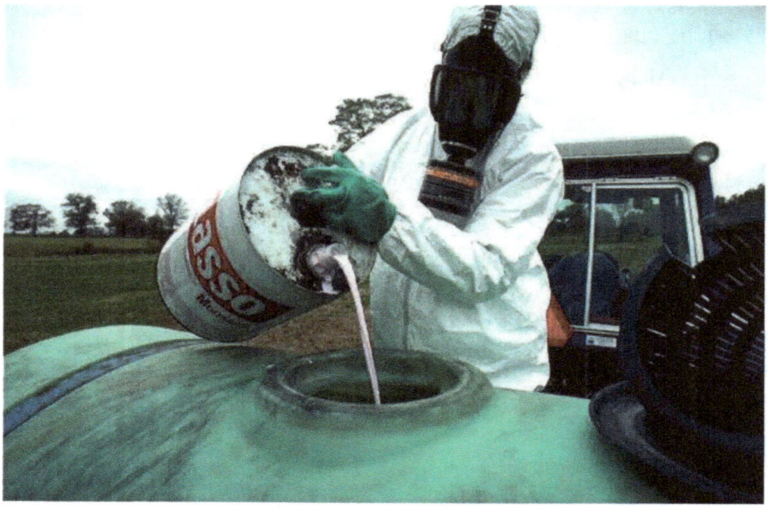

Preparing to spray a hazardous pesticide

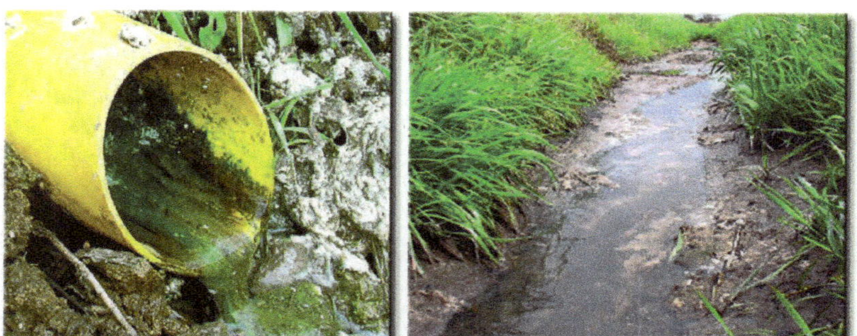

Drainage of fertilizers and pesticides into a stream.

The **impact of pesticides** consists of the effects of pesticides on non-target species. Over 98% of sprayed insecticides and 95% of herbicides reach a destination other than their target species, because they are sprayed or spread across entire agricultural fields. Runoff can carry pesticides into aquatic environments while wind can carry them to other fields, grazing areas, human settlements and undeveloped areas, potentially affecting other species. Other problems emerge from poor production, transport and storage practices. Over time, repeated application increases pest resistance, while its effects on other species can facilitate the pest's resurgence.

Each pesticide or pesticide class comes with a specific set of environmental concerns. Such undesirable effects have led many pesticides to be banned, while regulations have limited and/or reduced the use of others. Over time, pesticides have generally become less persistent and more species-specific, reducing their environmental footprint. In addition the amounts of pesticides applied per hectare have declined, in some cases by 99%. However, the global spread of pesticide use, including the use of older/obsolete pesticides that have been banned in some jurisdictions, has increased overall.

Agriculture and the Environment

The arrival of humans in an area, to live or to conduct agriculture, necessarily has environmental impacts. These range from simple crowding out of wild plants in favor of more desirable cultivars to larger scale impacts such as reducing biodiversity by reducing food availability of native species, which can propagate across food chains. The use of agricultural chemicals such as fertilizer and pesticides magnify those impacts. While advances in agrochemistry have reduced those impacts, for example by the replacement of long-lived chemicals with those that reliably degrade, even in the best case they remain substantial. These effects are magnified by the use of older chemistries and poor management practices.

While concern ecotoxicology began with acute poisoning events in the late 19th century; public concern over the undesirable environmental effects of chemicals arose in the early 1960s with the publication of Rachel Carson's book, *Silent Spring*. Shortly thereafter, DDT, originally used to combat malaria, and its metabolites were shown to cause population-level effects in raptorial birds. Initial studies in industrialized countries focused on acute mortality effects mostly involving birds or fish.

Data on pesticide usage remain scattered and/or not publicly available (3). The common practice of incident registration is inadequate for understanding the entirety of effects.

Since 1990, research interest has shifted from documenting incidents and quantifying chemical exposure to studies aimed at linking laboratory, mesocosm and field experiments. The proportion of effect-related publications has increased. Animal studies mostly focus on fish, insects, birds, amphibians and arachnids.

Since 1993, the United States and the European Union have updated pesticide risk assessments, ending the use of acutely toxic organophosphate and carbamate insecticides. Newer pesticides aim at efficiency in target and minimum side effects in nontarget organisms. The phylogenetic proximity of beneficial and pest species complicates the project.

One of the major challenges is to link the results from cellular studies through many levels of increasing complexity to ecosystems.

Specific Pesticide Effects

Pesticide environmental effects	
Pesticide/class	**Effect(s)**
Organochlorine DDT/DDE	Egg shell thinning in raptorial birds
	Endocrine disruptor
	Thyroid disruption properties in rodents, birds, amphibians and fish
	Acute mortality attributed to inhibition of acetylcholine esterase activity
:DDT	Carcinogen
	Endocrine disruptor
:DDT/Diclofol, Dieldrin and Toxaphene	Juvenile population decline and adult mortality in wildlife reptiles
:DDT/Toxaphene/Parathion	Susceptibility to fungal infection
Triazine	Earthworms became infected with monocystid gregarines
:Chlordane	Interact with vertebrate immune systems
Carbamates, the phenoxy herbicide 2,4-D, and atrazine	Interact with vertebrate immune systems
Anticholinesterase	Bird poisoning
	Animal infections, disease outbreaks and higher mortality.
Organophosphate	Thyroid disruption properties in rodents, birds, amphibians and fish
	Acute mortality attributed to inhibition of acetylcholine esterase activity
	Immunotoxicity, primarily caused by the inhibition of serine hydrolases or esterases
	Oxidative damage
	Modulation of signal transduction pathways
	Impaired metabolic functions such as thermoregulation, water and/or food intake and behavior, impaired development, reduced reproduction and hatching success in vertebrates.
Carbamate	Thyroid disruption properties in rodents, birds, amphibians and fish
	Impaired metabolic functions such as thermoregulation, water and/or food intake and behavior, impaired development, reduced reproduction and hatching success in vertebrates.
	Interact with vertebrate immune systems
	Acute mortality attributed to inhibition of acetylcholine esterase activity

Phenoxy herbicide 2,4-D	Interact with vertebrate immune systems
Atrazine	Interact with vertebrate immune systems
	Reduced northern leopard frog (Rana pipiens) populations because atrazine killed phytoplankton, thus allowing light to penetrate the water column and periphyton to assimilate nutrients released from the plankton. Periphyton growth provided more food to grazers, increasing snail populations, which provide intermediate hosts for trematode.
Pyrethroid	Thyroid disruption properties in rodents, birds, amphibians and fish
Thiocarbamate	Thyroid disruption properties in rodents, birds, amphibians and fish
Triazine	Thyroid disruption properties in rodents, birds, amphibians and fish
Triazole	Thyroid disruption properties in rodents, birds, amphibians and fish
	Impaired metabolic functions such as thermoregulation, water and/or food intake and behavior, impaired development, reduced reproduction and hatching success in vertebrates.
Nicotinoid	Respiratory, cardiovascular, neurological, and immunological toxicity in rats and humans
	Disrupt biogenic amine signaling and cause subsequent olfactory dysfunction, as well as affecting foraging behavior, learning and memory.
Imidacloprid, Imidacloprid/ pyrethroid λ-cyhalothrin	Impaired foraging, brood development, and colony success in terms of growth rate and new queen production.
Thiamethoxa	High honey bee worker mortality due to homing failure (risks for colony collapse remain controversial)
Spinosyns	Affect various physiological and behavioral traits of beneficial arthropods, particularly hymenopterans
Bt corn/Cry	Reduced abundance of some insect taxa, predominantly susceptible Lepidopteran herbivores as well as their predators and parasitoids.
Herbicide	Reduced food availability and adverse secondary effects on soil invertebrates and butterflies
	Decreased species abundance and diversity in small mammals.
Benomyl	Altered the patch-level floral display and later a two-thirds reduction of the total number of bee visits and in a shift in the visitors from large-bodied bees to small-bodied bees and flies
Herbicide and planting cycles	Reduced survival and reproductive rates in seed-eating or carnivorous birds

Air

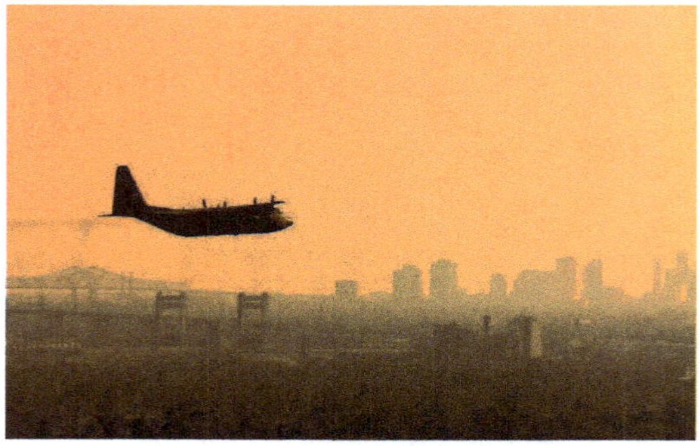

Spraying a mosquito pesticide over a city

Pesticides can contribute to air pollution. Pesticide drift occurs when pesticides suspended in the air as particles are carried by wind to other areas, potentially contaminating them.Pesticides that are applied to crops can volatilize and may be blown by winds into nearby areas, potentially posing a threat to wildlife. Weather conditions at the time of application as well as temperature and relative humidity change the spread of the pesticide in the air. As wind velocity increases so does the spray drift and exposure. Low relative humidity and high temperature result in more spray evaporating. The amount of inhalable pesticides in the outdoor environment is therefore often dependent on the season. Also, droplets of sprayed pesticides or particles from pesticides applied as dusts may travel on the wind to other areas, or pesticides may adhere to particles that blow in the wind, such as dust particles. Ground spraying produces less pesticide drift than aerial spraying does. Farmers can employ a buffer zone around their crop, consisting of empty land or non-crop plants such as evergreen trees to serve as windbreaks and absorb the pesticides, preventing drift into other areas. Such windbreaks are legally required in the Netherlands.

Pesticides that are sprayed on to fields and used to fumigate soil can give off chemicals called volatile organic compounds, which can react with other chemicals and form a pollutant called tropospheric ozone. Pesticide use accounts for about 6 percent of total tropospheric ozone levels.

Water

In the United States, pesticides were found to pollute every stream and over 90% of wells sampled in a study by the US Geological Survey. Pesticide residues have also been found in rain and groundwater. Studies by the UK government showed that pesticide concentrations exceeded those allowable for drinking water in some samples of river water and groundwater.

Pesticide impacts on aquatic systems are often studied using a hydrology transport model to study movement and fate of chemicals in rivers and streams. As early as the 1970s quantitative analysis of pesticide runoff was conducted in order to predict amounts of pesticide that would reach surface waters.

There are four major routes through which pesticides reach the water: it may drift outside of the intended area when it is sprayed, it may percolate, or leach, through the soil, it may be carried to the water as runoff, or it may be spilled, for example accidentally or through neglect. They may also be carried to water by eroding soil. Factors that affect a pesticide's ability to contaminate water include its water solubility, the distance from an application site to a body of water, weather, soil type, presence of a growing crop, and the method used to apply the chemical.

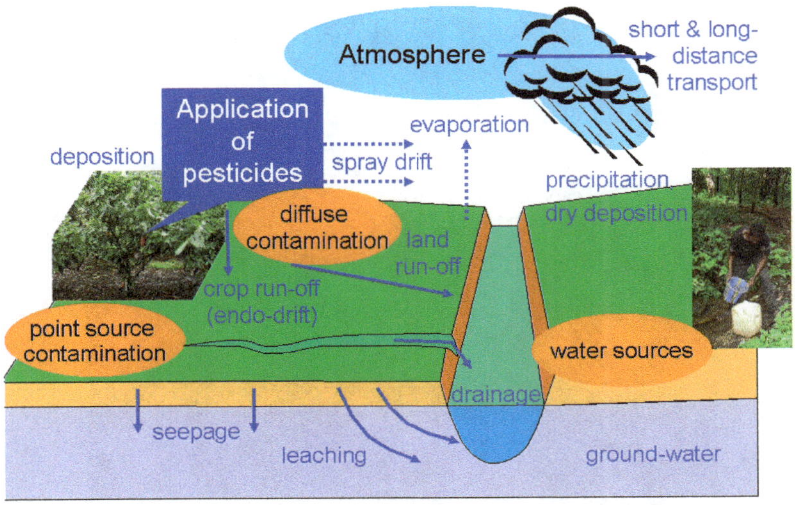

Pesticide pathways.

Maximum limits of allowable concentrations for individual pesticides in public bodies of water are set by the Environmental Protection Agency in the US. Similarly, the government of the United Kingdom sets Environmental Quality Standards (EQS), or maximum allowable concentrations of some pesticides in bodies of water above which toxicity may occur. The European Union also regulates maximum concentrations of pesticides in water.

Soil

Many of the chemicals used in pesticides are persistent soil contaminants, whose impact may endure for decades and adversely affect soil conservation.

The use of pesticides decreases the general biodiversity in the soil. Not using the chemicals results in higher soil quality, with the additional effect that more organic matter in the soil allows for higher water retention. This helps increase yields for farms in drought years, when organic farms have had yields 20-40% higher than their conventional counterparts. A smaller content of organic matter in the soil increases the amount of pesticide that will leave the area of application, because organic matter binds to and helps break down pesticides.

Degradation and sorption are both factors which influence the persistence of pesticides in soil. Depending on the chemical nature of the pesticide, such processes control directly the transportation from soil to water, and in turn to air and our food. Breaking down organic substances, degradation, involves interactions among microorganisms in the soil. Sorption affects bioaccumulation of pesticides which are dependent on organic matter in the soil. Weak organic acids have been shown to be weakly sorbed by soil, because of pH and mostly acidic structure. Sorbed chemicals have been shown to be less accessible to microorganisms. Aging mechanisms are poorly understood but as residence times in soil increase, pesticide residues become more resistant to degradation and extraction as they lose biological activity.

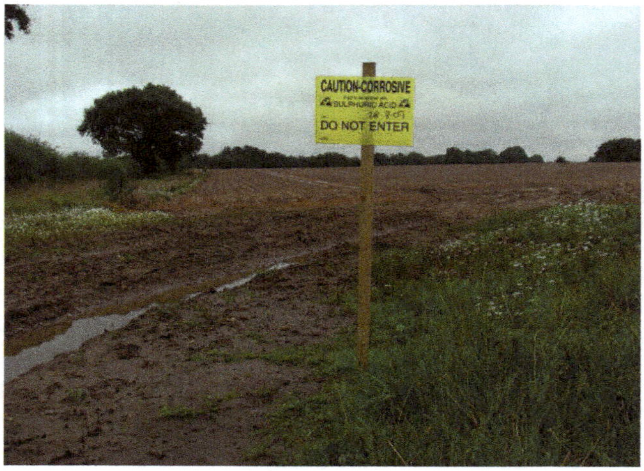

Caution against entering a field sprayed with sulphuric acid.

Effect on Plants

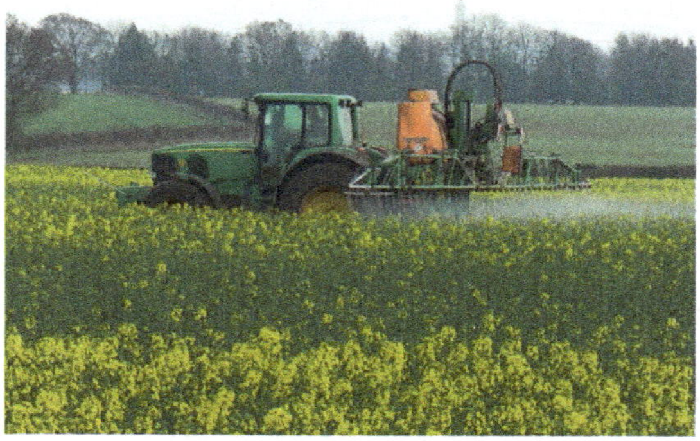

Crop spraying.

Nitrogen fixation, which is required for the growth of higher plants, is hindered by pesticides in soil. The insecticides DDT, methyl parathion, and especially pentachlorophenol have been shown to interfere with legume-rhizobium chemical signaling. Reduction of this symbiotic chemical signaling results in reduced nitrogen fixation and thus reduced crop yields. Root nodule formation in these plants saves the world economy $10 billion in synthetic nitrogen fertilizer every year.

Pesticides can kill bees and are strongly implicated in pollinator decline, the loss of species that pollinate plants, including through the mechanism of Colony Collapse Disorder, in which worker bees from a beehive or western honey bee colony abruptly disappear. Application of pesticides to crops that are in bloom can kill honeybees, which act as pollinators. The USDA and USFWS estimate that US farmers lose at least $200 million a year from reduced crop pollination because pesticides applied to fields eliminate about a fifth of honeybee colonies in the US and harm an additional 15%.

On the other side, pesticides have some direct harmful effect on plant including poor root hair development, shoot yellowing and reduced plant growth.

Effect on Animals

Many kinds of animals are harmed by pesticides, leading many countries to regulate pesticide usage through Biodiversity Action Plans.

Animals including humans may be poisoned by pesticide residues that remain on food, for example when wild animals enter sprayed fields or nearby areas shortly after spraying.

Pesticides can eliminate some animals' essential food sources, causing the animals to relocate, change their diet or starve. Residues can travel up the food chain; for example, birds can be harmed when they eat insects and worms that have consumed pesticides. Earthworms digest organic matter and increase nutrient content in the top layer of soil. They protect human health by ingesting decomposing litter and serving as bioindicators of soil activity. Pesticides have had harmful effects on growth and reproduction on earthworms. Some pesticides can bioaccumulate, or build up to toxic levels in the bodies of organisms that consume them over time, a phenomenon that impacts species high on the food chain especially hard.

Birds

The US Fish and Wildlife Service estimates that 72 million birds are killed by pesticides in the United States each year. Bald eagles are common examples of nontarget organisms that are impacted by pesticide use. Rachel Carson's book *Silent Spring* dealt with damage to bird species due to pesticide bioaccumulation. There is evidence that birds are continuing to be harmed by pesticide use. In the farmland of the United Kingdom, populations of ten different bird species declined by 10 million breeding individuals between 1979 and 1999, allegedly from loss of plant and invertebrate species on which the birds feed. Throughout Europe, 116 species of birds were threatened as of 1999. Reductions in bird populations have been found to be associated with times and areas in which pesticides are used. DDE-induced egg shell thinning has especially affected European and North

American bird populations. In another example, some types of fungicides used in peanut farming are only slightly toxic to birds and mammals, but may kill earthworms, which can in turn reduce populations of the birds and mammals that feed on them.

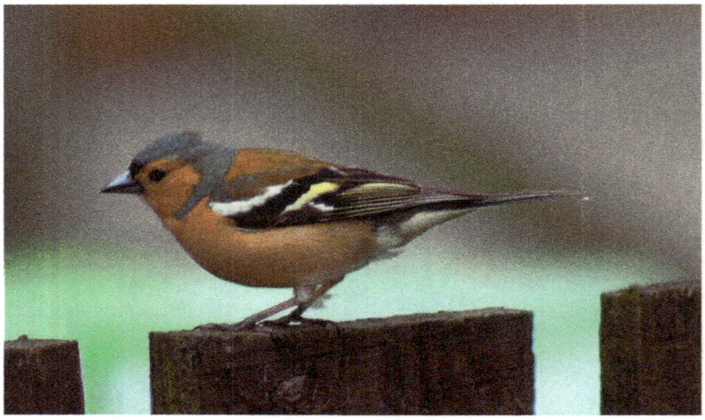

In England, the use of pesticides in gardens and farmland has seen a reduction in the number of common chaffinches.

Some pesticides come in granular form. Wildlife may eat the granules, mistaking them for grains of food. A few granules of a pesticide may be enough to kill a small bird.

The herbicide paraquat, when sprayed onto bird eggs, causes growth abnormalities in embryos and reduces the number of chicks that hatch successfully, but most herbicides do not directly cause much harm to birds. Herbicides may endanger bird populations by reducing their habitat.

Aquatic Life

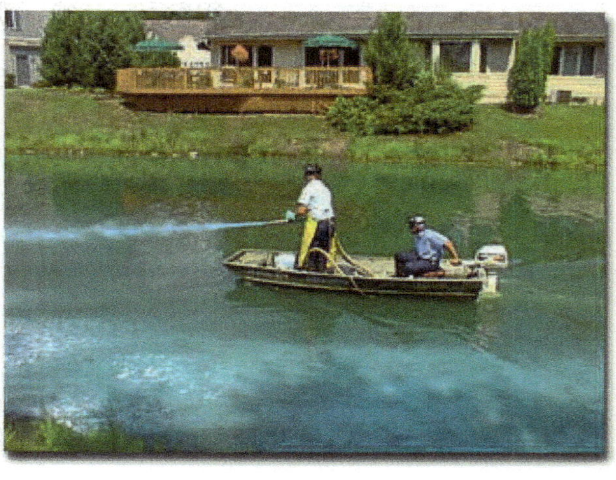

Using an aquatic herbicide

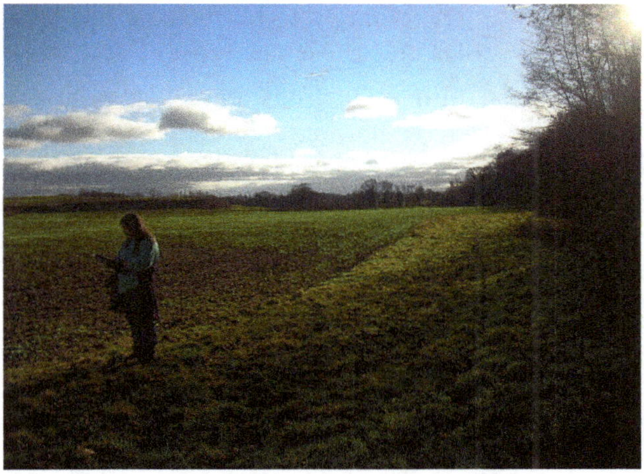

Wide field margins can reduce fertilizer and pesticide pollution in streams and rivers.

Fish and other aquatic biota may be harmed by pesticide-contaminated water. Pesticide surface runoff into rivers and streams can be highly lethal to aquatic life, sometimes killing all the fish in a particular stream.

Application of herbicides to bodies of water can cause fish kills when the dead plants decay and consume the water's oxygen, suffocating the fish. Herbicides such as copper sulfite that are applied to water to kill plants are toxic to fish and other water animals at concentrations similar to those used to kill the plants. Repeated exposure to sublethal doses of some pesticides can cause physiological and behavioral changes that reduce fish populations, such as abandonment of nests and broods, decreased immunity to disease and decreased predator avoidance.

Application of herbicides to bodies of water can kill plants on which fish depend for their habitat.

Pesticides can accumulate in bodies of water to levels that kill off zooplankton, the main source of food for young fish.Pesticides can also kill off insects on which some fish feed, causing the fish to travel farther in search of food and exposing them to greater risk from predators.

The faster a given pesticide breaks down in the environment, the less threat it poses to aquatic life. Insecticides are typically more toxic to aquatic life than herbicides and fungicides.

Amphibians

In the past several decades, amphibian populations have declined across the world, for unexplained reasons which are thought to be varied but of which pesticides may be a part.

Pesticide mixtures appear to have a cumulative toxic effect on frogs. Tadpoles from ponds containing multiple pesticides take longer to metamorphose and are smaller when they do, decreasing their ability to catch prey and avoid predators. Exposing tadpoles to the organochloride endosulfan at levels likely to be found in habitats near fields sprayed with the chemical kills the tadpoles and causes behavioral and growth abnormalities.

The herbicide atrazine can turn male frogs into hermaphrodites, decreasing their ability to reproduce.Both reproductive and nonreproductive effects in aquatic reptiles and amphibians have been reported. Crocodiles, many turtle species and some lizards lack sex-distinct chromosomes until after fertilization during organogenesis, depending on temperature. Embryonic exposure in turtles to various PCBs causes a sex reversal. Across the United States and Canada disorders such as decreased hatching success, feminization, skin lesions, and other developmental abnormalities have been reported.

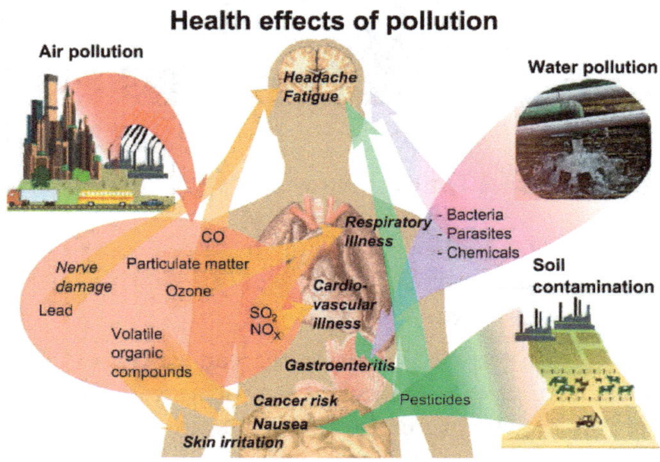

Pesticides are implicated in a range of impacts on human health due to pollution

Humans

Pesticides can enter the body through inhalation of aerosols, dust and vapor that contain pesticides; through oral exposure by consuming food/water; and through skin exposure by direct contact. Pesticides secrete into soils and groundwater which can end up in drinking water, and pesticide spray can drift and pollute the air.

The effects of pesticides on human health depend on the toxicity of the chemical and the length and magnitude of exposure.Farm workers and their families experience the greatest exposure to agricultural pesticides through direct contact. Every human contains pesticides in their fat cells.

Children are more susceptible and sensitive to pesticides, because they are still developing and have a weaker immune system than adults. Children may be more exposed due to their closer proximity to the ground and tendency to put unfamiliar objects in their mouth. Hand to mouth contact depends on the child's age, much like lead exposure. Children under the age of six months are more apt to experience exposure from breast milk and inhalation of small particles. Pesticides tracked into the home from family members increase the risk of exposure. Toxic residue in food may contribute to a child's exposure.The chemicals can bioaccumulate in the body over time.

Exposure effects can range from mild skin irritation to birth defects, tumors, genetic changes, blood and nerve disorders, endocrine disruption, coma or death. Developmental effects have been associated with pesticides. Recent increases in childhood cancers in throughout North America, such as leukemia, may be a result of somatic cell mutations. Insecticides targeted to disrupt insects can have harmful effects on mammalian nervous systems. Both chronic and acute alterations have been observed in exposees. DDT and its breakdown product DDE disturb estrogenic activity and possibly lead to breast cancer. Fetal DDT exposure reduces male penis size in animals and can produce undescended testicles. Pesticide can affect fetuses in early stages of development, in utero and even if a parent was exposed before conception. Reproductive disruption has the potential to occur by chemical reactivity and through structural changes.

Persistent Organic Pollutants

Persistent organic pollutants (POPs) are compounds that resist degradation and thus remain in the environment for years. Some pesticides, including aldrin, chlordane, DDT, dieldrin, endrin, heptachlor, hexachlorobenzene, mirex and toxaphene, are considered POPs. Some POPs have the ability to volatilize and travel great distances through the atmosphere to become deposited in remote regions. Such chemicals may have the ability to bioaccumulate and biomagnify and can bioconcentrate (i.e. become more concentrated) up to 70,000 times their original concentrations. POPs can affect non-target organisms in the environment and increase risk to humans by disruption in the endocrine, reproductive, and immune systems.

Pest Resistance

Pests may evolve to become resistant to pesticides. Many pests will initially be very susceptible to pesticides, but following mutations in their genetic makeup become resistant and survive to reproduce.

Resistance is commonly managed through pesticide rotation, which involves alternating among pesticide classes with different modes of action to delay the onset of or mitigate existing pest resistance.

Pest Rebound and Secondary Pest Outbreaks

Non-target organisms can also be impacted by pesticides. In some cases, a pest insect that is controlled by a beneficial predator or parasite can flourish should an insecticide application kill both pest and beneficial populations. A study comparing biological pest control and pyrethroid insecticide for diamondback moths, a major cabbage family insect pest, showed that the pest population rebounded due to loss of insect predators, whereas the biocontrol did not show the same effect. Likewise, pesticides sprayed to control mosquitoes may temporarily depress mosquito populations, however they may result in a larger population in the long run by damaging natural controls. This phenomenon, wherein the population of a pest species rebounds to equal or greater numbers than it had before pesticide use, is called pest resurgence and can be linked to elimination of its predators and other natural enemies.

Loss of predator species can also lead to a related phenomenon called secondary pest outbreaks, an increase in problems from species that were not originally a problem due to loss of their predators or parasites. An estimated third of the 300 most damaging insects in the US were originally secondary pests and only became a major problem after the use of pesticides. In both pest resurgence and secondary outbreaks, their natural enemies were more susceptible to the pesticides than the pests themselves, in some cases causing the pest population to be higher than it was before the use of pesticide.

Eliminating Pesticides

Many alternatives are available to reduce the effects pesticides have on the environment. Alternatives include manual removal, applying heat, covering weeds with plastic, placing traps and lures, removing pest breeding sites, maintaining healthy soils that breed healthy, more resistant plants, cropping native species that are naturally more resistant to native pests and supporting biocontrol agents such as birds and other pest predators. In the United States, conventional pesticide use peaked in 1979, and by 2007, had been reduced by 25 percent from the 1979 peak level, while US agricultural output increased by 43 percent over the same period.

Biological controls such as resistant plant varieties and the use of pheromones, have been successful and at times permanently resolve a pest problem. Integrated Pest Management (IPM) employs chemical use only when other alternatives are ineffective. IPM causes less harm to humans and the environment. The focus is broader than on a specific pest, considering a range of pest control alternatives. Biotechnology can also be an innovative way to control pests. Strains can be genetically modified (GM) to increase their resistance to pests. However the same techniques can be used to increase pesticide resistance and was employed by Monsanto to create glyphosate-resistant strains of major crops. In 2010, 70% of all the corn that was planted was resistant to glyphosate; 78% of cotton, and 93% of all soybeans.

HEALTH EFFECTS OF PESTICIDES

Health effects of pesticides may be acute or delayed in those who are exposed. A 2007 systematic review found that “most studies on non-Hodgkin lymphoma and leukemia showed positive associations with pesticide exposure” and thus concluded that cosmetic use of pesticides should be decreased. Strong evidence also exists for other negative outcomes from pesticide exposure including neurological problems, birth defects, fetal death, and neurodevelopmental disorder.

According to The Stockholm Convention on Persistent Organic Pollutants, 9 of the 12 most dangerous and persistent chemicals are pesticides.

Acute Effects

Acute health problems may occur in workers that handle pesticides, such as abdominal pain, dizziness, headaches, nausea, vomiting, as well as skin and eye problems. In China, an estimated half million people are poisoned by pesticides each year, 500 of whom die. Pyrethrins, insecticides commonly used in common bug killers, can cause a potentially deadly condition if breathed in.

Long-term Effects

Cancer

Many studies have examined the effects of pesticide exposure on the risk of cancer. Associations have been found with: leukemia, lymphoma, brain, kidney, breast, prostate, pancreas, liver, lung, and skin cancers. This increased risk occurs with both residential and occupational exposures. Increased rates of cancer have been found among farm workers who apply these chemicals. A mother's occupational exposure to pesticides during pregnancy is associated with an increases in her child's risk of leukemia, Wilms' tumor, and brain cancer. Exposure to insecticides within the home and herbicides outside is associated with blood cancers in children.

Neurological

Evidence links pesticide exposure to worsened neurological outcomes. The risk of developing Parkinson's disease is 70% greater in those exposed to even low levels of pesticides. People with Parkinson's were 61% more likely to report direct pesticide application than were healthy relatives. Both insecticides and herbicides significantly increased the risk of Parkinson's disease. There are also concerns that long-term exposures may increase the risk of dementia.

The United States Environmental Protection Agency finished a 10-year review of the organophosphate pesticides following the 1996 Food Quality Protection Act, but did little to account for developmental neurotoxic effects, drawing strong criticism from within the agency and from outside researchers.Comparable studies have not been done with newer pesticides that are replacing organophosphates.

Reproductive Effects

Strong evidence links pesticide exposure to birth defects, fetal death and altered fetal growth. In the United States, increase in birth defects is associated with conceiving in the same period of the year when agrochemicals are in elevated concentrations in surface water. Agent Orange, a 50:50 mixture of 2,4,5-T and 2,4-D, has been associated with bad health and genetic effects in Malaya and Vietnam. It was also found that offspring that were at some point exposed to pesticides had a low birth weight and had developmental defects.

Fertility

A number of pesticides including dibromochlorophane and 2,4-D has been associated with impaired fertility in males. Pesticide exposure resulted in reduced fertility in males, genetic alterations in sperm, a reduced number of sperm, damage to germinal epithelium and altered hormone function.

Other

Some studies have found increased risks of dermatitis in those exposed.

Additionally, studies have indicated that pesticide exposure is associated with long-term health problems such as respiratory problems, including asthma, memory disorders and depression. Summaries of peer-reviewed research have examined the link between pesticide exposure and neurologic outcomes and cancer, perhaps the two most significant things resulting in organophosphate-exposed workers.

According to researchers from the National Institutes of Health (NIH), licensed pesticide applicators who used chlorinated pesticides on more than 100 days in their lifetime were at greater risk of diabetes. One study found that associations between specific pesticides and incident diabetes ranged from a 20 percent to a 200 percent increase in risk. New cases of diabetes were reported by 3.4 percent of those in the lowest pesticide use category compared with 4.6 percent of those in the highest category. Risks were greater when users of specific pesticides were compared with applicators who never applied that chemical.

Route of Exposure

People can be exposed to pesticides by a number of different routes including: occupation, in the home, at school and in their food.

There are concerns that pesticides used to control pests on food crops are dangerous to people who consume those foods. These concerns are one reason for the organic food movement. Many food crops, including fruits and vegetables, contain pesticide residues after being washed or peeled. Chemicals that are no longer used but that are resistant to breakdown for long periods may remain in soil and water and thus in food.

The United Nations Codex Alimentarius Commission has recommended international standards for maximum residue limits (MRLs), for individual pesticides in food.

In the EU, MRLs are set by DG-SANCO.

In the United States, levels of residues that remain on foods are limited to tolerance levels that are established by the U.S. Environmental Protection Agency and are considered safe. The EPA sets the tolerances based on the toxicity of the pesticide and its breakdown products, the amount and frequency of pesticide application, and how much of the pesticide (i.e., the residue) remains in or on food by the time it is marketed and prepared. Tolerance levels are obtained using scientific risk assessments that pesticide manufacturers are required to produce by conducting toxicological studies, exposure modeling and residue studies before a particular pesticide can be registered, however, the effects are tested for single pesticides, and there is little information on possible synergistic effects of exposure to multiple pesticide traces in the air, food and water.

Strawberries and tomatoes are the two crops with the most intensive use of soil fumigants. They are particularly vulnerable to several type of diseases, insects, mites, and parasitic worms. In 2003, in California alone, 3.7 million pounds (1,700 metric tons) of metham sodium were used on tomatoes. In recent years other farmers have demonstrated that it is possible to produce strawberries and tomatoes without the use of harmful chemicals and in a cost-effective way.

Exposure routes other than consuming food that contains residues, in particular pesticide drift, are potentially significant to the general public.

Some pesticides can remain in the environment for prolonged periods of time. For example, most people in the United States still have detectable levels of DDT in their bodies even though it was banned in the US in 1972.

Prevention

Pesticides exposure cannot be studied in placebo controlled trials as this would be unethical. A definitive cause effect relationship therefore cannot be established. Consistent evidence can and has been gathered through other study designs. The precautionary principle is thus frequently used in environmental law such that absolute proof is not required before efforts to decrease exposure to potential toxins are enacted.

The American Medical Association recommend limiting exposure to pesticides. They came to this conclusion due to the fact that surveillance systems currently in place are inadequate to determine problems related to exposure. The utility of applicator certification and public notification programs are also of unknown value in their ability to prevent adverse outcomes.

Epidemiology

The World Health Organization and the UN Environment Programme estimate that each year, 3 million workers in agriculture in the developing world experience severe poisoning from pesticides, about 18,000 of whom die. According to one study, as many as 25 million workers in developing countries may suffer mild pesticide poisoning yearly. Detectable levels of 50 different pesticides were found in the blood of a representative sample of the U.S. population.

Society and Culture

Concerns regarding conflict of interests regarding the research base have been raised. A number of researchers involved with pesticides have been found to have undisclosed ties to industry including: Richard Doll or the Imperial Cancer Research Fund in England and Hans-Olov Adami of the Karolinska Institute in Sweden.

Other Animals

A number of pesticides including clothianidin, dinotefuran, imidacloprid are toxic to bees. Exposure to pesticides may be one of the contributory factors to colony collapse disorder. A study in North Carolina indicated that more than 30 percent of the quail tested were made sick by one aerial insecticide application. Once sick, wild birds may neglect their young, abandon their nests, and become more susceptible to predators or disease.

REFERENCES

1. George Tyler Miller (1 January 2004). Sustaining the Earth: An Integrated Approach. Thomson/Brooks/Cole. pp. 211–216. ISBN 978-0-534-40088-0.
2. Tashkent (1998), Part 1. Conditions and provisions for developing a national strategy for biodiversity conservation. Biodiversity Conservation National Strategy and Action Plan of Republic of Uzbekistan. Prepared by the National Biodiversity Strategy Project Steering Committee with the Financial Assistance of The Global Environmental Facility (GEF) and Technical Assistance of United Nations Development Programme (UNDP). Retrieved on September 17, 2007.
3. Damalas, C. A.; Eleftherohorinos, I. G. (2011). Pesticide Exposure, Safety Issues, and Risk Assessment Indicators. International Journal of Environmental Research and Public Health. **8** *(12): 1402–19.* doi:10.3390/ijerph8051402. PMC 3108117. PMID 21655127.
4. Lamberth, C.; Jeanmart, S.; Luksch, T.; Plant, A. (2013). Current Challenges and Trends in the Discovery of Agrochemicals. Science. **341** *(6147): 742–6. doi:10.1126/science.1237227. PMID 23950530.*
5. Kohler, H. -R.; Triebskorn, R. (2013). Wildlife Ecotoxicology of Pesticides: Can We Track Effects to the Population Level and Beyond?. *Science.* **341** *(6147): 759–765. doi:10.1126/science.1237591.*
6. Rattner, B. A. (2009). History of wildlife toxicology. Ecotoxicology. **18** *(7): 773–783.* doi:10.1007/s10646-009-0354-x.
7. Turusov, V; Rakitsky, V; Tomatis, L (2002). Dichlorodiphenyltrichloroethane (DDT): Ubiquity, persistence, and risks. Environmental Health Perspectives. **110** *(2): 125–8. doi:10.1289/ehp.02110125. PMC 1240724. PMID 11836138.*
8. ^ Jump up to:[a] [b] [c] [d] Fleischli, M. A.; Franson, J. C.; Thomas, N. J.; Finley, D. L.; Riley, W. (2004). Avian Mortality Events in the United States Caused by Anticholinesterase Pesticides: A Retrospective Summary of National Wildlife Health Center Records from 1980 to 2000. Archives of Environmental Contamination and Toxicology. **46** *(4).* doi:10.1007/s00244-003-3065-y.
9. Crain, D. A.; Guillette Jr, L. J. (1998). Reptiles as models of contaminant-induced endocrine disruption. Animal Reproduction Science. **53** *(1–4): 77–86.* doi:10.1016/s0378-4320(98)00128-6. PMID 9835368.
10. Galloway, T. S.; Depledge, M. H. (2001). Immunotoxicity in Invertebrates:

Measurement and Ecotoxicological Relevance. Ecotoxicology. **10**: 5–23. doi:10.1023/A:1008939520263.

11. Dzugan, S. A.; Rozakis, G. W.; Dzugan, K. S.; Emhof, L; Dzugan, S. S.; Xydas, C; Michaelides, C; Chene, J; Medvedovsky, M (2011). Correction of steroidopenia as a new method of hypercholesterolemia treatment. Neuro endocrinology letters. **32** *(1): 77–81. PMID 21407165.*
12. Galloway, T.; Handy, `R. (2003). Immunotoxicity of Organophosphorous Pesticides. Ecotoxicology. **12**: 345–363. doi:10.1023/A:1022579416322.
13. Story, P.; Cox, M. (2001). "Review of the effects of organophosphorus and carbamate insecticides on vertebrates. Are there implications for locust management in Australia?". *Wildlife Research.* **28** *(2): 179.* doi:10.1071/WR99060.
14. Rohr, J. R.; Schotthoefer, A. M.; Raffel, T. R.; Carrick, H. J.; Halstead, N.; Hoverman, J. T.; Johnson, C. M.; Johnson, L. B.; Lieske, C.; Piwoni, M. D.; Schoff, P. K.; Beasley, V. R. (2008). Agrochemicals increase trematode infections in a declining amphibian species. Nature. **455** *(7217): 1235–1239.* doi:10.1038/nature07281. PMID 18972018.
15. Lin, P. C.; Lin, H. J.; Liao, Y. Y.; Guo, H. R.; Chen, K. T. (2013). Acute poisoning with neonicotinoid insecticides: A case report and literature review. Basic & Clinical Pharmacology & Toxicology. **112** *(4): 282–6. doi:10.1111/bcpt.12027. PMID 23078648.*
16. Gill, R. J.; Ramos-Rodriguez, O.; Raine, N. E. (2012). Combined pesticide exposure severely affects individual- and colony-level traits in bees. Nature. **491** *(7422): 105–108.* doi:10.1038/nature11585. PMC 3495159. PMID 23086150.
17. Henry, M.; Beguin, M.; Requier, F.; Rollin, O.; Odoux, J. -F.; Aupinel, P.; Aptel, J.; Tchamitchian, S.; Decourtye, A. (2012). A Common Pesticide Decreases Foraging Success and Survival in Honey Bees. Science. **336** *(6079): 348–350. doi:10.1126/science.1215039. PMID 22461498.*
18. Cresswell, J. E.; Thompson, H. M. (2012). Comment on A Common Pesticide Decreases Foraging Success and Survival in Honey Bees. Science. **337** *(6101): 1453. doi:10.1126/science.1224618. PMID 22997307.*
19. Biondi, A.; Mommaerts, V.; Smagghe, G.; Viñuela, E.; Zappalà, L.; Desneux, N. (2012). The non-target impact of spinosyns on beneficial arthropods. Pest Management Science. **68** *(12): 1523–1536. doi:10.1002/ps.3396.*
20. Freemark, K. (1995). Impacts of agricultural herbicide use on terrestrial wildlife in temperate landscapes: A review with special reference to North America. Agriculture, Ecosystems & Environment. **52** *(2–3): 67–91.* doi:10.1016/0167-8809(94)00534-L.
21. Cahill, J. F.; Elle, E.; Smith, G. R.; Shore, B. H. (2008). Disruption of a Belowground Mutualism Alters Interactions Between Plants and Their Floral Visitors. Ecology. **89** *(7): 1791–1801. doi:10.1890/07-0719.1.*
22. Newton, I. (2004). The recent declines of farmland bird populations in Britain: An appraisal of causal factors and conservation actions. Ibis. **146** *(4): 579–600. doi:10.1111/j.1474-919X.2004.00375.x.*

23. Cornell University. Pesticides in the environment. Pesticide fact sheets and tutorial, . Pesticide Safety Education Program. Retrieved on 2007-10-11.
24. National Park Service. US Department of the Interior. (August 1, 2006), Sequoia & Kings Canyon National Park: Air quality -- Airborne synthetic chemicals. Nps.gov. Retrieved on September 19, 2007.
25. US Environmental Protection Agency (September 11th, 2007), Pesticide registration (PR) notice 2001-X Draft: Spray and dust drift label statements for pesticide products. Epa.gov. Retrieved on September 19, 2007.
26. Environment Canada (September–October 2001), Agricultural pesticides and the atmosphere. Retrieved on 2007-10-12.
27. Palmer, WE, Bromley, PT, and Brandenburg, RL. Wildlife & pesticides - Peanuts. North Carolina Cooperative Extension Service. Retrieved on 2007-10-11.
28. Science Daily (November 19, 1999), Evergreens help block spread of pesticide from crop fields. Sciencedaily.com. Retrieved on September 19, 2007.
29. UC IPM Online. (August 11, 2006), What's up, Doc? Maybe less air pollution. Statewide IPM Program, Agriculture and Natural Resources, University of California. Ipm.ucdavis.edu. Retrieved on 2007-10-15.
30. Gilliom, RJ, Barbash, JE, Crawford, GG, Hamilton, PA, Martin, JD, Nakagaki, N, Nowell, LH, Scott, JC, Stackelberg, PE, Thelin, GP, and Wolock, DM (February 15, 2007), The Quality of our nation's waters: Pesticides in the nation's streams and ground water, 1992–2001. Chapter 1, Page 4. US Geological Survey. Retrieved on September 13, 2007.
31. Kellogg RL, Nehring R, Grube A, Goss DW, and Plotkin S (February 2000), Environmental indicators of pesticide leaching and runoff from farm fields Archived June 18, 2002, at the Wayback Machine.. United States Department of Agriculture Natural Resources Conservation Service. Retrieved on 2007-10-03.
32. Bingham, S (2007), Pesticides in rivers and groundwater. Environment Agency, UK. Retrieved on 2007-10-12.
33. Hogan,, CM, Patmore L, Latshaw, G, Seidman, H, et al. (1973), Computer modeling of pesticide transport in soil for five instrumented watersheds, U.S. Environmental Protection Agency Southeast Water laboratory, Athens, Ga. by ESL Inc., Sunnyvale, California.
34. States of Jersey (2007), Environmental protection and pesticide use. Retrieved on 2007-10-10.
35. Papendick, RI; Elliott, LF; Dahlgren, RB (1986). Environmental consequences of modern production agriculture: How can alternative agriculture address these issues and concerns?. *American Journal of Alternative Agriculture.* **1** *(1): 3–10.* doi:10.1017/s0889189300000722.
36. Pedersen, TL (June 1997), Pesticide residues in drinking water. extoxnet.orst. edu. Retrieved on September 15, 2007.

37. Bingham, S (2007), Pesticides exceeding environmental quality standards (EQS). The Environment Agency, UK. Retrieved on 2007-10-12.

38. U.S. Environmental Protection Agency (2007), Sources of common contaminants and their health effects. Epa.gov. Retrieved on 2007-10-10.

39. Johnston, AE (1986). Soil organic-matter, effects on soils and crops. Soil Use Management. **2** *(3): 97–105. doi:10.1111/j.1475-2743.1986.tb00690.x.*

40. Lotter DW, Seidel R, Liebhardt W (2003). The performance of organic and conventional cropping systems in an extreme climate year. American Journal of Alternative Agriculture. **18** *(03): 146–154.* doi:10.1079/AJAA200345.

41. Arias-Estévez, Manuel; Eugenio López-Periago; Elena Martínez-Carballo; Jesús Simal-Gándara; Juan-Carlos Mejuto; Luis García-Río (February 2008). The mobility and degradation of pesticides in soils and the pollution of groundwater resources (PDF). Agriculture, Ecosystems & Environment. **123**: 247–260. doi:10.1016/j.agee.2007.07.011. ISSN 0167-8809. Retrieved 2011-11-10.

42. Rockets, Rusty (June 8, 2007), Down On The Farm? Yields, Nutrients And Soil Quality. Scienceagogo.com. Retrieved on September 15, 2007.

43. Fox, JE; Gulledge, J; Engelhaupt, E; Burrow, ME & McLachlan, JA (2007). Pesticides reduce symbiotic efficiency of nitrogen-fixing rhizobia and host plants. Proceedings of the National Academy of Sciences of the USA. **104** *(24): 10282–10287. doi:10.1073/pnas.0611710104. PMC 1885820. PMID 17548832.*

44. Hackenberg D (2007-03-14). Letter from David Hackenberg to American growers from March 14, 2007. Plattform Imkerinnen — Austria. Archived from the original on 2007-06-04. Retrieved 2007-03-27.

45. Wells, M (March 11, 2007). Vanishing bees threaten US. www.bbc.co.uk. BBC News. Retrieved 2007-09-19.

46. Haefeker, Walter (2000-08-12). Betrayed and sold out – German bee monitoring. Retrieved 2007-10-10.

47. Zeissloff, Eric (2001). Schadet imidacloprid den bienen (in German). Retrieved 2007-10-10.

48. Walley F, Taylor A and Lupwayi (2006) Herbicide effects on pulse crop nodulation and nitrogen fixation. FarmTech 2006 Proceedings 121-123.

49. Yasmin, S.; d'Souza, D. (2010). Effects of Pesticides on the Growth and Reproduction of Earthworm: A Review. Applied and Environmental Soil Science. **2010**: 1–9. doi:10.1155/2010/678360.

50. Fimrite, Peter (June 27, 2011). Suit says EPA fails to shield species from poisons. The San Francisco Chronicle.

51. Kerbs JR, Wilson JD, Bradbury RB, and Siriwardena GM (August 12, 1999), The second silent spring. Commentary in Nature, Volume 400, Pages 611-612.

52. Vos, J. G.; Dybing, E; Greim, H. A.; Ladefoged, O; Lambré, C; Tarazona, J. V.; Brandt, I; Vethaak, A. D. (2000). Health effects of endocrine-disrupting chemicals on wildlife, with special reference to the European situation. Critical

Reviews in Toxicology. **30** *(1): 71–133.* doi:10.1080/10408440091159176. PMID 10680769.

53. Helfrich, LA, Weigmann, DL, Hipkins, P, and Stinson, ER (June 1996), Pesticides and aquatic animals: A guide to reducing impacts on aquatic systems. Virginia Cooperative Extension. Retrieved on 2007-10-14.

54. Toughill K (1999), The summer the rivers died: Toxic runoff from potato farms is poisoning P.E.I. Archived January 18, 2008, at the Wayback Machine. Originally published in Toronto Star Atlantic Canada Bureau. Retrieved on September 17, 2007.

55. Pesticide Action Network North America (June 4, 1999), Pesticides threaten birds and fish in California. PANUPS. Retrieved on 2007-09-17.

56. Cone M (December 6, 2000), A wind-borne threat to Sierra frogs: A study finds that pesticides used on farms in the San Joaquin Valley damage the nervous systems of amphibians in Yosemite and elsewhere. L.A. Times Retrieved on September 17, 2007.

57. Science Daily (February 3, 2006), Pesticide combinations imperil frogs, probably contribute to amphibian decline. Sciencedaily.com. Retrieved on 2007-10-16.

58. Raloff, J (September 5, 1998) Common pesticide clobbers amphibians. Science News, Volume 154, Number 10, Page 150. Retrieved on 2007-10-15.

59. California Department of Pesticide Regulation (2008), What are the Potential Health Effects of Pesticides? Community Guide to Recognizing and Reporting Pesticide Problems. Sacramento, CA. Pages 27-29.

60. Lorenz, Eric S. (2009). Potential Health Effects of Pesticides (PDF). Ag Communications and Marketing: 1–8. Retrieved February 2014. Check date values in: |access-date= (help)

61. Du Toit, D. F. (1992). Pancreatic transplantation. South African medical. **81** *(8): 432–3. PMID 1566222.*

62. Crawford, S. L.; Fiedler, E. R. (1992). Childhood physical and sexual abuse and failure to complete military basic training. Military medicine. **157** *(12): 645–8. PMID 1470375.*

63. Hodgson, E; Levi, P. E. (1996). Pesticides: An important but underused model for the environmental health sciences. Environmental Health Perspectives. 104 Suppl 1: 97–106. doi:10.1289/ehp.96104s197. PMC 1469573. PMID 8722114.

64. Ritter L, Solomon KR, and Forget J, Stemeroff M, and O'Leary C. Persistent organic pollutants: An Assessment Report on: DDT, Aldrin, Dieldrin, Endrin, Chlordane, Heptachlor, Hexachlorobenzene, Mirex, Toxaphene, Polychlorinated Biphenyls, Dioxins and Furans. Prepared for The International Programme on Chemical Safety (IPCS), within the framework of the Inter-Organization Programme for the Sound Management of Chemicals (IOMC). Retrieved on September 16, 2007.

65. Centers for Disease Control and Prevention. Pesticides. cdc.gov. Retrieved on September 15, 2007.

66. Graeme Murphy (December 1, 2005), Resistance Management - Pesticide RotationArchived October 13, 2007, at the Wayback Machine.. Ontario Ministry of Agriculture, Food and Rural Affairs. Retrieved on September 15, 2007.

67. Muckenfuss AE, Shepard BM, Ferrer ER, Natural mortality of diamondback moth in coastal South Carolina Clemson University, Coastal Research and Education Center.

68. Howell V. Daly; John T. Doyen; Alexander H. Purcell (1 January 1998). Introduction to Insect Biology and Diversity. Oxford University Press. pp. 279–300. ISBN 978-0-19-510033-4.

69. "Take Action! How to Eliminate Pesticide Use." (2003) National Audubon Society. Pages 1-3.

70. United States Environmental Protection Agency. 2011. Pesticides industry sales and usage 2006 and 2007 market estimates. Archived copy (PDF). Archived from the original (PDF) on 2015-03-18. Retrieved 2014-07-24.

71. USDA ERS. 2013. Table 1. Indices of farm output, input and total factor productivity for the United States, 1948-2011. (last update 9/27/2013) http://www.ers.usda.gov/data-products/agricultural-productivity-in-the-us.aspx#28247

72. Lewis, W. J., J. C. van Lenteren, Sharad C. Phatak, and J. H. Tumlinson, III. A total system approach to sustainable pest management. The National Academy of Sciences 13 August 1997. Web of Science.

73. Thad Godish (2 November 2000). Indoor Environmental Quality. CRC Press. pp. 325–326. ISBN 978-1-4200-5674-7.

74. Acreage NASS National Agricultural Statistics Board annual report, June 30, 2010. Retrieved August 26, 2012.

CHAPTER 6

Aquatic Toxicology

Chapter Contents

INTRODUCTION

Aquatic toxicology is the study of the effects of manufactured chemicals and other anthropogenic and natural materials and activities on aquatic organisms at various levels of organization, from subcellular through individual organisms to communities and ecosystems. Aquatic toxicology is a multidisciplinary field which integrates toxicology, aquatic ecology and aquatic chemistry.

This field of study includes freshwater, marine water and sediment environments. Common tests include standardized acute and chronic toxicity tests lasting 24–96 hours (acute test) to 7 days or more (chronic tests). These tests measure endpoints such as survival, growth, reproduction, that are measured at each concentration in a gradient, along with a control test. Typically using selected organisms with ecologically relevant sensitivity to toxicants and a well-established literature background. These organisms can be easily acquired or cultured in lab and are easy to handle.

While basic research in toxicology began in multiple countries in the 1800s, it was not until around the 1930s that the use of acute toxicity testing, especially on fish, was established. Over the next two decades, the effects of chemicals and wastes on non-human species became more of a public issue and the era of the *pickle-jar bioassays* began as efforts increased to standardize toxicity testing techniques.In the United States of America, the passage of the Federal Water Pollution Control Act of 1947 marked the first comprehensive legislation for the control of water pollution and was followed by the Federal Water Pollution Control Act in 1956. In 1962, public and governmental interests were renewed, in large part due to the publication of Rachel Carson's *Silent Spring*, and three years later the Water Quality Act was passed which directed states to develop water quality standards. Public awareness, as well as scientific and governmental concern, continued to grow throughout the 1970s and by the end of the decade research had expanded to include hazard evaluation and risk analysis. In the subsequent decades, aquatic toxicology has continued to expand and internationalize so that there is now a strong application of toxicity testing for environmental protection.

AQUATIC TOXICITY TESTS

Aquatic toxicology tests (assays): toxicity tests are used to provide qualitative and quantitative data on adverse (deleterious) effects on aquatic organisms from a toxicant. Toxicity tests can be used to assess the potential for damage to an aquatic environment and provide a database that can be used to assess the risk associated within a situation for a specific toxicant. Aquatic toxicology tests can be performed in the field or in the laboratory. Field experiments generally refer to multiple species exposure and laboratory experiments generally refer to single species exposure. A dose response relationship is most commonly used with a sigmoidal curve to quantify the toxic effects at a selected end-point or criteria for effect (i.e. death or other adverse effect to the organism). Concentration is on the x-axis and percent inhibition or response is on the y-axis.

The criteria for effects, or endpoints tested for, can include lethal and sublethal effects (see Toxicological effects).

There are different types of toxicity tests that can be performed on various test species. Different species differ in their susceptibility to chemicals, most likely due to differences in accessibility, metabolic rate, excretion rate, genetic factors, dieteary factors, age, sex, health and stress level of the organism. Common standard test species are the fathead minnow (Pimephales promelas), daphnids (*Daphnia magna*, *D. pulex*, *D. pulicaria*, *Ceriodaphnia dubia*), midge (Chironomus tentans, C. ruparius), rainbow trout (Oncorhynchus mykiss), sheepshead minnow (Cyprinodon variegatu), mysids (Mysidopsis), oyster (Crassotreas), scud (Hyalalla Azteca), grass shrimp (Palaemonetes pugio), mussels (Mytilus). As defined by ASTM, these species are routinely selected on the basis of availability, commercial, recreational, and ecological importance, past successful use, and regulatory use.

A variety of acceptable standardized test methods have been published. Some of the more widely accepted agencies to publish methods are: the American Public Health Association, U.S. Environmental Protection Agency, American Society for Testing and Materials, International Organization for Standardization, Environment Canada, and Organization for Economic Cooperation and Development. Standardized tests offer the ability to compare results between laboratories.

There are many kinds of toxicity tests widely accepted in the scientific literature and regulatory agencies. The type of test used depends on many factors: Specific regulatory agency conducting the test, resources available, physical and chemical characteristics of the environment, type of toxicant, test species available, laboratory vs. field testing, end-point selection, and time and resources available to conduct the assays are some of the most common influencing factors on test design.

Exposure Systems

Exposure systems are four general techniques the controls and test organisms are exposed to the dealing with treated and diluted water or the test solutions.

Static- a static test exposes the organism in still water. The toxicant is added to the water in order to obtain the correct concentrations to be tested. The control and test organisms are placed in the test solutions and the water is not changed for the entirety of the test.

Recirculation- a recirculation test exposes the organism to the toxicant in a similar manner as the static test, except that the test solutions are pumped through an apparatus (i.e. filter) to maintain water quality, but not reduce the concentration of the toxicant in the water. The water is circulated through the test chamber continuously, similar to an aerated fish tank. This type of test is expensive and it is unclear whether or not the filter or aerator has an effect on the toxicant.

Renewal- a renewal test also exposes the organism to the toxicant in a similar manner as the static test because it is in still water. However, in a renewal test the test solution is renewed periodically (constant intervals) by transferring the organism to a fresh test chamber with the same concentration of toxicant.

Flow-through- a flow through test exposes the organism to the toxicant with a flow into the test chambers and then out of the test chambers. The once-through flow can either be intermittent or continuous. A stock solution of the correct concentrations of contaminant must be previously prepared. Metering pumps or diluters will control the flow and the volume of the test solution, and the proper proportions of water and contaminant will be mixed.

Types of Tests

Acute tests are short-term exposure tests (hours or days) and generally use lethality as an endpoint. In acute exposures, organisms come into contact with higher doses of the toxicant in a single event or in multiple events over a short period of time and usually produce immediate effects, depending on absorption time of the toxicant. These tests are generally conducted on organisms during a specific time period of the organism's life cycle, and are considered partial life cycle tests. Acute tests are not valid if mortality in the control sample is greater than 10%. Results are reported in EC50, or concentration that will affect fifty percent of the sample size.

Chronic tests are long-term tests (weeks, months years), relative to the test organism's life span (>10% of life span), and generally use sub-lethal endpoints. In chronic exposures, organisms come into contact with low, continuous doses of a toxicant. Chronic exposures may induce effects to acute exposure, but can also result in effects that develop slowly. Chronic tests are generally considered full life cycle tests and cover an entire generation time or reproductive life cycle ("egg to egg"). Chronic tests are not considered valid if mortality in the control sample is greater than 20%. These results are generally reported in NOECs (No observed effects level) and LOECs (Lowest observed effects level).

Early life stage tests are considered as subchronic exposures that are less than a complete reproductive life cycle and include exposure during early, sensitive life stages of an organism. These exposures are also called critical life stage, embryo-larval, or egg-fry tests. Early life stage tests are not considered valid if mortality in the control sample is greater than 30%.

Short-term sublethal tests are used to evaluate the toxicity of effluents to aquatic organisms. These methods are developed by the EPA, and only focus on the most sensitive life stages. Endpoints for these test include changes in growth, reproduction and survival. NOECs, LOECs and EC50s are reported in these tests.

Bioaccumulation tests are toxicity tests that can be used for hydrophobic chemicals that may accumulated in the fatty tissue of aquatic organisms. Toxicants with low solubilities in water generally can be stored in the fatty tissue due to the high lipid content in this tissue. The storage of these toxicants within the organism may lead to cumulative toxicity. Bioaccumulation tests use bioconcentration factors (BCF) to predict concentrations of hydrophobic contaminants in organisms. The BCF is the ratio of the average concentration of test chemical accumulated in the tissue of the test organism (under steady state conditions) to the average measured concentration in the water.

Freshwater tests and saltwater tests have different standard methods, especially as set by the regulatory agencies. However, these tests generally include a control (negative and/or positive), a geometric dilution series or other appropriate logarithmic dilution series, test chambers and equal numbers of replicates, and a test organism. Exact exposure time and test duration will depend on type of test (acute vs. chronic) and organism type. Temperature, water quality parameters and light will depend on regulator requirements and organism type.

Effluent toxicity tests are tests conducted under the Clean Water Act, National Pollutant Discharge Elimination System (NPDES) permit program and are used by dischargers of contaminated effluent to monitor the quality of effluent into receiving waters. Acute Effluent Toxicity Tests are used to monitor the quality of industrial effluent monthly using acute toxicity tests. Effluent is used to perform static-acute multi concentration toxicity tests with *Ceriodaphnia dubia* and *Pimephales promelas*. The test organisms are exposed for 48 hours under static conditions with five concentrations of the effluent. Short-term Chronic Effluent Toxicity Tests are used to monitor the quality of municipal wastewater treatment plants effluent quarterly using short-term chronic toxicity tests. The goal of this test is to ensure that the wastewater is not chronically toxic. The major deviation in the short-term chronic effluent toxicity tests and the acute effluent toxicity tests is that the short-term chronic test lasts for seven days and the acute test lasts for 48 hours.

Sediment Tests

At some point most chemicals originating from both anthropogenic and natural sources accumulate in sediment. For this reason, sediment toxicity can play a major role in the adverse biological effects seen in aquatic organisms, especially those inhabiting benthic habitats. A recommended approach for sediment testing is to apply the Sediment Quality Triad (SQT) which involves simultaneously examining sediment chemistry, toxicity, and field alterations so that more complete information can be gathered. Collection, handling, and storage of sediment can have an effect on bioavailability and for this reason standard methods have been developed to suit this purpose.

Toxicological Effects

Toxicity can be broken down into two broad categories of direct and indirect toxicity. Direct toxicity results from a toxicant acting at the site of action in or on the organism. Indirect toxicity occurs with a change in the physical, chemical, or biological environment.

Lethality is most common effect used in toxicology and used as an endpoint for acute toxicity tests. While conducting chronic toxicity tests sublethal effects are endpoints that are looked at. These endpoints include behavioral, physiological, biochemical, histological changes.

There are a number of effects that occur when an organism is simultaneously exposed to two or more toxicants. These effects include additive effects, synergistic effects, potentiation effects, and antagonistic effects. An additive effect occurs when combined effect is equal to a combination or sum of the individual effects. A synergistic effect occurs when the combination of effects is much greater than the two individual effects added together. Potentiation is an effect that occurs when an individual chemical has no effect is added to a toxicant and the combination has a greater effect than just the toxicant alone. Finally, an antagonistic effect occurs when a combination of chemicals has less of an effect than the sum of their individual effects.

IMPORTANT AQUATIC TOXICOLOGY RESOURCES

- American Society for Testing and Materials (ASTM International) – A consensus organization, representing 135 countries, that develops and delivers international voluntary standard methods for aquatic toxicity testing.
- Standard Methods for the Examination of Water and Wastewater – A compilation of techniques for the examination of water, jointly published by the American

Public Health Association (APHA), the American Water Works Association (AWWA), and the Water Pollution Control Federation (WPCF).

- Ecotox – A database maintained by the U.S. Environmental Protection Agency (EPA) that offers single chemical toxicity information for both aquatic and terrestrial purposes.
- Society of Environmental Toxicology and Chemistry (SETAC) – A nonprofit, worldwide society working to promote scientific research to further our understanding of environmental stressors, environmental education, and the use of science in environmental policy.
- United States Environmental Protection Agency (EPA) – A federal agency working to protect human and environmental health. Among many other functions, the U.S. EPA produces guidance manuals outlining aquatic toxicity test procedures.
- Organisation for Economic Co-operation and Development (OECD) – A forum for governments to work together to promote policies for the betterment of people's social and economic well-being around the world. One way in which they accomplish this is through the development of aquatic toxicity test guidelines.
- Environment Canada (EC) – A diverse organization working to protect Canada's water resources and the natural environment through the coordination of environmental policies and programs with the federal government.

TERMINOLOGY

- Median Lethal Concentration (LC50) – The chemical concentration that is expected to kill 50% of a group of organisms.
- Median Effective Concentration (EC50) – The chemical concentration that is expected to have one or more specified effects in 50% of a group of organisms.
- Critical Body Residue (CBR) – An approach that routinely examines whole-body chemical concentrations of an exposed organism that is associated with an adverse biological response.
- Baseline toxicity – Refers to narcosis which is a depression in biological activity due to toxicants being present in the organism.
- Biomagnification – The process by which the concentration of a chemical in the tissues of an organism increases as it passes through several levels in the food web.
- Lowest Observed Effect Concentration (LOEC) – The lowest test concentration that has a statistically significant effect over a specified exposure time.
- No Observed Effect Concentration (NOEC) – The highest test concentration for which no effect is observed relative to a control over a specified exposure time.
- Maximum Acceptable Toxicant Concentration (MATC) – An estimated value that represents the highest "no-effect" concentration of a specific substance within the range including the NOEC and LOEC.
- Application Factor (AF) – An empirically derived "safe" concentration of a

chemical.

- Biomonitoring – The consistent use of living organisms to analyze environmental changes over time.
- Effluent – Liquid, industrial discharge that usually contain varying chemical toxicants.
- Quantitative Structure-Activity Relationship (QSAR) – A method of modeling the relationship between biological activity and the structure of organic chemicals.
- Mode of Action – A set of common behavioral or physiological signs that represent a type of adverse response.
- Mechanism of Action – The detailed events that take place at the molecular level during an adverse biological response.
- KOW – The octanol-water partition coefficient which represents the ratio of the concentration of octanol to the concentration of chemical in the water.
- Bioconcentration Factor (BCF) – The ratio of the average chemical concentration in the tissues of the organism under steady-state conditions to the average chemical concentration measured in the water to which the organisms are exposed.

All terms were derived from Rand.

SIGNIFICANCE TO REGULATORY WORLD

In the United States aquatic toxicology plays an important role in the NPDES wastewater permit program. In addition to analytical testing for known pollutants, aquatic, whole effluent toxicity tests have been standardized and are performed routinely as a tool for evaluating the potential harmful effects of effluents discharged into surface waters.

For the Clean Water Act under United States Environmental Protection Agency there are water quality criteria and water quality standards derived from aquatic toxicity tests.

SEDIMENT QUALITY GUIDELINES

While sediment quality guidelines are not meant for regulation, they provide a way to rank and compare sediment quality developed by National Oceanic and Atmospheric Administration(NOAA). These sediment quality guidelines are summarized in NOAA's Screening Quick Reference Tables (SQuiRT) for many different chemicals.

REFERENCES

1. Rand, Gary M.; Petrocelli, Sam R. (1985). Fundamentals of aquatic toxicology: Methods and applications. Washington: Hemisphere Publishing. ISBN 0-89116-382-4.
2. "Final Report: Interlaboratory Variability Study of EPA Short-term Chronic and Acute Whole Effluent Toxicity Test Methods, Vol 1." U.S. Environmental Protection Agency (EPA), 2001

3. "Methods for Measuring the Acute Toxicity of Effluents and Receiving Waters to Freshwater and Marine Organisms, Fifth Edition." U.S. Environmental Protection Agency (EPA), 2002
4. "Water Quality Standards History" U.S. Environmental Protection Agency (EPA) Received 2012-06-06
5. "Whole Effluent Toxicity." U.S. Environmental Protection Agency (EPA)
6. "About ASTM" American Society for Testing and Materials International, Retrieved 2012-06-07
7. "ECOTOX Database" U.S. Environmental Protection Agency (EPA)
8. https://www.setac.org/
9. "About the Organisation for Economic Co-operation and Development (OECD)" Organisation for Economic Co-operation and Development, Retrieved 2012-06-07
10. "About Environment Canada" Environment Canada, Retrieved 2012-06-07
11. "Guidelines for Deriving Numerical National Water Quality Criteria for the Protection Of Aquatic Organisms and Their Uses" U.S. Environmental Protection Agency
12. "Sediment Quality Guidelines developed for the National Status and Trends Program" Archived June 12, 2013, at the Wayback Machine. National Status & Trends, 1999
13. "SQuiRT" National Oceanic and Atmospheric Administration, 2008

CHAPTER 7

Radioactive Contamination

Chapter Contents

- **Introduction**
- **Sources of Contamination**
- **Decontamination**
- **Contamination Hazards**
- **Health Effects of Contamination**

If radioactive material is not in a sealed source container, it might be spread onto other objects. Contamination occurs when material that contains radioactive atoms is deposited on materials, skin, clothing, or any place where it is not desired. It is important to remember that radiation does not spread or get "on" or "in" people; rather, it is radioactive ***contamination*** that can be spread.

INTRODUCTION

Radioactive contamination, also called **radiological contamination**, is the deposition of, or presence of radioactive substances on surfaces or within solids, liquids or gases (including the human body), where their presence is unintended or undesirable (from the International Atomic Energy Agency - IAEA - definition).

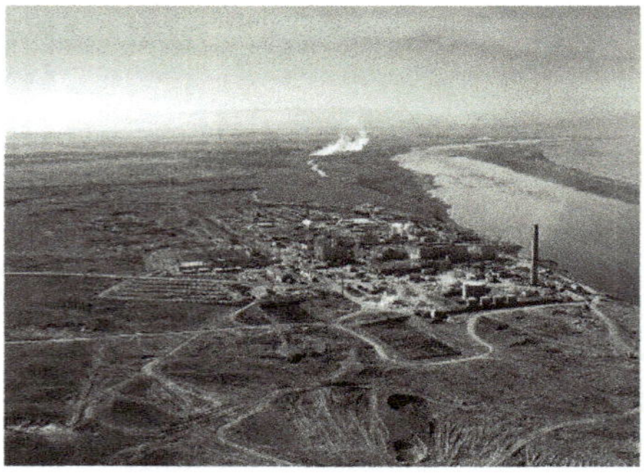

The Hanford site represents two-thirds of the United States' high-level radioactive waste by volume. Nuclear reactors line the riverbank at the Hanford Site along the Columbia River in January 1960.

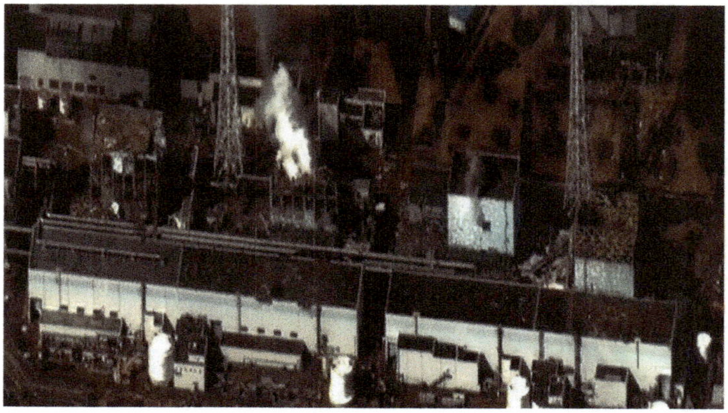

As of 2013, the Fukushima nuclear disaster site remains highly radioactive, with some 160,000 evacuees still living in temporary housing, and some land will be unfarmable for centuries. The difficult cleanup job will take 40 or more years, and cost tens of billions of dollars.

Such contamination presents a hazard because of the radioactive decay of the contaminants, which emit harmful ionising radiation such as alpha particles or beta particles, gamma rays or neutrons. The degree of hazard is determined by the concentration of the contaminants, the energy of the radiation being emitted, the type of radiation, and the proximity of the contamination to organs of the body. It is important to be clear that the contamination gives rise to the radiation hazard, and the terms radiation and contamination are not interchangeable.

Contamination may affect a person, a place, an animal, or an object such as clothing. Following an atmospheric nuclear weapon discharge or a nuclear reactor containment breach, the air, soil, people, plants, and animals in the vicinity will become contaminated by nuclear fuel and fission products. A spilled vial of radioactive material like uranyl nitrate may contaminate the floor and any rags used to wipe up the spill. Cases of widespread radioactive contamination include the Bikini Atoll, the Rocky Flats Plant in

Colorado, the Fukushima Daiichi nuclear disaster, the Chernobyl disaster, and the area around the Mayak facility in Russia.

SOURCES OF CONTAMINATION

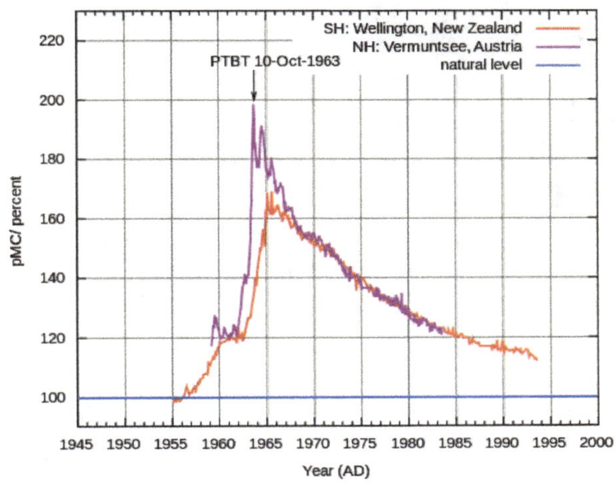

Global airborne contamination Atmospheric nuclear weapon tests almost doubled the concentration of ^{14}C in the Northern Hemisphere. Plot of atmospheric ^{14}C, New Zealandand Austria. The New Zealand curve is representative for the Southern Hemisphere, the Austrian curve is representative for the Northern Hemisphere. .

Radioactive contamination is typically the result of a spill or accident during the production, or use of, radionuclides (radioisotopes); these have unstable nuclei which are subject to radioactive decay.

Less typically, nuclear fallout is the distribution of radioactive contamination by a nuclear explosion. The amount of radioactive material released in an accident is called the *source term*.

Contamination may occur from radioactive gases, liquids or particles. For example, if a radionuclide used in nuclear medicine is spilled (accidentally or, as in the case of the Goiânia accident, through ignorance), the material could be spread by people as they walk around. Radioactive contamination may also be an inevitable result of certain processes, such as the release of radioactive xenon in nuclear fuel reprocessing. In cases that radioactive material cannot be contained, it may be diluted to safe concentrations. For a discussion of environmental contamination by alpha emitters please see actinides in the environment.

Contamination does not include residual radioactive material remaining at a site after the completion of decommissioning. Therefore, radioactive material in sealed and designated containers is not properly referred to as contamination, although the units of measurement might be the same.

Containment

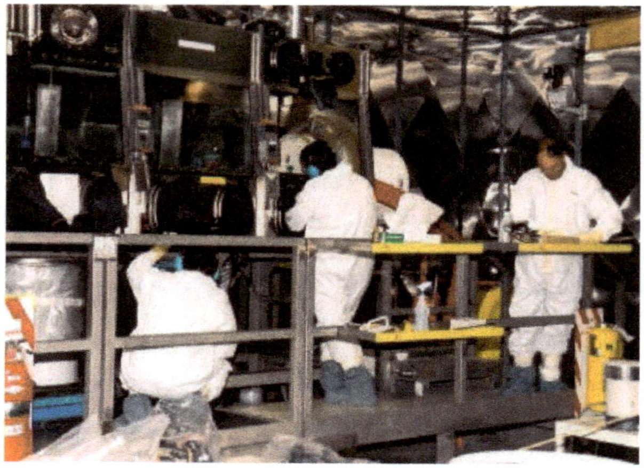

Large industrial glovebox in the nuclear industry.

Containment is the primary way of preventing contamination being released into the environment or coming into contact or being ingested by humans.

Being within the intended Containment differentiates radioactive *material* from radioactive *contamination*. When radioactive materials are concentrated to a detectable level outside a containment, the area affected is generally referred to as "contaminated".

There are a large number of techniques for containing radioactive material so that it does not spread beyond the containment and become contamination. In the case of liquids this is by the use of high integrity tanks or containers, usually with a sump system so that leakage can be detected by radiometric or conventional instrumentation.

Where material is likely to become airborne, then extensive use is made of the glovebox, which is a common technique in hazardous laboratory and process operations in many industries. The gloveboxes are kept under a slight negative pressure and the vent gas is filtered in high efficiency filters, which are monitored by radiological instrumentation to ensure they are functioning correctly.

Naturally Occurring Radioactivity

A variety of radionuclides occur naturally in the environment. Elements like uranium and thorium, and their decay products, are present in rock and soil. Potassium-40, a primordial nuclide, makes up a small percentage of all potassium and is present in the human body. Other nuclides, like carbon-14, which is present in all living organisms, are continuously created by cosmic rays.

These levels of radioactivity pose little danger but can confuse measurement. A particular problem is encountered with naturally generated radon gas which can affect instruments which are set to detect contamination close to normal background levels and can cause false alarms. Because of this skill is required by the operator of radiological survey equipment to differentiate between background radiation and the radiation which emanates from contamination.

Naturally occurring radioactive materials (NORM) can be brought to the surface or concentrated by human activities like mining and oil and gas extraction.

Control and Monitoring of Contamination

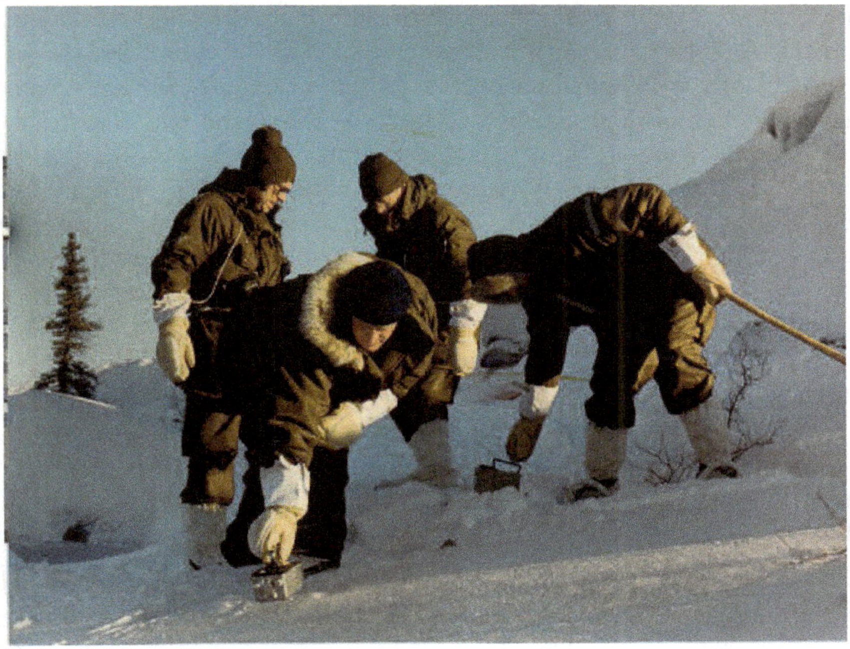

G-M counters being used as gamma survey monitors, seeking radioactive satellite debris.

Radioactive contamination may exist on surfaces or in volumes of material or air, and specialist techniques are used to measure the levels of contamination by detection of the emitted radiation.

Contamination Monitoring

Contamination monitoring depends entirely upon the correct and appropriate deployment and utilisation of radiation monitoring instruments.

Surface Contamination

Surface contamination may either be fixed or "free". In the case of fixed contamination, the radioactive material cannot by definition be spread, but its radiation is still measurable. In the case of free contamination there is the hazard of contamination spread to other surfaces such as skin or clothing, or entrainment in the air. A concrete surface contaminated by radioactivity can be shaved to a specific depth, removing the contaminated material for disposal.

For occupational workers controlled areas are established where there may be a contamination hazard. Access to such areas is controlled by a variety of barrier techniques, sometimes involving changes of clothing and foot wear as required. The contamination within a controlled area is normally regularly monitored. Radiological protection instrumentation (RPI) plays a key role in monitoring and detecting any potential contamination spread, and combinations of hand held survey instruments and permanently installed area monitors such as Airborne particulate monitors and area gamma monitors are often installed. Detection and measurement of surface contamination of personnel and plant is normally by Geiger counter, scintillation counter or proportional counter. Proportional counters and dual phosphor scintillation counters can discriminate between alpha and beta contamination, but the Geiger counter cannot. Scintillation detectors are generally preferred for hand held monitoring instruments, and are designed with a large detection window to make monitoring of large areas faster. Geiger detectors tend to have small windows, which are more suited to small areas of contamination.

Exit Monitoring

The spread of contamination by personnel exiting controlled areas in which nuclear material is used or processed is monitored by specialised installed exit control instruments such as frisk probes, hand contamination monitors and whole body exit monitors. These are used to check that persons exiting controlled areas do not carry contamination on their body or clothes.

In the United Kingdom the HSE has issued a user guidance note on selecting the correct portable radiation measurement instrument for the application concerned. This covers all radiation instrument technologies, and is a useful comparative guide for selecting the correct technology for the contamination type.

The UK NPL publishes a guide on the alarm levels to be used with instruments for checking personnel exiting controlled areas in which contamination may be encountered. Surface contamination is usually expressed in units of radioactivity per unit of area for alpha or beta emitters. For SI, this is becquerels per square meter (or Bq/m^2). Other units such as picoCuries per 100 cm^2 or disintegrations per minute per square centimeter (1 dpm/cm^2 = 167 Bq/m^2) may be used.

Airborne Contamination

The air can be contaminated with radioactive isotopes in particulate form, which poses a particular inhalation hazard. Respirators with suitable air filters, or completely self-contained suits with their own air supply can mitigate these dangers.

Airborne contamination is measured by specialist radiological instruments that continuously pump the sampled air through a filter. Airborne particles accumulate on the filter and can be measured in a number of ways:

- The filter paper is periodically manually removed to an instrument such as a "scaler" which measures any accumulated radioactivity.
- The filter paper is static and is measured in situ by a radiation detector.
- The filter is a slowly moving strip and is measured by a radiation detector. These are commonly called "moving filter" devices and automatically advance the filter to present a clean area for accumulation, and thereby allow a plot of airborne concentration over time.

Commonly a semiconductor radiation detection sensor is used that can also provide spectrographic information on the contamination being collected.

A particular problem with airborne contamination monitors designed to detect alpha particles is that naturally occurring radon can be quite prevalent and may appear as contamination when low contamination levels are being sought. Modern instruments consequently have "radon compensation" to overcome this effect.

See the article on Airborne particulate radioactivity monitoring for more information.

Internal human Contamination

Radioactive contamination can enter the body through ingestion, inhalation, absorption, or injection. This will result in a committed dose of radiation.

For this reason, it is important to use personal protective equipment when working with radioactive materials. Radioactive contamination may also be ingested as the result of eating contaminated plants and animals or drinking contaminated water or milk from exposed animals. Following a major contamination incident, all potential pathways of internal exposure should be considered.

DECONTAMINATION

Cleaning up contamination results in radioactive waste unless the radioactive material can be returned to commercial use by reprocessing. In some cases of large areas of contamination, the contamination may be mitigated by burying and covering the contaminated substances with concrete, soil, or rock to prevent further spread of the contamination to the environment. If a person's body is contaminated by ingestion or by injury and standard cleaning cannot reduce the contamination further, then the person may be permanently contaminated.

Contamination control products have been used by the U.S. Department of Energy (DOE) and the commercial nuclear industry for decades to minimize contamination on radioactive equipment and surfaces and fix contamination in place. "Contamination control products" is a broad term that includes fixatives, strippable coatings, and decontamination gels. A *fixative* product functions as a permanent coating to stabilize residual loose/ transferable radioactive contamination by fixing it in place; this aids in preventing the spread of contamination and reduces the possibility of the contamination becoming airborne, reducing workforce exposure and facilitating future deactivation and decommissioning (D&D) activities. *Strippable coating* products are loosely adhered paint-like films and are used for their decontamination abilities. They are applied to surfaces with loose/ transferable radioactive contamination and then, once dried, are peeled off, which removes the loose/transferable contamination along with the product. The residual radioactive contamination on the surface is significantly reduced once the strippable coating is removed. Modern strippable coatings show high decontamination efficiency and can rival traditional mechanical and chemical decontamination methods. *Decontamination gels* work in much the same way as other strippable coatings. The results obtained through the use of contamination control products is variable and depends on the type of substrate, the selected contamination control product, the contaminants, and the environmental conditions (e.g., temperature, humidity, etc.).

Some of the largest areas committed to be decontaminated are in the Fukushima Prefecture, Japan. The national government is under pressure to clean up radioactivity due to the Fukushima nuclear accident of March 2011 from as much land as possible so that some of the 110,000 displaced people can return. Stripping out the key radioisotope threatening health (caesium-137) from low level waste could also dramatically decrease the volume of waste requiring special disposal. A goal is to find techniques that might be able to strip out 80 to 95% of the caesium from contaminated soil and other materials, efficiently and without destroying the organic content in the soil. One being investigated is termed hydrothermal blasting. The caesium is broken away from soil particles and then precipitated with ferric ferricyanide (Prussian blue). It would be the only component of the waste requiring special burial sites.The aim is to get annual exposure from the contaminated environment down to one millisievert (mSv) above background. The most contaminated area where radiation doses are greater than 50 mSv/year must remain off limits, but some areas that are currently less than 5 mSv/year may be decontaminated allowing 22,000 residents to return.

To help with protection of people living in geographical areas which have been radioactively contaminated the International Commission on Radiological Protection has published a guide: "Publication 111 - Application of the Commission's Recommendations to the Protection of People Living in Long-term Contaminated Areas after a Nuclear Accident or a Radiation Emergency".

CONTAMINATION HAZARDS

- Elements which contain at least one stable isotope.
- Radioactive elements: the most stable isotope is very long-lived, with half-life of over four million years.
- Radioactive elements: the most stable isotope has half-life between 800 and 34.000 years.
- Radioactive elements: the most stable isotope has half-life between one day and 103 years.
- Highly radioactive elements: the most stable isotope has half-life between several minutes and one day.
- Extremely radioactive elements: the most stable isotope has half-life less than several minutes.

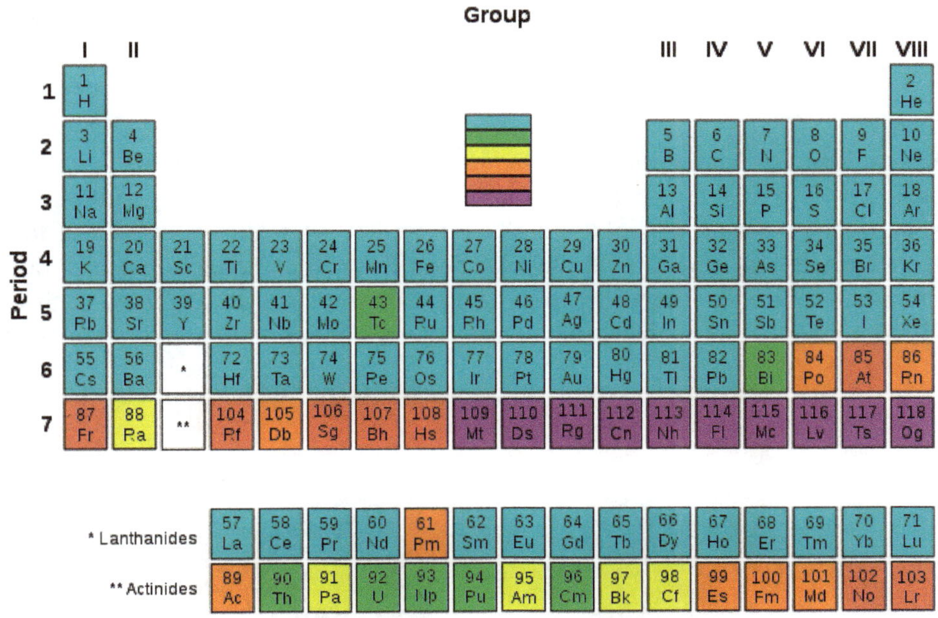

Periodic table with elements colored according to the half-life of their most stable isotope.

Low-level Contamination

The hazards to people and the environment from radioactive contamination depend on the nature of the radioactive contaminant, the level of contamination, and the extent of the spread of contamination. Low levels of radioactive contamination pose little risk, but can still be detected by radiation instrumentation. If a survey or map is ade of a contaminated area, random sampling locations may be labeled with their activity in becquerels or curies on contact. Low levels may be reported in counts per minute using a scintillation counter.

In the case of low-level contamination by isotopes with a short half-life, the best course of action may be to simply allow the material to naturally decay. Longer-lived isotopes should be cleaned up and properly disposed of, because even a very low level of radiation can be life-threatening when in long exposure to it.

Facilities and physical locations that are deemed to be contaminated may be cordoned off by a health physicist and labeled “Contaminated area.” Persons coming near such an area would typically require anti-contamination clothing (“anti-Cs”).

High-Level Contamination

High levels of contamination may pose major risks to people and the environment. People can be exposed to potentially lethal radiation levels, both externally and internally, from the spread of contamination following an accident (or a deliberate initiation) involving large quantities of radioactive material. The biological effects of external exposure to radioactive contamination are generally the same as those from an external radiation source not involving radioactive materials, such as x-ray machines, and are dependent on the absorbed dose.

When radioactive contamination is being measured or mapped *in situ*, any location that appears to be a point source of radiation is likely to be heavily contaminated. A highly contaminated location is colloquially referred to as a "hot spot." On a map of a contaminated place, hot spots may be labeled with their "on contact" dose rate in mSv/h. In a contaminated facility, hot spots may be marked with a sign, shielded with bags of lead shot, or cordoned off with warning tape containing the radioactive trefoil symbol.

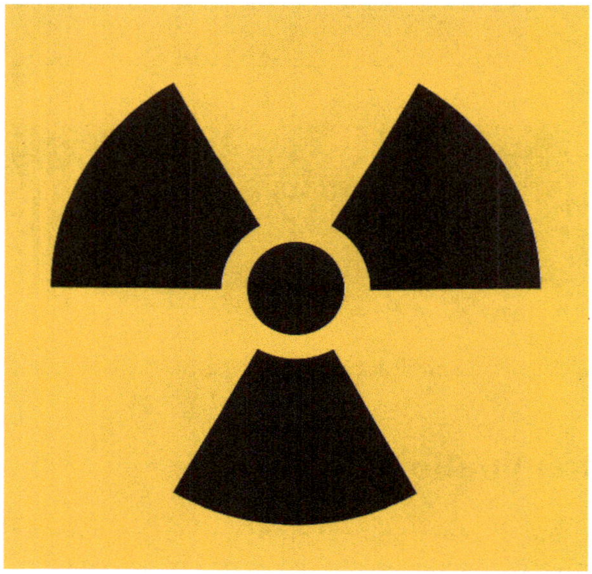

The radiation warning symbol (*trefoil*)

The hazard from contamination is the emission of ionising radiation. The principal radiations which will be encountered are alpha, beta and gamma, but these have quite different characteristics. They have widely differing penetrating powers and radiation effect, and the accompanying diagram shows the penetration of these radiations in simple terms. For an understanding of the different ionising effects of these radiations and the weighting factors applied, see the article on absorbed dose.

Radiation monitoring involves the measurement of radiation dose or radionuclide contamination for reasons related to the assessment or control of exposure to radiation or radioactive substances, and the interpretation of the results. The methodological and technical details of the design and operation of environmental radiation monitoring programmes and systems for different radionuclides, environmental media and types of facility are given in IAEA Safety Standards Series No. RS–G-1.8 and in IAEA Safety Reports Series No. 64.

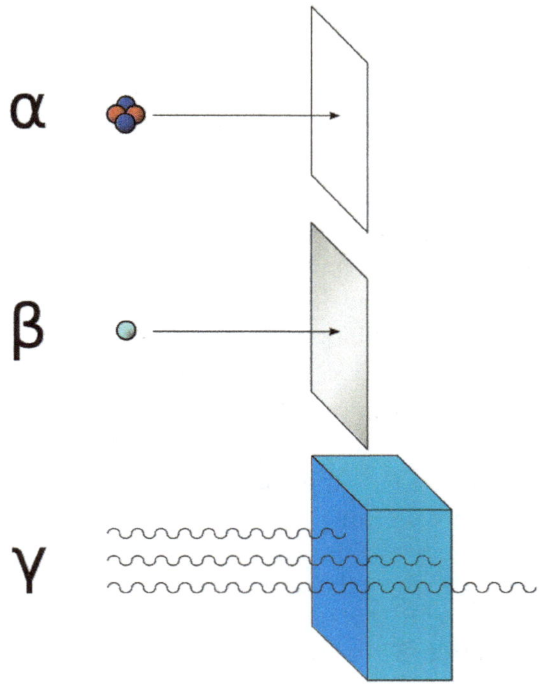

Alpha radiation consists of helium-4 nucleus and is readily stopped by a sheet of paper. Beta radiation, consisting of electrons, is halted by an aluminium plate. Gamma radiation is eventually absorbed as it penetrates a dense material. Lead is good at absorbing gamma radiation, due to its density.

HEALTH EFFECTS OF CONTAMINATION

Biological Effects

Radioactive contamination by definition emits ionizing radiation, which can irradiate the human body from an external or internal origin.

External Irradiation

This is due to radiation from contamination located outside the human body. The source can be in the vicinity of the body or can be on the skin surface. The level of health risk is dependent on duration and the type and strength of irradiation. Penetrating radiation such as gamma rays, X-rays, neutrons or beta particles pose the greatest risk from an external source. Low penetrating radiation such as alpha particles have a low external risk due to the shielding effect of the top layers of skin. See the article on sievert for more information on how this is calculated.

Internal Irradiation

Radioactive contamination can be ingested into the human body if it is airborne or is taken in as contamination of food or drink, and will irradiate the body internally. The art and science of assessing internally generated radiation dose is Internal dosimetry.

The biological effects of ingested radionuclides depend greatly on the activity, the biodistribution, and the removal rates of the radionuclide, which in turn depends on its chemical form, the particle size, and route of entry. Effects may also depend on the chemical toxicity of the deposited material, independent of its radioactivity. Some radionuclides may be generally distributed throughout the body and rapidly removed, as is the case with tritiated water.

Some organs concentrate certain elements and hence radionuclide variants of those elements. This action may lead to much lower removal rates. For instance, the thyroid gland takes up a large percentage of any iodine that enters the body. Large quantities of inhaled or ingested radioactive iodine may impair or destroy the thyroid, while other tissues are affected to a lesser extent. Radioactive iodine-131 is a common fission product; it was a major component of the radioactivity released from the Chernobyl disaster, leading to nine fatal cases of pediatric thyroid cancer and hypothyroidism. On the other hand, radioactive iodine is used in the diagnosis and treatment of many diseases of the thyroid precisely because of the thyroid's selective uptake of iodine.

The radiation risk proposed by the International Commission on Radiological Protection (ICRP) predicts that an effective dose of one sievert (100 rem) carries a 5.5% chance of developing cancer. Such a risk is the sum of both internal and external radiation dose.

The ICRP states Radionuclides incorporated in the human body irradiate the tissues over time periods determined by their physical half-life and their biological retention within the body. Thus they may give rise to doses to body tissues for many months or years after the intake. The need to regulate exposures to radionuclides and the accumulation of radiation dose over extended periods of time has led to the definition of committed dose quantities. The ICRP further states For internal exposure, committed effective doses are generally determined from an assessment of the intakes of radionuclides from bioassay measurements or other quantities (e.g., activity retained in the body or in daily excreta). The radiation dose is determined from the intake using recommended dose coefficients.

The ICRP defines two dose quantities for individual committed dose:

Committed Equivalent Dose, $H_T(t)$ is the time integral of the equivalent dose rate in a particular tissue or organ that will be received by an individual following intake of radioactive material into the body by a Reference Person, where t is the integration time in years. This refers specifically to the dose in a specific tissue or organ, in a similar way to external equivalent dose.

Committed Effective Dose, $E(t)$ is the sum of the products of the committed organ or tissue equivalent doses and the appropriate tissue weighting factors W_T, where t is the integration time in years following the intake. The commitment period is taken to be 50 years for adults, and to age 70 years for children.This refers specifically to the dose to the whole body, in a similar way to external effective dose.

Social and Psychological Effects

A 2015 report in *Lancet* explained that serious impacts of nuclear accidents were often not directly attributable to radiation exposure, but rather social and psychological effects. The consequences of low-level radiation are often more psychological than radiological. Because damage from very-low-level radiation cannot be detected, people exposed to it are left in anguished uncertainty about what will happen to them. Many believe they have been fundamentally contaminated for life and may refuse to have children for fear of birth defects. They may be shunned by others in their community who fear a sort of mysterious contagion.

Forced evacuation from a radiological or nuclear accident may lead to social isolation, anxiety, depression, psychosomatic medical problems, reckless behavior, even suicide. Such was the outcome of the 1986 Chernobyl nuclear disaster in the Ukraine. A comprehensive 2005 study concluded that "the mental health impact of Chernobyl is the largest public health problem unleashed by the accident to date". Frank N. von Hippel, a U.S. scientist, commented on the 2011 Fukushima nuclear disaster, saying that fear of ionizing radiation could have long-term psychological effects on a large portion of the population in the contaminated areas. Evacuation and long-term displacement of affected populations create problems for many people, especially the elderly and hospital patients.

Such great psychological danger does not accompany other materials that put people at risk of cancer and other deadly illness. Visceral fear is not widely aroused by, for example, the daily emissions from coal burning, although, as a National Academy of Sciences study found, this causes 10,000 premature deaths a year in the US population of 317,413,000. Medical errors leading to death in U.S. hospitals are estimated to be between 44,000 and 98,000. It is "only nuclear radiation that bears a huge psychological burden — for it carries a unique historical legacy".

REFERENCES

1. Richard Schiffman (12 March 2013). Two years on, America hasn't learned lessons of Fukushima nuclear disaster. The Guardian.
2. Martin Fackler (June 1, 2011). Report Finds Japan Underestimated Tsunami Danger. New York Times.
3. International Atomic Energy Agency (2007). IAEA Safety Glossary: Terminology Used in Nuclear Safety and Radiation Protection (PDF). Vienna: IAEA. ISBN 92-0-100707-8.
4. Atmospheric $\delta^{14}C$ record from Wellington". Trends: A Compendium of Data on Global Change. Carbon Dioxide Information Analysis Center. Oak Ridge National Laboratory. 1994. Retrieved 2007-06-11.
5. Levin, I.; et al. (1994). $\delta^{14}C$ record from Vermunt". Trends: A Compendium of Data on Global Change. Carbon Dioxide Information Analysis Center.
6. Radiocarbon dating. University of Utrecht. Retrieved 2008-02-19.
7. http://www.hse.gov.uk/pubns/irp7.pdf

8. Operational Monitoring Good Practice Guide "The Selection of Alarm Levels for Personnel Exit Monitors" Dec 2009 - National Physical Laboratory, Teddington UK
9. Dennis Normile, "Cooling a Hot Zone," Science, 339 (1 March 2013) pp. 1028-1029.
10. ICRP Protection of people living in long term contaminated areas
11. International Atomic Energy Agency (2005). Environmental and Source Monitoring for Purposes of Radiation Protection, IAEA Safety Standards Series No. RS–G-1.8 (PDF). Vienna: IAEA.
12. International Atomic Energy Agency (2010). Programmes and Systems for Source and Environmental Radiation Monitoring. Safety Reports Series No. 64. Vienna: IAEA. p. 234. ISBN 978-92-0-112409-8.
13. ICRP publication 103 - Paragraph 83.
14. ICRP Publication 103 paragraph 140
15. ICRP publication 103 - Paragraph 144.
16. ICRP publication 103 - Glossary.
17. Arifumi Hasegawa, Koichi Tanigawa, Akira Ohtsuru, Hirooki Yabe, Masaharu Maeda, Jun Shigemura, et al. Health effects of radiation and other health problems in the aftermath of nuclear accidents, with an emphasis on Fukushima, The Lancet, 1 August 2015.
18. Andrew C. Revkin (March 10, 2012). "Nuclear Risk and Fear, from Hiroshima to Fukushima". New York Times.
19. Frank N. von Hippel (September–October 2011). The radiological and psychological consequences of the Fukushima Daiichi accident. Bulletin of the Atomic Scientists. vol. 67 no. 5. pp. 27–36.

CHAPTER 8

Aquatic Toxicology Databases

Chapter Contents

TOXICOLOGICAL DATABASES

Toxicological databases are large compilations of data derived from aquatic and environmental toxicity studies. Data is aggregated from a large number of individual studies in which toxic effects to aquatic and terrestrial organisms was determined from different chemicals. These databases are then used by toxicologists, chemists, regulatory agencies and scientists to investigate and predict the likelihood that an organic or inorganic chemicals will cause an adverse effect (i.e. toxicity) to exposed organisms. In aquatic toxicology multiple databases exist and each generally pertains to a single aspect of aquatic toxicology such as a PCBs, tissue residues or sediment toxicity for example. A multitude of other informational and regulatory databases are maintained by the U.S. EPA , USGS , United States Army Corps of Engineers databases and the National Oceanic and Atmospheric Administration. Databases pertaining specifically to aquatic toxicology are less prolific and the three major U.S. databases are described here.

These databases are invaluable resources in the field of aquatic toxicology because the likelihood of a chemical to cause toxicity is highly variable across the broad spectrum of contaminants in the environment. This is because the likelihood that adverse effects to an organism will be realized is dependent on the concentration of that substance in the target tissues of the organism, the physicochemical properties of that chemical and the duration of exposure to the organism. Tools that enable the capability to predict the toxicity of specific chemicals to particular organisms or groups of organisms is essential to regulators and researches in the field of toxicology.

AVAILABLE DATABASES

Toxicity/Residue Database

The Toxicity/Residue Database is maintained by the U.S. EPA and is a data base for the prediction of toxicity of organic and inorganic chemicals to aquatic organisms. This data base was developed by the EPA Duluth office and became operational in 1999. The data base is derived from more than 500 peer reviewed references and is a collection of their findings on roughly 200 chemicals and 190 species both marine and fresh water. Data regarding organism response endpoints or effects are measured as the concentration of chemical in the tissue of the test organism at the time which effects such as lethality, metabolic depression, increased respiration etc., is reached. More than 3,000 effects may be queried from a small piece of downloaded software to gather survival, growth or reproductive endpoint effect data.

Environmental Residue Effects Database

The Environmental Residue Effects Database (ERED) is a database maintained by the U.S. Army Corps of Engineers that pairs data regarding the bioaccumulation of toxicants in tissue (via tissue residue)to endpoint effects such as mortality, growth, or physiological and biochemical responses. Response data also include low effect detected (LOED) and no effect detected (NOED) concentrations. This database is derived from 2329 peer reviewed references regarding 413 chemicals. The data base covers literature from 1964 to the present and compiles more than 15,000 overall records. This database is updated with 300 or more records every year on average. The ERED database is specific to sediment toxicity and the effects of contaminates in dredged materials on fresh water organisms. It is intended to be used to evaluate the potential for contaminate concentrations of dredged sediment to have unacceptable adverse effects on aquatic organisms. Although the ERED database was designed as a tool for the Army Corps of Engineers to manage adverse effects of dredging it is widely applicable to sediment toxicity studies and management.

THE ECOTOX DATABASE

ECOTOX is considered to be more comprehensive in that it holds results from toxicity tests of single chemicals on aquatic and terrestrial plants and animals. Data can be found on both freshwater and marine taxa. ECOTOX collects data from previously EPA established databases AQUIRE, TERRATOX, and PHYTOTOX which individually provide aquatic, terrestrial species and plant data respectively. Data large is collected from peer reviewed literature however some amount of data is sourced from grey literature. Using the Quick Database Query function enables searches by chemical, taxonomic name, effect, and publication year. Data from ECOTOX is used to provide reference parameters to current toxicity studies and severs as a regulatory guideline.

ECOTOX Source Data Screening

Data resulting from toxicity studies that is integrated in to the ECOTOX database is subjected to a screening and quality assurance criteria developed by the EPA and the Office of Pesticide Programs. (OPP). In order for study results to be accepted by the EPA and OPP the toxicity study must follow or consist of the following:

- The toxic effects are related to single chemical exposure;
- The toxic effects are on an aquatic or terrestrial plant or animal species;
- There is a biological effect on live, whole organisms;
- A concurrent environmental chemical concentration/dose or application rate is reported; and
- There is an explicit duration of exposure.

In addition to the criteria listed above, the following criteria, which are discussed in further detail in Attachment I, are applied by OPP as a further screen of acceptability:

- Toxicology information is reported for a chemical of concern to OPP;
- The article is published in the English language;
- The study is presented as a full article;
- The paper is a publicly available document;
- The paper is the primary source of the data
- A calculated endpoint is reported;
- Treatment(s) are compared to an acceptable control;
- The location of the study (e.g., laboratory vs. field) is reported; and
- The tested species is reported and verified.

USES IN REGULATIONS

The ECOTOX, ERED (sediment) and Toxicity Residue Databases are used by many regulatory agencies such as state environmental quality agencies and the EPA to determine regulatory environmental toxicant concentration levels. Under the Clean Water Act the EPA has used the ECOTOX database among other information to set wastewater toxicant concentration standards for industry as well as water quality standards for all contaminants in surface waters. Under the CWA, individual states must regulate water quality criteria at or below the concentrations set forth by the EPA. Sediment toxicant concentrations, however, are generally not regulated in the same way. The determination of sediment quality criteria and sediment toxicity testing is highly complex and is often regulated by states or some state run environmental agency. Sediment toxicity evaluations of contaminated sediments are very site specific and toxicant effect levels are often much more variable than those of surface waters. For this reason it may be nearly impossible to develop feasible acceptable sediment concentration regulations that apply to all aquatic systems or regions.

Rather than regulations Acceptable concentrations or sediment quality guidelines have been developed and are used in risk assessments and the management of dredged materials. "Sediment quality guidelines," as defined at the 2002 Society of Environmental Toxicology and Chemistry (SETAC) Pellston Workshop, are numerical chemical concentrations intended to be either protective of biological resources, or predictive of adverse effects to those resources, or both. SQGs for assessing sediment quality relative to the potential for adverse effects on sediment-dwelling organisms have been derived using both mechanistic and empirical approaches.

PSA FAILURE POST-RADICAL PROSTATECTOMY

- See PSA Failure

Probability of positive bone scan with rising PSA:

- **MSKCC**, 2005 - PMID 15774789 — "Pattern of prostate-specific antigen (PSA) failure dictates the probability of a positive bone scan in patients with an increasing PSA after radical prostatectomy." Dotan ZA et al. J Clin Oncol. 2005 Mar 20;23(9):1962-8.
- Article provides a handy nomogram.

Workup

Bone scan: not recommended. Chance of positive bone scan is <5% until PSA reaches 30-40. (PMID 9751361)

Prostate re-biopsy is not necessary and The PSA level or threshold seemed to be 1.5 ng/mL.

- **ASTRO consensus panel** - PMID 10561174 — "Consensus statements on radiation therapy of prostate cancer: guidelines for prostate re-biopsy after radiation and for radiation therapy with rising prostate-specific antigen levels after radical prostatectomy. American Society for Therapeutic Radiology and Oncology Consensus Panel." Cox et al. J Clin Oncol 1999 17:1155-1163.
- The panel judged that prostate re-biopsy is not necessary as standard follow-up care and that the absence of a rising PSA level after radiation therapy is the most rigorous end point of total tumor eradication.
- The panel noted that most data indicate the PSA level at time of salvage radiation may make a prognostic difference in outcome. The PSA level or threshold, based on the data presented, seemed to be 1.5 ng/mL.
- Based on the data presented at this conference, the dose should be 64 Gy or slightly higher with standard fractionation (1.8 or 2.0 Gy per fraction).

- There is no standard role for androgen suppression therapy in patients with or without radiation therapy for rising PSA values after prostatectomy.

ProstaScint: (indium 111-capromab pendetide)

- **ProstaScint study group** (1987-95)
- PMID 11920467, 2002 — "Clinical utility of indium 111-capromab pendetide immunoscintigraphy in the detection of early, recurrent prostate carcinoma after radical prostatectomy." Raj GV et al. Cancer. 2002 Feb 15;94(4):987-96.
- 255 pts with rising PSA (but < 4 ng/mL) after prostatectomy, who had negative bone scans and negative nodes, underwent ProstaScint scan.
- Uptake in 72%; 31% in prostatic fossa only. Avg PSA 1.1 (all pts). Serum PSA did not correlate with pattern of positive scan.

Outcome

Predictors of progression after salvage RT include Gleason Score 8-10, pre-RT PSA >2, negative surgical margins, PSA-DT <10 months and seminal vesicle invasion.

- **Duke/Harvard; 2011** (1988-2008) PMID 21437885 -- "Salvage radiation in men after prostate-specific antigen failure and the risk of death." (Cotter SE, Cancer. 2011 Mar 22. doi: 10.1002/cncr.25993. [Epub ahead of print])
    - Retrospective. 519 men treated with RP at Duke, with PSA failure. Median F/U 11.3 years
    - Outcome: Salvage RT reduction in all-cause mortality (HR 0.5, SS)
    - Conclusion: Salvage RT is associated with a decreased risk in mortality
- **Johns Hopkins; 2008** (1982-2004) PMID 18560003 -- "Prostate cancer-specific survival following salvage radiotherapy vs observation in men with biochemical recurrence after radical prostatectomy." (Trock BJ, JAMA. 2008 Jun 18;299(23):2760-9.)
    - Retrospective. Compared cohorts of pts who had biochemical failure after RP (n=635) from those who had 1) no salvage treatment (397 pts), 2) salvage RT alone (160), or 3) salvage RT + hormones (78).
    - Median f/u 6 yrs after recurrence. Death from prostate cancer in 18% (116 pts). Risk of death with observation, 22% (89 deaths); following salvage RT, 11% (18 deaths); following RT + hormones, 12% (9 deaths). Salvage RT with 3-fold increase in PC-specific survival (HR=0.32) and OS. Addition of hormonal therapy not associated with additional increase in survival.
    - Increase in survival with RT was limited to pts with PSA doubling time < 6 months. Salvage RT after 2 yrs provided no survival advantage. Men who did not achieve bNED after salvage RT did not experience an increase in survival.

- Multi-institutional
  - **2004** PMID 15026399 -- *Salvage radiotherapy for recurrent prostate cancer after radical prostatectomy.* **(2004 Stephenson AJ**, JAMA)
    - Retrospective review of 501 patients at 5 US academic tertiary centers who received salvage RT; median follow-up 45 months
    - 4-year PFS was 45%
    - No risk factors 4-year PFP was 77%
    - Multivariate predictors of progression:
      - Gleason Score 8-10 (HR 2.6)
      - Pre-RT post-relapse PSA >2.0 (HR 2.3)
      - Negative surgical margins (HR 1.9)
      - PSA-DT <10 months (HR 1.7)
      - Seminal vesicle invasion (HR 1.4)
    - Conclusion: "The Authors conducted a multicenter analysis of 501 patients undergoing salvage radiotherapy for an increasing PSA level after radical prostatectomy in order to reliably identify prognostic variables associated with a durable response.
      - In this cohort, a Gleason score of 8 to 10, preradiotherapy PSA level greater than 2.0 ng/mL, negative surgical margins, PSADT of 10 months or less, and seminal vesicle invasion were significant predictors of disease progression despite salvage radiotherapy.
      - In their multivariable analysis, only preradiotherapy PSA level greater than 2.0 ng/mL had a significant association with progression after salvage radiotherapy. However, patients receiving treatment at very low PSA levels (<0.6 ng/mL) had an improved outcome compared with patients with a preradiotherapy PSA level between 0.61 and 2.0 ng/mL. But the use of very low PSA thresholds risks overtreating patients whose PSA level is detectable due to residual benign prostatic tissue.
      - A patient with positive margins who relapses is more likely to benefit from salvage radiotherapy than a patient with negative margins, whose PSA level is more likely to represent distant disease.
        - patients with Gleason scores of 4 to 7 and a rapid PSADT, 67% will have a durable response to early salvage radiotherapy if they have **positive surgical margins**,

        - compared with 22% for those having **negative margins**.
    - Patients with a Gleason score of 4 to 7 and a slow PSADT (>10 months) had a 4-year PFP greater than 70% when radiation was delivered early, when the PSA level was lower.
- Gives flowchart to predict progression-free probability after salvage RT based on Gleason score, Pre-RT PSA, Surgical margins, and PSADT.
- **2007 Update** PMID 17513807 -- "Predicting the outcome of salvage radiation therapy for recurrent prostate cancer after radical prostatectomy." (Stephenson AJ, J Clin Oncol. 2007 May 20;25(15):2035-41.)
    - Updates previous report with larger cohort and longer follow up; 1540 pts from 17 centers, median f/u 53 months.
    - Median pre-RT PSA 1.1, median doubling time 6.9 months. Median 64.8 Gy.
    - 6-yr PFP 32%. By pre-RT PSA: 6-yr PFP 48% for PSA <0.50, 40% 0.51-1.00, 28% 1.01-1.5, 18% >1.5.
    - PSA response: nadir of ≤0.10 achieved in 59% following RT
    - Nomogram and flowchart to predict PFP.
- **2016: New Contemporary Update** PMID 27528718 -- "Contemporary Update of a Multi-Institutional Predictive Nomogram for Salvage Radiotherapy After Radical Prostatectomy." (Tendulkar RD, J Clin Oncol. 2016 Aug 15. [Epub ahead of print])
    - New cohort, including 2460 pts from 10 centers. Median f/u 5 yrs. Median pre-SRT PSA 0.5
    - Includes pts with lower pre-SRT PSA values <= 0.20 (18% of pts) who were excluded from the previous cohorts.
    - On multivariable analysis, pre-SRT PSA, GS, EPE, SVI, surgical margins, ADT use, and SRT dose were associated with FFBF. Pre-SRT PSA, GS, SVI, surgical margins, and ADT use were associated with DM, whereas EPE and SRT dose were not.
    - Conclusion: "Early SRT at low PSA levels after RP is associated with improved FFBF and DM rates. Contemporary nomograms can estimate individual patient outcomes after SRT in the modern era."
- PMID 7513108 - "Evaluation of serum prostate-specific antigen velocity after radical prostatectomy to distinguish local recurrence from distant metastases." Partin et al. Urology. 1994 May;43(5):649-59.

- Proposed criteria to distinguish local recurrence from distant metastases for patients with an increasing PSA level after radical prostatectomy. A Gleason score of 8 to 10, seminal vesicle invasion, positive lymph nodes, and a rapid PSA velocity were associated with distant metastases. Local recurrence was more frequently observed in patients with low-grade and organ-confined disease, a slow PSA velocity, and a disease free interval greater than 3 years, suggesting that isolated local recurrence has a low metastatic potential.

■ **Virginia Commonwealth University and University of Florida** - PMID 15145145 — *Comparison Of Adjuvant Versus Salvage Radiotherapy Policies For Postprostatectomy Radiotherapy*. Hagan et al. Int. J. Radiation Oncology Biol. Phys., Vol. 59, No. 2, pp. 329–340, **2004**

- The Authors compared the long-term results of postprostatectomy radiotherapy (RT) from two institutions, one adapting a prospective policy of adjuvant RT (69 patients) and the other salvage RT (88 patients). The salvage group underwent RT after longer postoperative intervals (median, 40.3 vs. 2.9 months; $p < 0.0001$) and had higher prostate-specific antigen (PSA) values before starting RT (4.5 vs. 0.86 ng/mL; $p = 0.003$). Both groups were routinely treated to a minimal total dose of 60 Gy.

- Results: Of the 69 patients referred for adjuvant RT, 22 (32%) had nonzero PSA values before RT. Multivariable modeling of BRFS found **only the PSA value before RT to be statistically significant ($p < 0.0001$)**. RT after prostatectomy was equally effective in either setting when the pre-RT PSA level was <1 ng/mL. **When the PSA value before RT was >1 ng/mL, the 5-year BRFS for each group was inferior.**

- Conclusion: Durable biochemical control is re-established in approximately 50% of patients who undergo salvage treatment, and 70–80% of patients in adjuvant series have disease control. Although the adjuvant treatment policy was associated with significantly improved BRFS, this was attributable to low pre-RT PSA values. When the treatment groups were stratified for pre-RT PSA level, the differences in BRFS were not statistically significant. Patients with a rising PSA level after prostatectomy, regardless of their initial risk, should receive prompt referral for RT.

■ **University of Heidelberg (Germany)**, 2007 (1991-2004)

- PMID 17275204 — "Long-term results and predictive factors of three-dimensional conformal salvage radiotherapy for biochemical relapse after prostatectomy." Neuhof D et al. Int J Radiat Oncol Biol Phys. 2007 Jan 31. [Epub ahead of print]

- 171 pts. Median f/u 39 mos.

- PSA decreased after RT in 82.5%. 5-yr bRFS 35.1%. On multivar. analysis, only Gleason score and pre-RT PSA level were predictive of PSA recurrence.

- **Mayo**, 2000 (1987-96)
  - PMID 10687990 — "Radiotherapy for isolated serum prostate specific antigen elevation after prostatectomy for prostate cancer." Pisansky TM et al. J Urol. 2000 Mar;163(3):845-50.
  - 166 pts. Median f/u 52 mos.
  - 5-yr bRFS 46%. Predictors for relapse: SV invasion, tumor grade, pre-RT PSA.

Use of ProstaScint imaging:

- **University of Chicago, 2008** (1988-2005)
  - PMID 18234446 — "Salvage radiotherapy after postprostatectomy biochemical failure: does pretreatment radioimmunoscintigraphy help select patients with locally confined disease?" (Liawu SL, Int J Radiat Oncol Biol Phys. 2008 Aug 1;71(5):1316-21.)
  - Retrospective, 82 pts. Compared outcomes for patients undergoing salvage RT with or without the use of pre-RT ProstaScint (RIS) scans. All pts had persistently elevated or increasing post-op PSA >0.1. Median pre-RT PSA 0.637. 3% had negative CT scan and/or bone scan. 47 pts had pre-RT ProstaScint scan. Pts were not included on the study if they had a RIS scan showing distant disease. RT was to median dose 66 Gy and included prostate bed (91% with RIS, 83% without) or pelvis + prostate bed (6% and 17%).
  - Patients who had prostate bed-only uptake on RIS did not have improved outcomes, with biochemical control of 40% at 5 years. Positive margins were associated with improved control.
  - Patients

RT + HORMONAL THERAPY

Preliminary Trials:

- **RTOG 96-01** (1998-2003) -- Post-op RT +/- Casodex 150 mg x 2 years for pT3 with PSA elevation.
  - pT3N0 (or pT2N0 with positive surgical margin) with post-op PSA 0.2-4.0. Randomized to prostate bed RT 64.8 Gy +/- casodex beginning concurrent with RT.
- ASTRO 2010 Report with 7.1 years of follow up:
  - Freedom from PSA progression at 7 yrs: 57% vs. 40% ($p<0.01$)

- True across all Gleason scores

- Cumulative incidence of metastatic disease at 7 years: 7.4% vs. 12.6% ($p<0.04$)

- Not reporting survival yet given too few events

- Grade 3/4 Toxicity:

    - GI: 2.3% vs. 1.4%

    - Bladder: 5.9% vs 5.0%

    - Gynecomastia (predominantly grades 1/2): 89% vs. 15%

RADIATION VOLUME

Whole Pelvis vs Prostate Bed Only:

- **Stanford, 2007** (1985-2005) PMID 17459606 -- "Radiotherapy after prostatectomy: improved biochemical relapse-free survival with whole pelvic compared with prostate bed only for high-risk patients." (Spiotto MT, Int J Radiat Oncol Biol Phys. 2007 Sep 1;69(1):54-61.)
    - Retrospective. 160 pts, treated with adjuvant (21 pts) or salvage RT (139). Androgen suppression in 87. 114 pts considered ‹high risk' for LN+ based on: GS >= 8, PSA > 20, SV+, prostate capsule involvement, or pN+. Of the high risk group, 72 treated with WPRT and 42 with RT to prostate bed only.

    - Benefit of WPRT limited to high risk pts: 5-yr BRFS 47% (WPRT) vs 21% (PO). Benefit for androgen suppression when given concurrently with RT.

    - Conclusion: WPRT confers superior bRFS compared with PBRT for high-risk patients receiving adjuvant or salvage RT after radical prostatectomy. This advantage was observed only with concurrent TAS.

TIMING OF SALVAGE RT

Systematic Reviews:

- **2012: UCLA** PMID 22795730 -- "The timing of salvage radiotherapy after radical prostatectomy: a systematic review." (King CR, Int J Radiat Oncol Biol Phys. 2012 Sep 1;84(1):104-11.)
    - Review of 41 studies (published 1995-2012) including 5597 patients.

    - PSA level before SRT and RT dose associated with RFS. Average 2.6% loss of

RFS for each incremental 0.1 PSA at the time of SRT.

- Conclusion: "This study provides Level 2a evidence for initiating SRT at the lowest possible PSA. Dose escalation is also suggested by the data."

HIGH DOSE SALVAGE RT

high dose in this context refers to a dose >= 66 Gy

- **2012: MSKCC** (1988-2007) PMID 22300563 -- "Long-term outcomes after high-dose postprostatectomy salvage radiation treatment." (Goenka A, Int J Radiat Oncol Biol Phys. 2012 Sep 1;84(1):112-8.)
    - 285 pts treated with salvage RT. Median PSA before SRT 0.4. 60 pts (21%) had MRI-detected local recurrence. 42 pts had pathologic confirmation of local recurrence.
    - 95% were treated to a dose >= 66 Gy; 72% received >= 70 Gy. ADT used in 31%.
    - Median f/u 60 mo. 7-yr bRFS 37%, DMFS 77%. Predictors of recurrence: vascular invasion, negative margins, presalvage PSA > 0.4, no use of ADT, Gleason >= 7, and +SV. RT dose >= 70 Gy was not associated with improved biochemical control. PSA-DT < 3 months was the only indep. predictor of DM. Trend toward benefit of dose >= 70 Gy in decreasing clinical local failure in pts who had radiographically visible local disease at the time of SRT.
    - Conclusion: "Salvage RT provides effective long-term biochemical control and freedom from metastasis in selected patients presenting with detectable PSA after prostatectomy. Androgen-deprivation therapy was associated with improvement in biochemical progression-free survival. Clinical local failures were rare but occurred most commonly in patients with greater burden of disease at time of SRT as reflected by either radiographic imaging or a greater PSA level. Salvage radiation doses ≥70 Gy may ultimately be most beneficial in these patients, but this needs to be further studied."

PSA MEASUREMENTS DURING RT

- PMID 12240547 — "The value of PSA measurements at 30 Gy, 50 Gy and 60 Gy for dose limitation in patients with radiotherapy for PSA increase after radical prostatectomy." Wiegel T et al. Strahlenther Onkol. 2002 Aug;178(8):422-5.
    - 41 pts treated to 66.6 Gy. At 30 Gy, 26% of those who would eventually respond still had a rising PSA, but at 50 and 60 Gy, 93% had decreasing PSA. In those who would fail, 75% and 88% had rising PSA at 50 and 60 Gy.

- PMID 11483332 — "Serum PSA evaluations during salvage radiotherapy for post-prostatectomy biochemical failures as prognosticators for treatment outcomes." Do T et al. Int J Radiat Oncol Biol Phys. 2001 Aug 1;50(5):1220-5.
    - 41 patients with biochemical failure after RP had PSA were treated to 59.4-66.6 Gy without hormone therapy. PSA checked at 30 Gy and 45 Gy.
    - Rising PSA at 45 Gy significantly predicted for poor outcome. PSA at 30 Gy did not significantly predict for disease outcome.

TOXICITY

- **Mayo, 2009** (1987-2003) PMID 19766337 -- "Late toxicity after postprostatectomy salvage radiation therapy." (Peterson JL, Radiother Oncol. 2009 Nov;93(2):203-6.)
    - Retrospective. 308 pts treated at Mayo-Rochester or Mayo-Jacksonville. Median RT dose 64.8 Gy; no IMRT. Hormonal therapy in 19%.
    - Late complication (any grade) in 14% by 5 yrs. Grade 3-4 complication: 4 pts (0.7%). GU toxicity: 3.9% gr 2 urethral strictures, 3 pts with gr 3 cystitis. GI: 1 pt with gr 4 rectal complication.

RADIATION INJURY

- **Toronto Sunnybrook** PMID 15936551 -- *Effect of androgen suppression on hemoglobin in prostate cancer patients undergoing salvage radiotherapy plus 2-year buserelin acetate for rising PSA after surgery.* (**2005 Chander S**, Int J Radiat Oncol Biol Phys.)
    - Conclusion: "Two-year AS resulted in a statistically significant drop in the mean Hb, but had no clinically apparent adverse effect. The pattern of Hb change was similar to that of testosterone change."

REFERENCES

1. https://archive.epa.gov/med/med_archive_03/web/html/pcbres.html
2. Bay, Steven. "Spiked Sediment Database". Society of Environmental Toxicology and Chemistry Sediment Advisory Group. Retrieved 18 May 2016.
3. Rand, Gary M. (1995). Fundamentals of aquatic toxicology: effects, environmental fate and risk assessment (3rd ed.). CRC Press. Retrieved 18 May 2016.
4. Elonen, Colleen. "Toxicity Residue Research". U.S. Environmental Protection Agency.
5. Bridges, Todd (1999). "Interpreting Bioaccumulation Data with the Environmental Residue-Effects Database" (PDF). Technical Notes Collection. Retrieved 18 May 2016.

6. «Evaluation Guidelines for Ecological Toxicity Data in the Open Literature". United States Environmental Protection Agency. EPA. Retrieved 24 May 2016.
7. Chapman, PM (1989). "Current approaches to developing sediment quality criteria". Environmental Toxicology and Chemistry. **8**: 589–599. doi:10.1002/etc.5620080706.
8. http://c.ymcdn.com/sites/www.setac.org/resource/resmgr/publications_and_resources/sqgsummary.pdf

Index